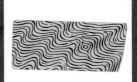

Echocardiography in Heart Failure

Look for these other titles in Catherine M. Otto's Practical Echocardiography Series

Donald C. Oxorn
Intraoperative Echocardiography

Linda Gillam & Catherine M. Otto
Advanced Approaches in Echocardiography

Mark Lewin & Karen Stout
Echocardiography in Congenital Heart Disease

Echocardiography in Heart Failure

PRACTICAL ECHOCARDIOGRAPHY SERIES

Martin St. John Sutton, MBBS, FRCP, FASE
John Bryfogle Professor of Medicine
University of Pennsylvania School of Medicine;
Director, Cardiovascular Imaging
Hospital of the University of Pennsylvania
Philadelphia, Pennsylvania

Susan E. Wiegers, MD, FASE
Professor of Medicine
Division of Cardiology
University of Pennsylvania
Philadelphia, Pennsylvania

ELSEVIER
SAUNDERS

1600 John F. Kennedy Blvd.
Ste 1800
Philadelphia, PA 19103-2899

ECHOCARDIOGRAPHY IN HEART FAILURE   ISBN: 978-1-4377-2695-4

Copyright © 2012 by Saunders, an imprint of Elsevier Inc.

Notices

Library of Congress Cataloging-in-Publication Data
Echocardiography in heart failure / [edited by] Martin St. John Sutton, Susan E. Wiegers.—1st ed.
   p.; cm.—(Practical echocardiography series)
Includes bibliographical references.
ISBN 978-1-4377-2695-4
 I. St. John Sutton, Martin, 1945- II. Wiegers, Susan E. III. Series: Practical echocardiography series.
[DNLM: 1. Heart Failure—ultrasonography—Handbooks. 2. Echocardiography—methods—Handbooks. WG 39]
 LC classification not assigned
 616.1′2307543—dc23
                                                                    2011033464

Senior Acquisitions Editor: Dolores Meloni
Editorial Assistant: Brad McIlwain
Publishing Services Manager: Pat Joiner-Myers
Senior Project Manager: Joy Moore
Designer: Steven Stave

To Clare, Eleanor Isabelle, and Eugenie Alice

To the Penn Cardiology Fellows

Contributors

Jacob Abraham, MD
Providence St. Vincent Heart Clinic Cardiology, St. Vincent Medical Center, Portland, Oregon
Evaluation of the Patient with Diastolic Dysfunction

Theodore Abraham, MD
Associate Professor, Cardiology, The Johns Hopkins University School of Medicine, Baltimore, Maryland
Evaluation of the Patient with Diastolic Dysfunction

Meryl S. Cohen, MD
Associate Professor of Pediatrics, University of Pennsylvania School of Medicine; Medical Director, Echocardiography Laboratory, and Associate Director, Cardiology Fellowship Program, The Children's Hospital of Philadelphia, Philadelphia, Pennsylvania
Heart Failure Caused by Congenital Heart Disease

Richard B. Devereux, MD
Professor of Medicine, Greenberg Division of Cardiology, Weill Cornell Medical College; Director, Echocardiography Laboratory, New York Presbyterian Hospital, New York, New York
Hypertensive Heart Failure

Maurice Enriquez-Sarano, MD, FACC
Professor of Medicine, Mayo Clinic College of Medicine; Consultant, Division of Cardiovascular Diseases, and Director, Valve Clinic, Mayo Clinic, Rochester, Minnesota
Echocardiographic Assessment of Patients with Systolic Heart Failure

Kristian Eskesen, MD
Fellow, Heart and Vascular Institute, The Johns Hopkins University School of Medicine, Baltimore, Maryland
Evaluation of the Patient with Diastolic Dysfunction

Judy Hung, MD
Associate Director, Cardiac Ultrasound Laboratory, Massachusetts General Hospital, Harvard Medical School, Boston, Massachusetts
Echocardiographic Assessment of Treatment for Systolic Congestive Heart Failure

Sean Jedrzkiewicz, MD
Lecturer, University of Toronto; Associate Staff, Division of Cardiology, Toronto General Hospital, University Health Network, Toronto, Ontario, Canada
Hypertrophic Cardiomyopathy

James N. Kirkpatrick, MD
Assistant Professor, Cardiovascular Medicine Division, University of Pennsylvania; Hospital of the University of Pennsylvania, Philadelphia, Pennsylvania
Echocardiographic Evaluation of Ventricular Support Devices

Bonnie Ky, MD, MSCE
Assistant Professor of Medicine and Epidemiology, Division of Cardiovascular Medicine, Center for Clinical Epidemiology and Biostatistics, University of Pennsylvania School of Medicine; Assistant Professor of Medicine and Epidemiology, Hospital of the University of Pennsylvania, Philadelphia, Pennsylvania
Role of Echocardiography in Patients Treated with Cardiotoxic Drugs

Fay Y. Lin, MD, MSc
Assistant Professor, Division of Cardiology, Department of Medicine, Weill-Cornell Medical Center; Attending Physician, New York Presbyterian Hospital, New York, New York
Hypertensive Heart Failure

Robert L. McNamara, MD, MHS

Associate Professor, Yale University; Director of Echocardiography, Yale-New Haven Hospital, New Haven, Connecticut
Echocardiographic Parameters Important for Decision Making

Tasneem Z. Naqvi, MD, FRCP

Professor of Medicine, Clinical Scholar, and Director, Non Invasive Cardiology, Keck School of Medicine, University of Southern California; Attending, Keck University Hospital of USC, Los Angeles, California
Distinguishing Systolic versus Diastolic Heart Failure A Practical Approach by Echocardiography

Anjali Tiku Owens, MD

Assistant Professor of Medicine, Division of Cardiovascular Medicine, University of Pennsylvania School of Medicine; Assistant Professor of Medicine, Heart Failure and Transplantation, Penn Heart and Vascular Center, Hospital of the University of Pennsylvania, Philadelphia, Pennsylvania
Echocardiography in the Patient with Right Heart Failure

Sorin Pislaru, MD, PhD

Assistant Professor of Medicine, Division of Cardiovascular Diseases, Mayo Clinic, Rochester, Minnesota
Echocardiographic Assessment of Patients with Systolic Heart Failure

Theodore J. Plappert, CVT

Center for Quantitative Echocardiography, Hospital of the University of Pennsylvania, Philadelphia, Pennsylvania
Echocardiographic Assessment of Heart Failure Resulting from Coronary Artery Disease

Atif N. Qasim, MD

Cardiology Fellow, Hospital of the University of Pennsylvania, Philadelphia, Pennsylvania
Echocardiography in Cardiac Transplantation

Amresh Raina, MD

Assistant Professor of Medicine, Temple University School of Medicine at West Penn Allegheny Health System; Attending Physician, Section of Heart Failure, Transplant and Pulmonary Hypertension, Allegheny General Hospital, Pittsburgh, Pennsylvania
Echocardiography in Cardiac Transplantation

Martin St. John Sutton, MBBS, FRCP, FASE

John Bryfogle Professor of Medicine, University of Pennsylvania School of Medicine; Director, Cardiovascular Imaging, Hospital of the University of Pennsylvania, Philadelphia, Pennsylvania
Echocardiographic Assessment of Heart Failure Resulting from Coronary Artery Disease, Echocardiography in the Patient with Right Heart Failure

Yan Wang, MBBS, RDCS

Echocardiography Technologist, Hospital of the University of Pennsylvania, Philadelphia, Pennsylvania
Echocardiographic Assessment of Heart Failure Resulting from Coronary Artery Disease

Rory B. Weiner, MD

Clinical and Research Fellow, Harvard Medical School; Fellow in Echocardiography and Cardiovascular Medicine, Massachusetts General Hospital, Boston, Massachusetts
Echocardiographic Assessment of Treatment for Systolic Congestive Heart Failure

Anna Woo, MD, SM, FACC

Associate Professor, University of Toronto; Staff Cardiologist and Director, Echocardiography Laboratory, University Health Network, Toronto General Hospital, Toronto, Ontario, Canada
Hypertrophic Cardiomyopathy

Foreword

Echocardiography is a core component of every aspect of clinical cardiology and now plays an essential role in daily decision making. Both echocardiographers and clinicians face unique challenges in interpretation of imaging and Doppler data and in integraton of these data with other clinical information. However, with the absorption of echocardiography into daily patient care, there are some voids in our collective knowledge base. First, clinicians caring for patients need to understand the value, strengths, and limitations of echocardiography relevant to their specific scope of practice. Second, echocardiographers need a more in-depth understanding of the clinical context of the imaging study. Finally, there often are unique aspects of data acquisition and analysis in different clinical situations, all of which are essential for accurate echocardiographic diagnosis. The books in the Practical Echocardiography Series are aimed at filling these knowledge gaps, with each book focusing on a specific clinical situation in which echocardiographic data are key for optimal patient care.

In addition to *Echocardiography in Heart Failure*, edited by Martin St. John Sutton, MBBS, FRCP, FASE, and Susan E. Wiegers, MD, FASE, other books in the series are *Intraoperative Echocardiography*, edited by Donald C. Oxorn, MD; *Echocardiography in Congenital Heart Disease*, edited by Mark Lewin, MD, and Karen Stout, MD; and *Advanced Approaches in Echocardiography*, edited by Linda Gillam, MD and myself. Information is presented as concise bulleted text accompanied by numerous illustrations and tables, providing a practical approach to data acquisition and analysis, including technical details, pitfalls, and clinical interpretation, and supplemented by web-based video case examples. Each volume in this series expands on the basic principles presented in the *Textbook of Clinical Echocardiography, Fourth Edition*, and can be used as a supplement to that text or can be used by physicians interested in a focused introduction to echocardiography in their area of clinical practice.

Over the past few decades there have been dramatic improvements in the therapy and clinical outcomes of adults with heart failure. In addition to the success of heart transplantation in selected patients, many others have benefited from improved pharmacologic and device therapy. In parallel with the complexity of the disease process and patient management, medical centers now frequently have dedicated inpatient and outpatient heart failure services. This book is intended to meet the needs of health care providers who care for adults with heart failure, spanning the spectrum of specialization from primary care providers to the expert in advanced heart failure and cardiac transplantation. Many other health care providers also contribute to the care of these patients, including cardiac surgeons, electrophysiologists, interventional cardiologists, nurse practitioner cardiac sonographers, pharmacists, social workers, and many others.

The editors of this volume, Drs. Martin St. John Sutton and Susan E. Wiegers, are both experts in echocardiography and in the clinical care of heart failure patients. They have put together an outstanding team of chapter authors whose expertise is reflected on every page of this book. Our hope is that the knowledge summarized in this book will contribute to the optimal care of all our patients with heart failure.

Catherine M. Otto, MD

Preface

Heart failure is a growing problem that currently involves between 5 and 6 million persons and costs in excess of 30 billion dollars each year in the United States alone. There are two reasons for the recent increase in the prevalence of heart failure. The first is in large part due to earlier diagnosis of systolic heart failure. The second is due to recognition of heart failure with normal ejection fraction as a clinical entity that comprises 30% to 40% of all heart failure, previously known as *diastolic heart failure*. Both of these have been achieved with Doppler echocardiography. Echocardiography plays an important role in assessing the efficacy of novel pharmacologic agents and guiding the selection of patients for devices and surgical interventions.

Echocardiography in Heart Failure should be used in conjunction with Dr. Catherine Otto's authoritative *Textbook of Clinical Echocardiography*. This title reviews the basic principles of heart failure and explains how Doppler echocardiography can be used to improve contemporary management and clinical outcomes of heart failure by optimizing image acquisition and interpretation.

This volume includes chapters on systolic heart failure and diastolic heart failure, ways to distinguish between the two conditions, and ways to use Doppler echocardiography for clinical decision making. In addition, there are informative chapters on cardiomyopathies, hypertensive heart failure, right and left ventricular remodeling, heart failure caused by cardiotoxic drugs, and heart failure presenting in childhood. Finally, there are chapters on pharmacologic treatment, ventricular assist devices, and orthotopic transplantation.

All chapters use a step-by-step approach to patient examination for each clinical diagnosis. Information is presented in bulleted points, each with a set of major principles followed by a list of key echocardiographic points. Potential pitfalls are identified, and emphasis is placed on avoiding errors in image acquisition and interpretation. Measurements and calculations are explained with specific examples. Each chapter is fully illustrated with detailed figure legends demonstrating each major step in order to guide the reader through the various teaching points. Pertinent cases are included where indicated, with self-assessment supplemented by web-based video case examples to help the reader to actively engage in the learning process, monitor his/her progress, consolidate the information, and identify areas where further study is required. Along with the correct answer to each question, there is a brief discussion of how that answer was determined and why the other potential answers are incorrect.

Echocardiography in Heart Failure will be of interest to practicing cardiologists involved with cardiac imaging and/or heart failure as well as sonographers for a quick but precise update on echocardiography in heart failure. It will also be of value for cardiology fellows and cardiac sonographer students learning the material for the first time. The self-assessment case studies will be helpful for those preparing for both the echocardiography examinations and the cardiology board examinations.

Martin St. John Sutton,
MBBS, FRCP, FASE
Susan E. Wiegers, MD, FASE

Contents

Video Contents

Glossary

2D two-dimensional
3D three-dimensional
4C 4-chamber
5-FU 5-fluorouracil
A area
A late diastolic wave/atrial filling
a′, A′, A_a late diastolic velocity
ACE angiotensin-converting enzyme
a_{dur} atrial wave velocity duration
AI aortic insufficiency
ALCAPA anomalous left coronary artery from the pulmonary artery
ALT alanine aminotransferase
AR aortic regurgitation
Ar-A difference in duration between pulmonary venous and mitral atrial filling velocities
ARB angiotensin II receptor blocker
ARVC arrhythmogenic right ventricular cardiomyopathy
AS aortic stenosis
AV aortic valve
AVB atrioventricular block
AVC aortic valve closure
BiVAD biventricular assist device
BNP brain natriuretic peptide
BP blood pressure
BSA body surface area
CABG coronary artery bypass grafting
CAD coronary artery disease
CAV chronic allograft vasculopathy
cc-TGA congenitally corrected transposition of the great arteries
CK creatine kinase
CMRI cardiac magnetic resonance imaging
CP constrictive pericarditis
CRT cardiac resynchronization therapy
CSA cross-sectional area
CSP cuff systolic pressure
CW continuous wave
D diastolic wave
D diastolic pulmonary vein flow velocity
DA cavity area in diastole

DHF diastolic heart failure
dia_{asc} diameter of the ascending aorta
dia_{in} diameter of inflow cannula
dia_{out} diameter of outflow cannula
dia_{pa} diameter of the pulmonary artery
dP/dt change in pressure over time
DT deceleration time
E mitral inflow early-filling wave/early diastolic wave/early rapid filling
e′, E′, E_a early diastolic velocity
E/A mitral inflow early-to-late diastolic velocity ratio
ECG electrocardiography/electrocardiogram
ECMO extracorporeal membrane oxygenation
EDA end-diastolic area
EDD end-diastolic dimension
E/E′ ratio of mitral inflow early filling wave to myocardial early diastolic velocity
EF ejection fraction
Em/E_m early diastolic relaxation
ERO effective regurgitant orifice
ESA end-systolic area
ESD end-systolic dimension
ET ejection time
E/Vp ratio of mitral inflow early-filling wave to early propagation velocity by color M-mode
FAC fractional area change
%FAC percent fractional area change
GFR glomerular filtration rate
GS global strain
h height
HF heart failure
HFNEF heart failure with normal ejection fraction
HR heart rate
IABP intra-aortic balloon pump
IAS interatrial septum
ICD implantable cardioverter-defibrillator
ICM ischemic cardiomyopathy
IVA isovolumic acceleration
IVC inferior vena cava
IVCD intraventricular conduction delay

IVCT isovolumic contraction time
IVRT isovolumic relaxation time
IVS interventricular septum
L length
L_0 resting length
LA left atrial/left atrium
LAD left anterior descending coronary artery
LAV left atrial volume
LAVI left atrial volume index
LV left ventricle/left ventricular
LVAD left ventricular assist device
LVEDD left ventricular end-diastolic dimension
LVEDP left ventricular end-diastolic pressure
LVESD left ventricular end-systolic dimension
LVEDVI left ventricular end-diastolic volume index
LVEF left ventricular ejection fraction
LVET left ventricular ejection time
LGE late gadolinium enhancement
LVIDd left ventricular diastolic internal dimension
LVH left ventricular hypertrophy
LVM left ventricular mass
LVMI left ventricular mass index
LVOT left ventricular outflow tract
LVPP left ventricular peak pressure
MI myocardial infarction
MIBI sestamibi
MPI myocardial performance index
MR mitral regurgitation
MRI magnetic resonance imaging
MRV mitral regurgitant volume
MV mitral valve
NICM nonischemic cardiomyopathy
NPV negative predictive value
NSVT nonsustained ventricular tachycardia
NYHA New York Heart Association
OHT orthotopic heart transplantation
PA pulmonary artery
PADP pulmonary artery diastolic pressure
PAP pulmonary artery pressure
PASP pulmonary artery peak systolic pressure
PE pericardial effusion
PHT pressure half-time
PI pulmonary insufficiency
PISA proximal isovelocity surface area
PLAX parasternal long-axis
PM papillary muscle
PPV positive predictive value
PR pulmonic regurgitation
PSAX parasternal short-axis
PV pulmonary vein
PVAD percutaneous ventricular assist device
PW pulsed wave
PWT posterior wall thickness
PWTd posterior wall diastolic thickness
Qp blood flow in the pulmonary circulation

Qs blood flow in the systemic circulation
RA right atrial/right atrium
RAP right atrial pressure
RCM restrictive cardiomyopathy
RF regurgitant fraction
RFP restrictive filling pattern
RHC right heart catheterization
ROA regurgitant orifice area
rpm rotations per minute
RV regurgitant volume
RV right ventricle/right ventricular
RVEF right ventricular ejection fraction
RVFAC right ventricular fractional area change
RVo regurgitant volume
RVOT right ventricular outflow tract
RV$_{VAD}$ regurgitant volume of ventricular assist device
RWMA regional wall motion abnormality
RWT relative wall thickness
S systolic wave
S systolic pulmonary vein flow velocity
S' systolic velocity
SA cavity area in systole
SAM systolic anterior motion
SAX short-axis
SBP systolic blood pressure
Sc circumferential wall stress
SCD sudden cardiac death
S/D systolic/diastolic ratio
SHF systolic heart failure
Sm meridional wall stress
Sm systolic annular motion
SPECT single-photon emission computed tomography
SPWMD septal-posterior wall motion delay
STd septal diastolic thickness
STE speckle tracking echocardiography
STEMI ST-segment elevation myocardial infarction
SV stroke volume
SVR surgical ventricular reconstruction
SWT septal wall thickness
TAPSE tricuspid annular plane systolic excursion
TDI tissue Doppler imaging
TEE transesophageal echocardiography
TGA transposition of the great arteries
TOF tetralogy of Fallot
TR tricuspid regurgitation
Ts-SD standard deviation of time to peak systolic velocity among 12 basal segments and mid-LV segments
TST total systolic time
TTE transthoracic echocardiography
TV tricuspid valve
v, V velocity

V volume
VAD ventricular assist device
VC vena contracta
V_{myo} myocardial volume

Vp propagation velocity
VSD ventricular septal defect
VTI velocity-time integral
V_{TR} tricuspid regurgitation jet velocity

Distinguishing Systolic versus Diastolic Heart Failure A Practical Approach by Echocardiography

Tasneem Z. Naqvi

Definition

Systolic heart failure is characterized by (1) signs and symptoms of dyspnea, easy fatigue and exercise intolerance, (2) a dilated left ventricle with or without a dilated right ventricle, (3) moderate to severe left ventricular systolic dysfunction associated with generalized left ventricular hypokinesis with or without segmental akinesis/dyskinesis, and (4) diastolic dysfunction that is often proportional to systolic dysfunction but may range from mild to severe. The right ventricle may be dilated and right ventricular systolic function may be normal to severely abnormal. Atrial enlargement is often proportional to ventricular enlargement, and atrioventricular valve regurgitation may range from mild to severe.

Diastolic heart failure is characterized by (1) signs or symptoms of shortness of breath, (2) normal or mildly abnormal systolic LV function, and (3) evidence of diastolic LV dysfunction out of proportion to systolic dysfunction. Normal or mildly abnormal systolic LV function implies both an LV ejection fraction (LVEF) greater than 50% and an LV end-diastolic volume index (LVEDVI) less than 97 mL/m^2. Echocardiographic techniques required for the diagnosis and management of systolic and diastolic heart failure are described below.

Left Ventricular Dimensions and Thickness

See Appendix for reference values.

KEY POINTS

- These values are measured in the parasternal long-axis (PLAX) (Figure 1-1) or parasternal short-axis (PSAX) view using 2D or M-mode.
- M-mode measurements should be made from leading edge to leading edge.
- Two-dimensional (2D) echocardiographic measurements should be made from trailing edge to leading edge.
- M-mode echocardiographic measurements are always slightly greater than 2D measurements because of these conventions.
- Measurement is made at the level of the LV minor axis, approximately at the mitral valve leaflet tips.
- LV mass is measured by M-mode at PLAX view or by 2D method at the midpapillary muscle level in the short-axis (SAX) view.
- These linear measurements can be made directly from 2D images or using 2D-targeted M-mode echocardiography (Figure 1-2; see also Figure 1-1).
- Ensure visualization of aortic and mitral valves.

- Maximize horizontal orientation of the interventricular septum.
- The M-mode cursor should be positioned perpendicular to the septum and LV posterior wall.

Limitations
- LV posterior chords, anterior aberrant chords, and the tricuspid apparatus may be misinterpreted as the LV posterior wall and inner and outer borders of the anterior interventricular septum (IVS), respectively (see Figure 1-1C, orange arrow).
- End-diastole can be defined at the onset of the QRS complex, but is preferably defined as the frame after mitral valve closure or the frame in the cardiac cycle in which the cardiac dimension is largest.
- The M-mode cursor may be difficult to align perpendicular to the LV walls.
- Left ventricular mass can be measured by the M-mode or 2D method (Figure 1-3).

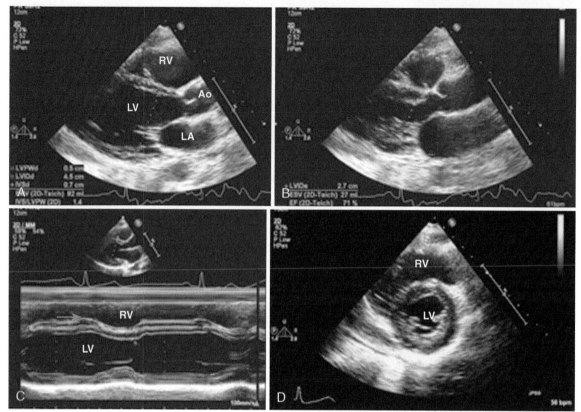

Figure 1-1. Measurement of left ventricular dimensions in the PLAX view in end-diastole (**A**) and end-systole (**B**) by 2D method. **C,** Measurement of LV dimensions by M-mode obtained from PLAX (**A** and **B**) or SAX (**D**) view. *Orange arrow* points at the RV chord that should not be included in the measurement of IVS thickness.

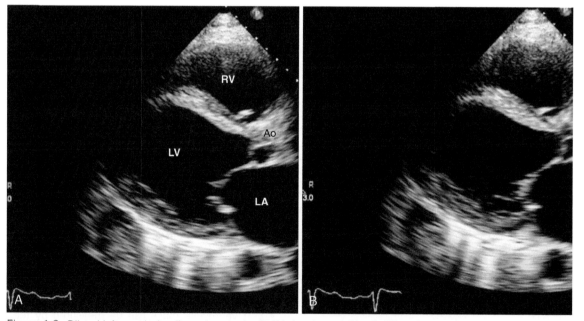

Figure 1-2. Dilated left ventricular dimensions in the PLAX view in end-diastole (**A**) and end-systole (**B**) in a patient with dilated NICM. Note enlargement of left atrium (>4.0 cm) and right ventricle (>3.3 cm).

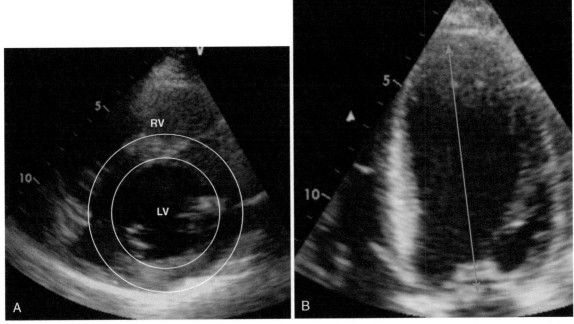

Figure 1-3. LV mass measurement is shown by 2D method. LV epicardium and LV endocardium are traced at end-diastole in mid–SAX view (**A**). LV end-diastolic length is measured from apical 4-chamber view (**B**).

Left Ventricular Systolic Function

Fractional Area Change

KEY POINTS

- Fractional area change is obtained from the PLAX view by the M-mode or 2D method as (LVEDD − LVESD)/LVEDD×100, where LVEDD is end-diastolic dimension and LVESD is end-systolic dimension (see Figure 1-1).
- It is easy to perform; however, it has technical limitations in the presence of segmental wall motion abnormalities and an abnormally shaped ventricle. 2D- and M-mode–derived ejection fraction by the Teichholz method are based on minor dimensions: (end-diastolic volume − end-systolic volume)/end-systolic volume where the end-diastolic volume $= 7/(2.4 + EDD) \times EDD^3$ and the end-systolic volume $= 7/(2.4 + ESD) \times ESD^3$. Because of geometric assumptions, these methods have been superseded by 2D volumetric methods.

Left Ventricular Volumes and Ejection Fraction (Table 1-1)

KEY POINTS

- The most commonly used 2D measurement for volume estimations is the biplane method of disks (modified Simpson's rule; Figures 1-4 and 1-5). Left-sided contrast agents used for endocardial border delineation are helpful and improve measurement reproducibility for suboptimal studies and correlation with other imaging techniques (Figure 1-6). These agents also help improve diagnosis of left ventricular thrombus (Figure 1-7).

- Left ventricular volumes are increased in systolic heart failure.

Limitations
- Difficult to quantify due to endocardial dropout.
- Foreshortening underestimates true LV volumes.
- Ejection fraction is often eyeballed without volume measurement.

TABLE 1-1 ECHOCARDIOGRAPHIC ASSESSMENT OF LEFT VENTRICULAR SYSTOLIC FUNCTION

Method	View	Pitfalls
Two-Dimensional Imaging		
Fractional shortening	PLAX or PSAX	*Geometric Assumptions* Based on a single cross section Ignores wall motion in nonmeasured segments
Ejection fraction	(LVEDV – LVESV) × 100/LVEDV	Dependent on load and heart rate (HR)
Modified Simpson's rule	4-chamber and 2-chamber	Foreshortening of apical views Poor visualization of anterior wall
Area-length method	4-chamber (LV area)2 × 0.85/LV end-diastolic length	Not appropriate for non-symmetrical LV Assumes cylindrical LV shape
Bullet method	Mid-SAX and apical 4- chamber	LV shape assumption
Wall motion score index	PLAX, PSAX, apical 4-, 2-, and 3-chamber Average endocardial thickening score of 16 or 17 segments	Reader and center variability Requires visualization of all segments
Exercise ejection fraction	As above	To detect incipient LV systolic dysfunction Usually eyeballed
Three-dimensional volumes	Full-volume apical view	Resolution is dependent on 2D image quality
Doppler Methods		
LV stroke volume	PLAX 2D and apical 5- or 3-chamber	Circular shape assumption of LV outflow tract (LVOT) Error in LVOT measurement Errors are squared
LV dP/dt (mm Hg/s)	MR CW Doppler $\Sigma \Delta t$ 1 m/s to 3 m/s, 32/Δt	Load independent Not always feasible
MPI	Apical 5-chamber	Somewhat load dependent No geometric assumption
Tissue Doppler	Apical views Objective data Less dependent on image quality Less dependent on reader expertise	Somewhat load dependent Requires parallel angle of insonation Affected by translation, tethering, and respiration
2D speckle tracking	*Longitudinal Strain* Not affected by Doppler angle *Radial Strain* Not affected by Doppler angle	Requires high frame rate Requires good 2D image resolution Decreased feasibility versus TDI

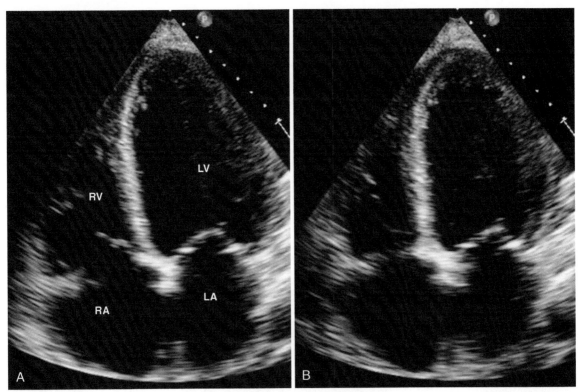

Figure 1-4. Reduced endocardial excursion and dilatation of four chambers in the same patient with dilated NICM in the apical 4-chamber view in end-diastole (**A**) and end-systole (**B**). Note enlargement of right ventricle and atrium.

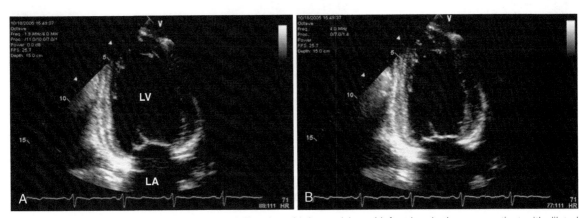

Figure 1-5. Reduced endocardial excursion and dilatation of left ventricle and left atrium in the same patient with dilated NICM in the apical 2-chamber view in end-diastole (**A**) and end-systole (**B**). Use inspiratory or expiratory breath hold if necessary to define endocardial borders.

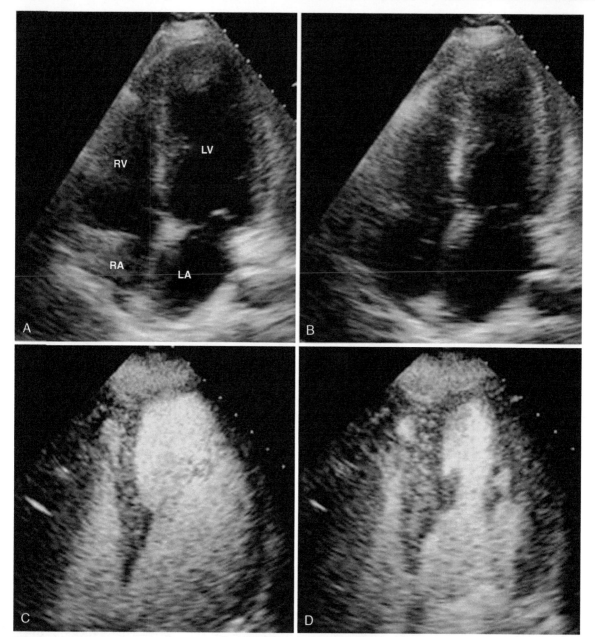

Figure 1-6. Apical 4-chamber views in end-diastole (**A**) and end-systole (**B**) before (**C**) and after (**D**) Definity contrast injection. Note clear delineation of endocardial borders in **C** and **D** compared to **A** and **B**.

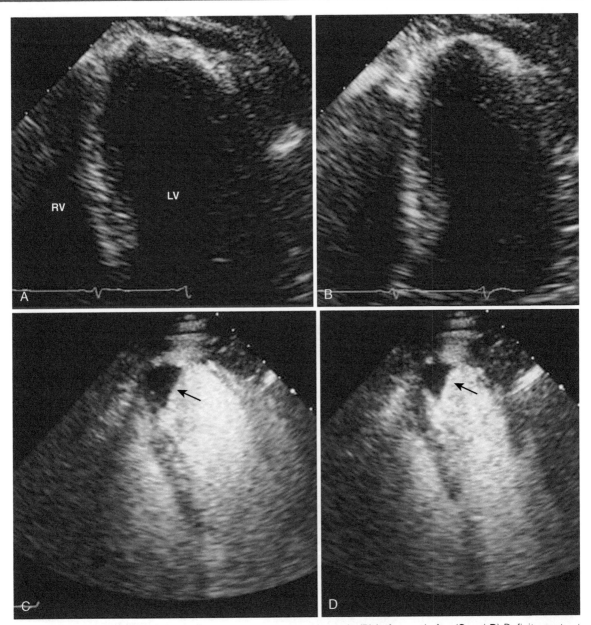

Figure 1-7. Apical 4-chamber views in end-diastole (**A**) and end-systole (**B**) before and after (**C** and **D**) Definity contrast injection. Note clear delineation of LV apical thrombus (*arrows*) in **C** and **D** after contrast injection.

Three-Dimensional (3D) Volumes and Ejection Fraction

KEY POINTS	
• More accurate than 2D assessment of LV volumes and ejection fraction.	**Limitations**
• Overcome the limitation of foreshortening.	• Image quality is dependent on 2D images.
	• Requires postprocessing.

Segmental Wall Motion

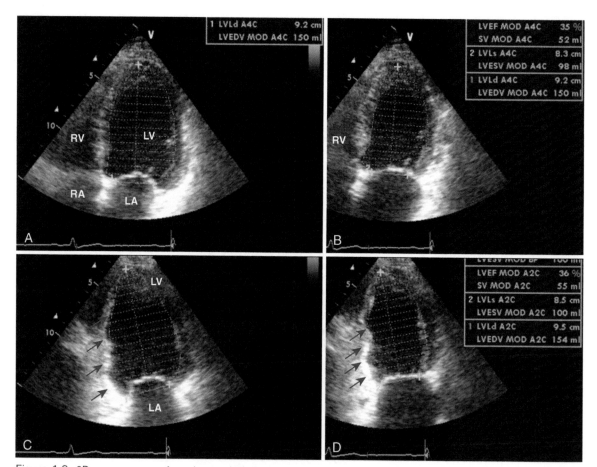

Figure 1-8. 2D measurements for volume calculations using biplane method of disks (modified Simpson's rule) in apical 4-chamber (**A** and **B**) and apical 2-chamber views (**C** and **D**) at end-diastole (**A** and **C**) and at end-systole (**B** and **D**) in a patient with dilated ICM. Papillary muscles should be excluded from the cavity in the tracing. Note thin and echodense basal to midinferior walls (*red arrows* in **C** and **D**) indicating prior inferior wall transmural infarct. Upper-normal LV diastolic (152 mL) and increased LV systolic (99 mL) volumes are present, which are characteristic of dilated ICM.

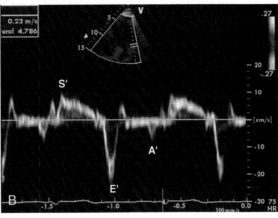

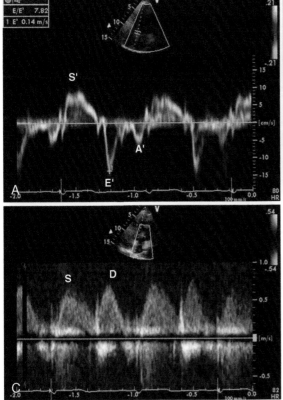

Figure 1-9. TDI velocities at septal annulus (**A**) and lateral annulus (**B**) and at the pulmonary veins (**C**) in a normal male adult age 30 years. A′, late diastolic velocity; D, diastolic pulmonary vein flow velocity; E′, early diastolic velocity; S, systolic pulmonary vein flow velocity; S′, systolic velocity.

LV Function Assessment by Tissue Doppler Imaging (Figure 1-9)

KEY POINTS	
• Tissue Doppler imaging (TDI) provides more objective data and is less dependent on reader expertise. • TDI systolic and diastolic velocities can be obtained reliably in basal and mid-myocardial segments by color-coded and pulsed wave (PW) Doppler techniques. Velocity of motion, displacement, and deformation can be measured in the longitudinal, radial, and circumferential planes. • Global normal strain by TDI echocardiography ranges from 16% to 19%.	**Limitations** • TDI systolic and diastolic velocities are age dependent. • TDI velocities are decreased by increasing wall thickness. • Requires parallel angle of insonation to area of interest. • Affected by translational and respiratory motion. • Significant variability. • No standardized guidelines. • Sample volume placement determines measurement precision.

LV Function Assessment by 2D Speckle Tracking (Figure 1-10)

KEY POINTS	
• Normal values for global longitudinal strain: 18.5% to 18.7%. • Normal values for global radial strain: 47% ± 7%. • Independent of cardiac translation and angle of insonation.	• Can measure radial, circumferential, and longitudinal strain as well as torsion. • Less variable than ejection fraction. • Feasible in approximately 80% of cases.

Continued

KEY POINTS—cont'd

- Twist is normal in diastolic heart failure (DHF) and markedly reduced in systolic heart failure (SHF) (SHF: 5 ± 2.8, DHF: 13 ± 6.8, control: 14 ± 5.8).
- Circumferential strain is normal in DHF (15% ± 5%) and markedly reduced in SHF (7% ± 3%) (control groups: 20% ± 3%).
- Longitudinal strain is reduced in SHF (–4%) and DHF (–12%).
- Radial strain is reduced in SHF (14% ± 8%) and DHF (28% ± 7%).
- In patients with preserved ejection fraction (50%), regional longitudinal strain of ≤13% compared to

other segments identified transmural myocardial infarction (MI) with 80% sensitivity and specificity (see Figure 1-10).

Limitations
- Requires harmonic imaging and high frame rate.
- Subject to image factors, including reverberation artifacts and attenuation.
- Requires technical proficiency in image processing.

Other Methods of Assessment of Left Ventricular Systolic Function

---

KEY POINTS

- LV systolic function can be measured from rate of change of pressure gradients between the left ventricle and left atrium using the initial slope of the mitral regurgitation envelope as LV *dP/dt*.
- A normal *dP/dt* is greater than 1200 mm Hg/s (Figure 1-11).

Limitations
- Not always feasible.
- Usual limitations of Doppler intercept angle.

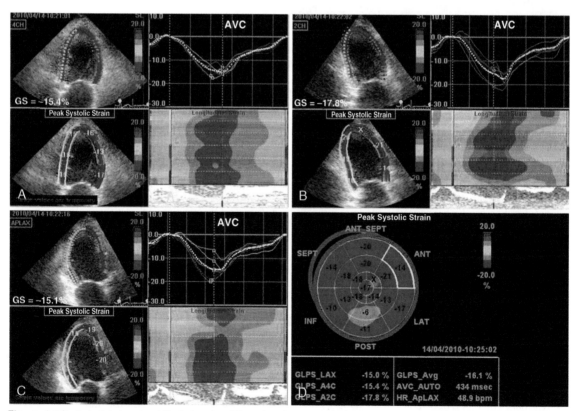

Figure 1-10. Apical 4-chamber (**A**), 2-chamber (**B**), and 3-chamber (**C**) 2D strain maps and segmental strain scores along with bull's-eye map (**D**) showing global strain (GS) and segmental strain values in the same patient as in Figure 1-8. Note reduced segmental strain values of –6 to –13% in the basal to midinferior and inferolateral segments consistent with transmural infarction. GS is mildly reduced at –16%. AVC, aortic valve closure.

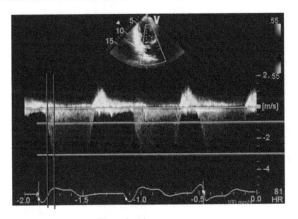

Figure 1-11. Measurement of left ventricular *dP/dt* from MR envelope. Time for LV-LA gradient to increase from 4 mm Hg to 36 mm Hg is measured by calculating the time interval between MR velocity of 1 m/s to MR velocity of 3 m/s (corresponding to LV-LA gradients of 4 mm Hg and 36 mm Hg, respectively). This time is then divided by 32 mm Hg (36 − 4 mm Hg) to calculate *dP/dt* in mm Hg/s.

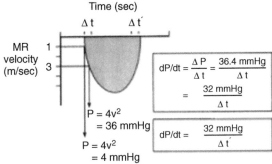

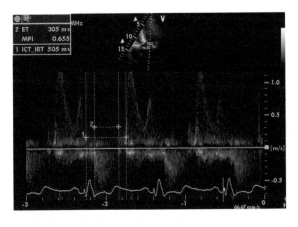

Figure 1-12. PW Doppler velocity curves of mitral inflow and left ventricular outflow. *A* is time from cessation to onset of mitral inflow (shown as 1); *B* is the left ventricular ET from onset to cessation of LV ejection (shown as 2). Myocardial performance index is (*A* − *B*)/*B*.

Methods Evaluating Combined Systolic and Diastolic Function

Myocardial Performance Index

KEY POINTS

- The myocardial performance index is defined as the sum of isovolumic contraction time (IVCT) and isovolumic relaxation time (IVRT) divided by ejection time (ET).
- It is useful in patients with primary myocardial systolic dysfunction.
- The myocardial performance index has prognostic value in various clinical settings because

it seems to be independent of heart rate (Figure 1-12).

Limitations
- Somewhat load dependent.
- Combined mitral inflow and aortic PW Doppler is difficult to obtain for accurate time intervals.

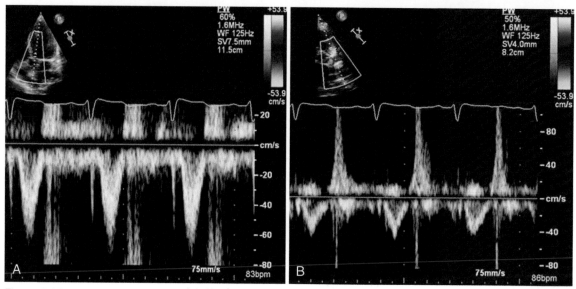

Figure 1-13. PW Doppler of the left ventricular outflow tract (**A**) and of the right ventricular outflow tract (**B**) in the same patient with NICM showing reduced peak ejection velocity and hence stroke volume for both left ventricle and right ventricle.

LV Stroke Volume

KEY POINTS	
• Can be measured by PW Doppler of LV outflow tract and LV outflow diameter (Figure 1-13).	**Limitations** • LV outflow diameter measurements may be imprecise, and error in measurement is squared. • Assumes spherical shape of LV outflow.

Left Ventricular Diastolic Function

Mitral Inflow PW Doppler

KEY POINTS

• PW sample volume is placed between the tips of the mitral valve leaflets or at the level of the mitral annulus.

• Ensure parallel alignment of the Doppler beam to blood flow.

• In dilated hearts, mitral inflow is often directed posterolaterally.

• Normal mitral inflow comprises an early-filling E wave and a late-filling A wave. Deceleration time of mitral inflow E wave is generally 170 to 180 ms (Figure 1-14).

• There is an age-associated change in mitral inflow pattern (Figures 1-15 and 1-16).

• Four major patterns of mitral inflow are seen with advancing diastolic dysfunction:

  • *Grade I Diastolic Dysfunction:* Mitral inflow filling shows an abnormal relaxation pattern with E/A ratio of less than 1, a prolonged mitral inflow E-wave deceleration time (DT), and a prolonged IVRT.

  • *Grade II Diastolic Dysfunction:* A pseudonormal phase is seen on mitral inflow that looks like a normal inflow filling pattern. This usually reverses to an abnormal relaxation pattern upon Valsalva maneuver (Figure 1-17). Even in the presence of an abnormal relaxation pattern on mitral inflow, a reduction in E/A ratio of greater than 0.5 upon Valsalva maneuver indicated elevated left atrial preload and grade II diastolic dysfunction (Figure 1-18).

• *Grade III Diastolic Dysfunction:* A markedly increased E-wave velocity is seen with a small A-wave velocity and E/A ratio of greater than 2.0. DT becomes short. This *restrictive mitral inflow pattern* is reversible upon preload reduction with the Valsalva maneuver or nitroglycerin or diuretic administration (Figure 1-19).

• *Grade IV Diastolic Dysfunction:* Same as grade III, except no change in filling pattern occurs with preload-reducing maneuvers (Figure 1-20). Advanced systolic dysfunction is often associated with grade IV diastolic dysfunction (Figure 1-21).

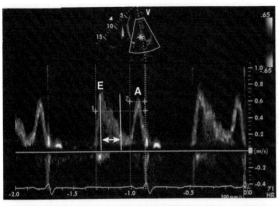

Figure 1-14. PW Doppler of mitral inflow showing appropriate filter, gain, scale, and sweep speed settings. The goal is to maximize Doppler signal on the screen to improve temporal and spatial resolution. A discrete electrocardiographic signal is shown at the bottom of the ultrasound panel to allow measurement of time intervals in relation to the QRS complex, such as time from onset of mitral inflow to onset of QRS complex, as well as duration of mitral inflow diastolic filling time as compared to cardiac cycle length measured as R-to-R interval. White arrow indicates deceleration time of E wave.

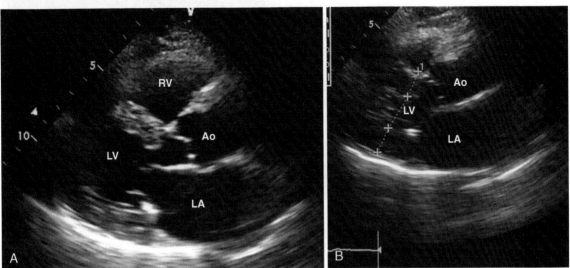

Figure 1-15. There is an age-associated increase in LV wall thickness, LA size, and LV mass. End-diastolic (A) and end-systolic (B) frames in the PLAX view in a 72-year-old female patient are shown.

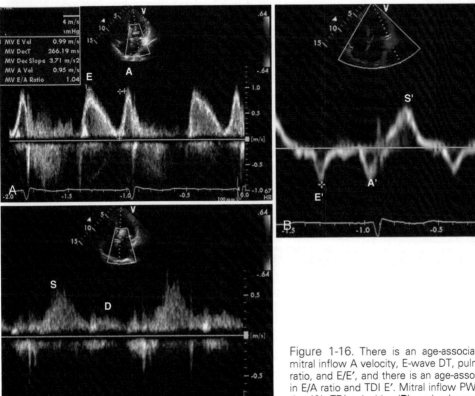

Figure 1-16. There is an age-associated increase in mitral inflow A velocity, E-wave DT, pulmonary vein S/D ratio, and E/E', and there is an age-associated decrease in E/A ratio and TDI E'. Mitral inflow PW Doppler velocities (A), TDI velocities (B), and pulmonary vein Doppler velocities (C) are shown in a 60-year-old male.

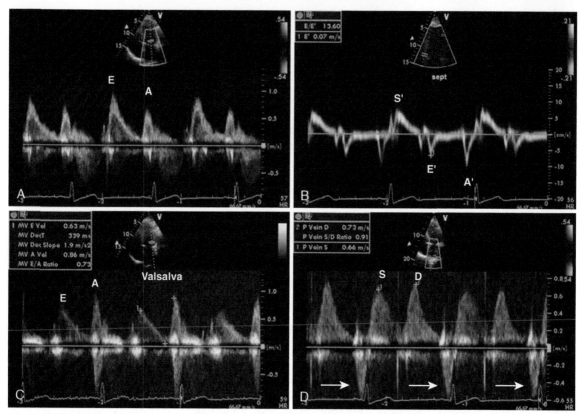

Figure 1-17. Mitral inflow PW Doppler (**A**) and TDI of medial annulus (**B**) in a 55-year-old female with exertional shortness of breath. Note E/A' ratio of 13 is inconclusive for left atrial pressure. **C,** Mitral inflow PW Doppler during Valsalva maneuver; **D,** pulmonary vein inflow. A greater than 0.5 reduction in E/A ratio, S/D ratio reversal on pulmonary vein flow, and prominent pulmonary vein atrial reversal (*white horizontal arrows* in **D**) all indicate elevated left ventricular end-diastolic pressure and left atrial pressure in this patient.

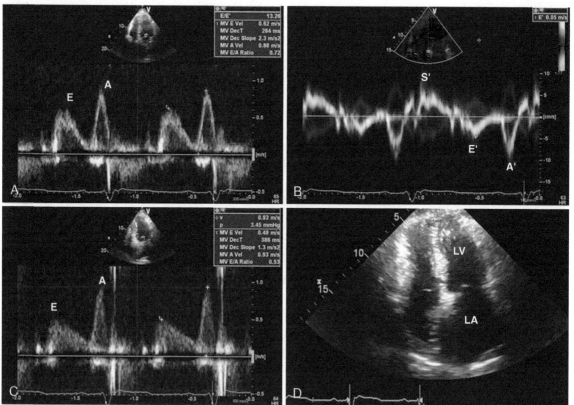

Figure 1-18. Mitral inflow PW Doppler (**A**) in this 60-year-old male with a history of coronary artery disease shows E and A reversal, suggesting grade I diastolic dysfunction. Evaluation of medial mitral annulus (**B**) shows E/E' of 13 (suggesting left atrial pressure is indeterminate). Valsalva maneuver leads to a further reduction in mitral inflow E/A ratio (**C**) by greater than 25%, suggesting there is elevation of left atrial pressure. Left atrium was markedly enlarged in the apical 4-chamber view (**D**) with a volume index of 42 mL/m².

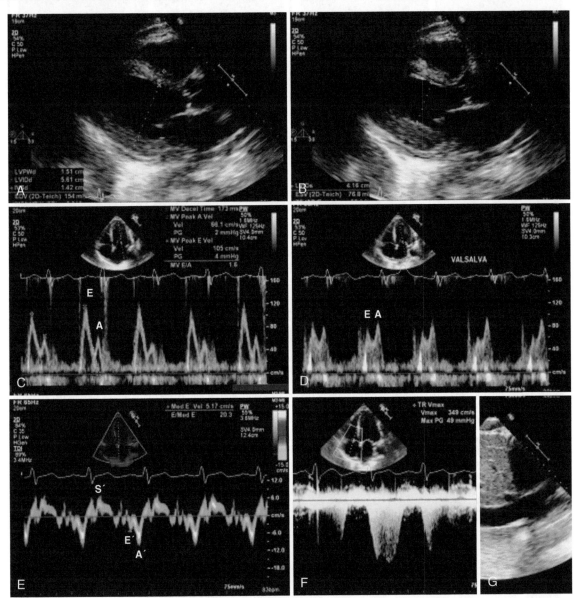

Figure 1-19. Left ventricular end-diastolic (**A**) and end-systolic (**B**) frames in the PLAX view in a 45-year-old male with a history of uncontrolled hypertension. IVS and posterior wall thicknesses are 1.42 and 1.51 cm, respectively, and LV end-diastolic and end-systolic diameters are 5.6 cm and 4.2 cm, respectively. Mitral inflow PW Doppler (**C**) shows E/A ratio of 1.6 and DT of 173 ms. Valsalva maneuver (**D**) decreased E/A ratio to 0.8. TDI of medial mitral annulus (**E**) showed reduced S′ for age and a markedly reduced E′ with E/E′ ratio of 20. RV-RA gradient (**F**) was 40 mm Hg, and IVC was dilated with a reduced respiratory variation (**G**). PAP was estimated at 55 mm Hg. LVEF was 51%. LA volume index was 38 mL/m². These findings of moderate left ventricular hypertrophy, increased LVESD, a 50% reduction in E/A ratio with a preload-reducing maneuver, and an increased E/E′ along with a reduced S′ suggest a combination of systolic and diastolic dysfunction. Diastolic dysfunction is grade III and is predominant in this patient with markedly elevated LVEDP and left atrial pressure. There is mild to moderate pulmonary hypertension secondary to predominant LV diastolic dysfunction.

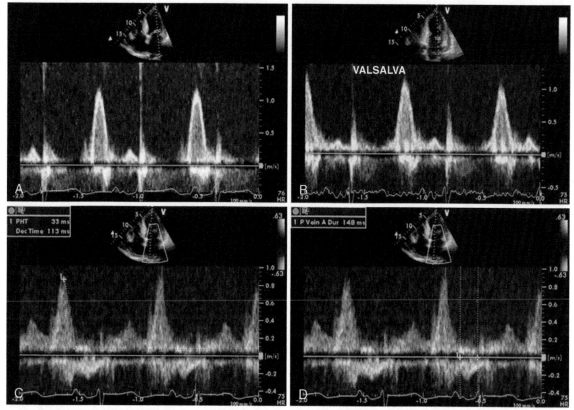

Figure 1-20. Restrictive cardiomyopathy with grade IV diastolic dysfunction. **A** and **B** are mitral inflow before (**A**) and after (**B**) Valsalva maneuver. No change in mitral inflow occurs with Valsalva maneuver. Pulmonary vein shows S/D ratio of 0.3 and short pulmonary vein DT. In addition, pulmonary vein A duration is greater than mitral inflow A duration.

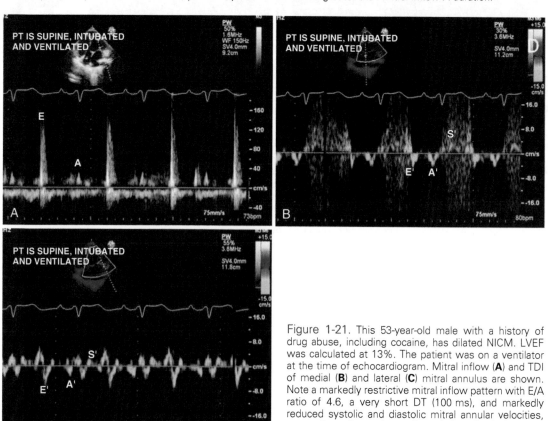

Figure 1-21. This 53-year-old male with a history of drug abuse, including cocaine, has dilated NICM. LVEF was calculated at 13%. The patient was on a ventilator at the time of echocardiogram. Mitral inflow (**A**) and TDI of medial (**B**) and lateral (**C**) mitral annulus are shown. Note a markedly restrictive mitral inflow pattern with E/A ratio of 4.6, a very short DT (100 ms), and markedly reduced systolic and diastolic mitral annular velocities, suggesting advanced systolic and diastolic dysfunction. E/E' is 53.

Pulmonary Vein PW Doppler

KEY POINTS

- A color flow–guided 2- to 3-mm PW Doppler sample volume from an apical 4-chamber position is placed 1 to 3 cm deep within the right superior pulmonary vein.
- Place the sample volume further into the pulmonary vein for a crisp atrial reversal signal.
- Sometimes better signals are obtained from apical 2- or 3-chamber views.
- Normal pulmonary vein inflow is composed of an early systolic-filling S wave and a diastolic-filling D wave. The DT of the D wave is greater than 170 to 180 ms.
- Four major patterns of pulmonary inflow are seen with advancing diastolic dysfunction:
  - *Grade I Diastolic Dysfunction:* Pulmonary inflow filling shows an S-dominant pattern. D-wave DT is normal and atrial reversal is minimal (see Figure 1-16).
  - *Grade II Diastolic Dysfunction:* A prominent pulmonary vein atrial reversal is seen with an S-dominant pattern.
  - *Grade III Diastolic Dysfunction:* S/D ratio reversal is present. Atrial reversal is usually prominent, and pulmonary vein atrial duration is greater than mitral inflow A duration. The DT of the D wave is less than 170 ms (see Figure 1-17).
  - *Grade IV Diastolic Dysfunction:* Same as grade III, except atrial reversal is often not seen due to mechanical atrial failure (see Figure 1-20).
- In the presence of atrial fibrillation, marked blunting of the pulmonary vein S wave with or without mitral regurgitation (MR) is the rule.

TDI of Mitral Annulus

KEY POINTS

- The TDI PW Doppler sample volume is placed at the medial (or septal) corner and then at the lateral corner of the mitral annulus in the apical 4-chamber view.
- Doppler beam alignment should be parallel to myocardial/annular motion.
- In patients with excessive respiratory excursion of the annulus, record these velocities during breath hold after expiration.
- Filters are set to exclude high-frequency signals, and the Nyquist limit is adjusted to a velocity range of 15 to 30 cm/s to eliminate the signals produced by transmitral flow and measured at sweep speed of at least 100 mm/s.
- The myocardial early motion wave shows a progressive decline in amplitude with increasing stage of diastolic dysfunction (see Figures 1-16 through 1-19 and 1-21).
- A markedly diminished early diastolic velocity (E′) is observed in patients with advanced restrictive cardiomyopathy.

Limitations

- Load dependent in patients with severe volume overload, such as end-stage renal and liver disease.
- Septal E′ may be less reliable in the presence of normal systolic function or in the presence of right ventricular diastolic dysfunction.

Color M-Mode Velocity Propagation

- Place the M-mode cursor, guided by color Doppler ultrasonography, in the middle of the LV aligned through the center of the mitral ring to the apex.
- Keep the color sector as narrow as possible.
- Use the zoom function to enlarge the image and maximize the sweep speed.
- The aliasing velocity is set to 0.5 to 0.7 m/s and the sweep speed at 100 to 200 mm/s.
- The color scale may be reduced to emphasize low-velocity flow, particularly in patients with poor LV function. Recording during held breathing or only at the end-expiratory phase can eliminate respiratory motion artifacts.

KEY POINTS

- More user dependent than TDI.
- Color Doppler of LV inflow is obtained in the apical 4-chamber view.
- Color Doppler is considered less load dependent than mitral inflow. Using the slope of the first aliasing contour, progressive LV diastolic dysfunction leads to progressive shortening of the slope. The normal value is considered to be greater than 50 cm/s.
- Because of the physiologic beat-to-beat variability of the PW TDI data, an averaged value from a few cardiac cycles should be obtained.

Assessment of Left Atrium

Assessment of Linear Dimensions

An increase in atrial size most commonly is related to increased wall tension as a result of increased filling pressure.

Linear Diameters

Anteroposterior Diameter. Measured by 2D-guided M-mode echocardiography or 2D obtained in the PLAX view: trailing edge of posterior aortic wall and inner edge of posterior LA wall (Figures 1-22 and 1-23).

Mediolateral Diameter. Midhorizontal diameter from the mid-interatrial septum (IAS) to the LA lateral wall (4-chamber view) (Figure 1-24).

Superoinferior Diameter. The distance of the perpendicular line measured from the middle of the plane of the mitral annulus to the superior aspect of the LA (see Figure 1-24).

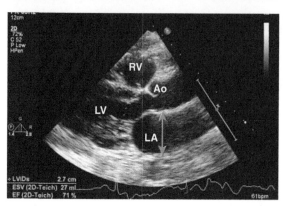

Figure 1-22. A normal-size left atrium, measured by 2D method (*arrow*), in the PLAX view is shown.

Left Atrial Volume
- LA volume is more reliable than linear dimensions due to asymmetrical LA enlargement (Figure 1-25; see also Figure 1-24).
- Avoid foreshortening.
- Maximize LA length.
- Avoid confluences of the pulmonary veins and left atrial appendage.

Ellipsoid Method
Biplane area-length method is calculated using the formula:

$$8/3\pi\,[(A_1) \times (A_2)/L]$$

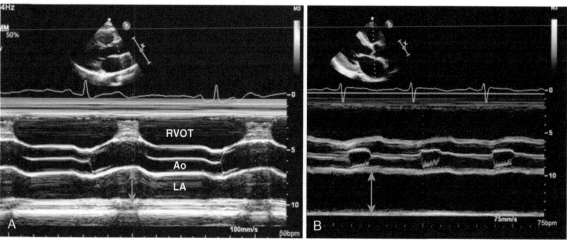

Figure 1-23. A normal left atrial diameter by 2D-guided M-mode is shown in the PLAX image (**A**). LV systolic dysfunction (**B**) leads to loss of normal aortic root motion during the cardiac cycle and enlargement of the left atrium. Angle correction can be used for more perpendicular M-mode alignment with the aortic root. RVOT, right ventricular outflow tract.

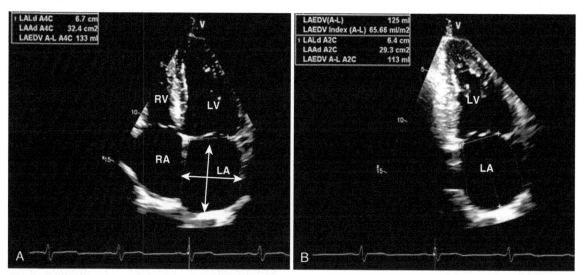

Figure 1-24. Measurement of left atrial horizontal and superoinferior dimensions as well as left atrial volume by the area-length (*L*) method in apical 4-chamber (**A**) and apical 2-chamber (**B**) views at ventricular end-systole and at maximum LA size. *L* is measured from the back wall to a line across the hinge points of the mitral valve. The shorter *L* from any of the views is used in the calculation.

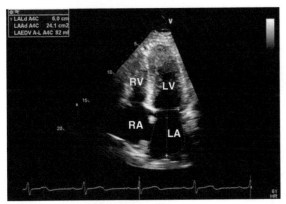

Figure 1-25. Measurement of left atrial volume from biplane method of disks (modified Simpson's method) using apical 4-chamber view at ventricular end-systole and maximum LA size. Four- and 2-chamber views are used for measurement.

where A_1 is the LA area on 4-chamber view, A_2 is the LA area on apical 2-chamber view, and L is the shorter of the major axes. Length (L) is measured from the back wall to a line across the hinge points of the mitral valve (see Figure 1-24).

Simpson's Method (Method of Disks)

The volume of the LA is calculated from the sum of the volumes of a series of stacked oval disks whose height is h and whose orthogonal minor and major axes are D_1 and D_2 (see Figure 1-25), using the formula:

$$\text{Volume: } \pi/4 \, (h) \Sigma(D_1)(D_2)$$

Noninvasive Assessment of Left Atrial and Left Ventricular Filling Pressures

Diagnostic evidence of diastolic LV dysfunction can be obtained invasively (LV end-diastolic pressure [LVEDP] >16 mm Hg or mean pulmonary capillary wedge pressure > 12 mm Hg) or noninvasively by TDI (E/E′ > 15). Multiple other parameters, including the mitral inflow E/A ratio, its reduction with the Valsalva maneuver, E-wave deceleration time, the pulmonary vein S/D ratio, the pulmonary vein D-wave DT, mitral inflow and pulmonary vein inflow duration, and E/velocity of propagation, can be used for assessing left atrial pressure (Table 1-2).

If TDI yields an E/E′ ratio suggestive of diastolic LV dysfunction (15 > E/E′ > 8), additional noninvasive investigations are required for diagnostic evidence of diastolic LV dysfunction. These can consist of blood flow Doppler of the mitral valve or pulmonary veins, echocardiographic measures of LV mass index or left atrial

TABLE 1-2 ASSESSMENT OF CARDIAC FILLING PRESSURES

Mitral regurgitation	To evaluate LA filling pressure [SBP – 4(MR velocity)²]
Tricuspid regurgitation	To evaluate pulmonary artery systolic pressure [4 × (tricuspid insufficiency jet velocity)² (m/s)]
Pulmonary regurgitation	Pulmonary artery diastolic pressure [4 × (pulmonary insufficiency jet velocity)² (m/s)] plus right atrial pressure
Left atrial pressure	Mitral inflow E-wave DT < 160 ms Mitral inflow E/A > 2.0 Pulmonary vein S < pulmonary vein D Pulmonary vein a_dur 30 ms > mitral inflow a_dur Mitral inflow E/A > 0.5 with Valsalva maneuver E/E′ > 15 E/Vp > 2.0 Pulmonary vein D wave DT < 160 ms

a_{dur}, atrial wave velocity duration; D, diastolic wave; E, mitral inflow early-filling wave; E/A, mitral inflow early-to-late diastolic velocity ratio; E/E′, ratio of mitral inflow early filling wave to myocardial early diastolic velocity; E/Vp, ratio of mitral inflow early-filling wave to early propagation velocity by color M-mode; S, systolic wave; SBP, systolic blood pressure.
To evaluate dP/dt: $\Sigma \, \Delta t$ from 1 m/s to 3 m/s, $32/\Delta t$

volume index, electrocardiographic evidence of atrial fibrillation, or plasma levels of natriuretic peptides. If plasma levels of natriuretic peptides are elevated, diagnostic evidence of diastolic LV dysfunction also requires additional noninvasive investigations such as TDI, blood flow Doppler of the mitral valve or pulmonary veins, echocardiographic measures of LV mass index or left atrial volume index, or electrocardiographic evidence of atrial fibrillation.

Assessment of Right Ventricle

Right Ventricular Size
Qualitative
- RV smaller than LV—normal.
- RV cavity area similar to that of LV—moderate enlargement, RV may share the apex of the heart.
- RV cavity area exceeds that of LV and RV is apex forming—severe RV enlargement.

Quantitative
- Midcavity diameter at end-diastole—PLAX view, SAX view (Figure 1-26), apical 4-chamber view (Figure 1-27).

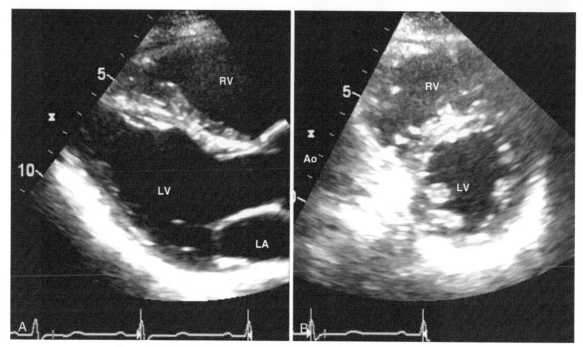

Figure 1-26. PLAX (**A**) and PSAX (**B**) views showing dilated right ventricle.

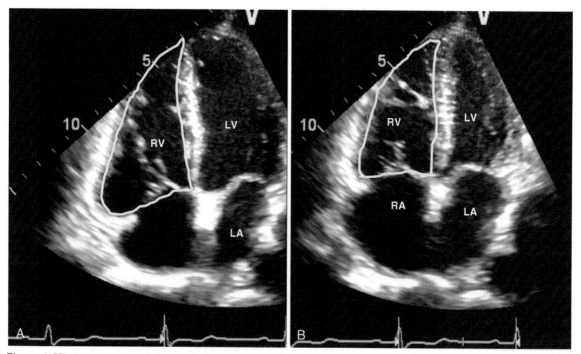

Figure 1-27. Assessment of right ventricular systolic function by fractional shortening. Endocardium is traced in the apical 4-chamber view, including trabeculation in end-diastole (**A**) and end-systole (**B**). Images demonstrate a decreased percent fractional area change (%FAC) of 30%; less than 35% indicates RV systolic dysfunction.

- Obtain a true non-foreshortened apical 4-chamber view, oriented to obtain the maximum RV dimension. RV longitudinal diameter can be measured from this view.

Right Ventricular Systolic Function

Given the complex geometry of the RV and the lack of standard methods for assessing RV volumes, RV systolic function is generally estimated qualitatively in clinical practice. Nevertheless, a number of echocardiographic techniques may be used to assess RV function. These are listed in Table 1-3.

Global RV Function
- Fractional area change (see Figure 1-27).
- RV ejection fraction (RVEF)—by 3D methods.
- Myocardial performance index (Figure 1-28).
- RV *dP/dt* (Figure 1-29).

Regional RV Function
- Tricuspid annular plane systolic excursion (TAPSE) (see Figure 1-28).
- Doppler-derived velocities of the annulus (systolic annular motion [Sm]) (see Figure 1-28).
- TDI-derived and two-dimensional strain.
- Myocardial acceleration during isovolumic contraction.

Assessment of Filling Pressure by Continuous Wave (CW) Doppler Signals (Table 1-4)

Assessment of Left Atrial Pressure

LA systolic pressure can be obtained by subtracting the peak systolic LV-LA gradient, calculated from the peak MR velocity ($4V^2$), from the systolic blood pressure, assuming there is no aortic stenosis or subclavian stenosis (Figure 1-30).

Limitation
- Peak MR velocity may not be visible in the presence of trace or mild MR.

The ascending limb of the MR signal can be used to calculate LV *dP/dt* ($32/\Delta t$, where t = time in ms between MR velocity of 1 m/s and 3 m/s).

Limitation
- Usually needs presence of mild to moderate regurgitation from MR signal on CW Doppler.

Assessment of Left Ventricular End-Diastolic Pressure
The LV-aortic end-diastolic pressure gradient can be calculated from the end-aortic regurgitation velocity as $4V^2$. This gradient is then subtracted from the diastolic blood pressure to get the LVEDP (Figure 1-31).

TABLE 1-3 ASSESSMENT OF RIGHT VENTRICULAR FUNCTION

Measurement	Location	Normal Values
TAPSE M-mode apical 4-chamber view	Tricuspid annulus	≥16 mm
Peak tricuspid valve (TV) annular velocity in systole (S_a) TDI apical 4-chamber view	Systole at lateral and medial TV annulus	≥10 cm/s
Fractional area change (FAC) 2D—apical 4-chamber view	FAC = (EDA – ESA)/EDA	>35%
Isovolumic acceleration (IVA) Tissue Doppler—lateral tricuspid annulus	IVA = TV peak isovolumic annular velocity/time to peak velocity	2.2 m/s^2
RV *dP/dt*	Tricuspid regurgitant jet by CW Doppler—time for the TR velocity to increase from 0.5 m/s to 2 m/s $\Delta P = (4V_2^2 - 4V_1^2)$ $= 15/\Delta t$	>400 mm Hg/s
Myocardial performance index (MPI) PW Doppler RV inflow and outflow	MPI = (time interval of TV closure – ET)/ET	≤0.4

EDA, end-diastolic area; ESA, end-systolic area.

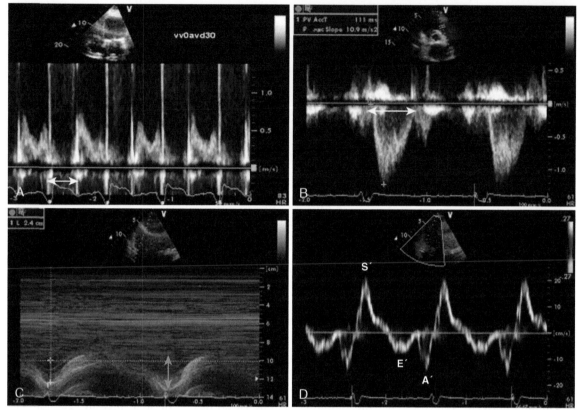

Figure 1-28. Calculation of right ventricular myocardial performance index (MPI) by PW Doppler: MPI = (TST − ET)/ET. Total systolic time (TST) is measured from the end of the tricuspid inflow A wave to the tricuspid inflow E wave (arrow in **A**). The TST encompasses IVCT, ET, and IVRT. In the PW Doppler method, the TST can also be measured by the duration of the TR CW Doppler signal. ET is measured from PW Doppler of RVOT (arrow in **B**). MPI of greater than 0.4 indicates RV systolic dysfunction. TAPSE is obtained by M-mode of the lateral tricuspid annulus (orange arrow in **C**). Normal distance between systole and diastole should be greater than 16 mm. Peak systolic velocity of the lateral tricuspid annulus is measured by placing PW TDI sample volume at the lateral tricuspid annulus (**D**). Peak S′ of tricuspid should be >10 cm/s.

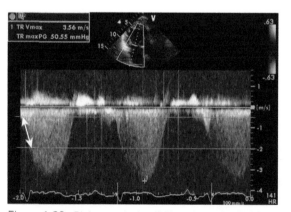

Figure 1-29. Right ventricular dP/dt can be estimated from the ascending limb of the TR CW Doppler signal using the time for the TR velocity to increase from 0.5 m/s to 2 m/s (arrow). $\Delta P = 4[V_2^2 - V_1^2]$. dP/dt = Δt from V_1 to V_2/ΔP. If Δt is 55 ms, RV dP/dt is 273 mm Hg/s.

TABLE 1-4 ASSESSMENT OF CARDIAC FILLING PRESSURES	
LA pressure	LV systolic pressure – LV-LA systolic gradient SBP – 4(peak mitral regurgitation jet velocity)² (m/s)
Peak PA pressure	RV systolic pressure + right atrial pressure [4 × (tricuspid insufficiency jet velocity)² (m/s)] + RA pressure
End-diastolic PA pressure	PA-RV late diastolic pressure gradient + RV diastolic pressure [4 × (late pulmonary insufficiency jet velocity)² (m/s)] + RA pressure
Mean PA pressure	PA-RV early diastolic pressure gradient + RV diastolic pressure [4 × (early pulmonary insufficiency jet velocity)² (m/s)] + RA pressure
LV end-diastolic pressure	Aortic diastolic pressure – end-diastolic aortic-LV pressure gradient Diastolic blood pressure – [4 × (late aortic insufficiency jet velocity)² (m/s)]

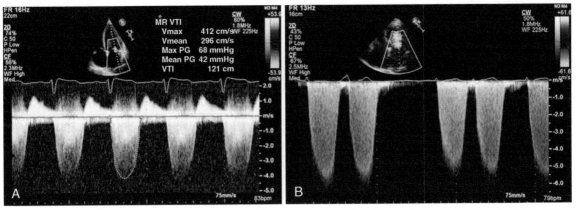

Figure 1-30. CW Doppler of MR in a patient with NICM in sinus rhythm (**A**) and in a patient with NICM and atrial fibrillation (**B**). Multiple measurements are averaged in a patient in atrial fibrillation to obtain peak and mean MR velocity. Subtracting the systolic LV-LA gradient, obtained from peak velocity ($4V^2$), from the systolic blood pressure gives an assessment of left atrial pressure.

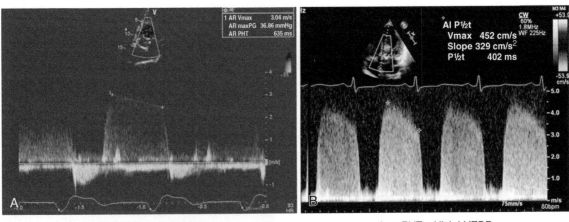

High PHT – Low LVEDP   Low PHT – High LVEDP

Figure 1-31. CW Doppler AI pressure half-time (PHT) in a patient with trace aortic regurgitation (**A**) and a patient with moderate aortic regurgitation (**B**). Pressure half-time (time for pressure gradient between aorta and LV to decrease to half in diastole) is longer when AI is insignificant and shortens when AI is significant.

Limitation

- End-diastolic aortic insufficiency (AI) velocity may not be visible in the presence of trace or mild aortic regurgitation or when aortic regurgitation is very eccentric.

LA pressure and LVEDP can also be calculated from a number of other Doppler parameters listed in Table 1-4.

Assessment of Right Ventricular and Right Atrial Pressures

The RV-RA gradient can be obtained from the peak tricuspid regurgitation (TR) velocity ($4V^2$) from the TR signal (Figure 1-32; see also Figures 1-19 and 1-29). Peak RV systolic pressure (peak pulmonary artery pressure [PAP] in the absence of pulmonic valve stenosis) can be estimated by adding right atrial pressure to the RV-RA gradient.

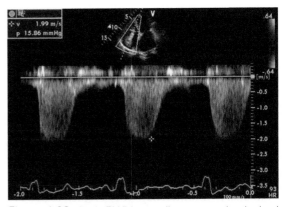

Figure 1-32. Peak RV-PA systolic pressure is obtained from the peak velocity of CW Doppler TR envelope. Pressure is obtained by Bernoulli equation as $4 \times V^2$. Normal resting values are usually a peak TR gradient of up to 2.8 m/s or a peak systolic pressure less than 35 mm Hg and less than 43 mm Hg during exercise.

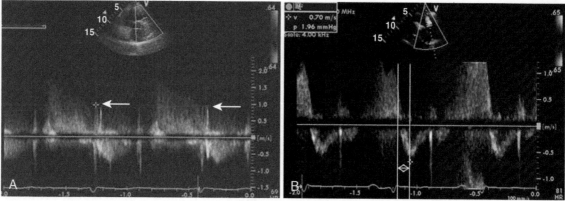

Figure 1-33. Doppler echocardiographic determination of PA diastolic pressure. CW Doppler signal of pulmonic regurgitation (PI) is shown in **A**. *White arrow* points to the velocity at end PI corresponding to the PA-RV diastolic pressure gradient. PA diastolic pressure is calculated as the sum of the RA pressure and the gradient between the PA end-diastolic pressure and the RV end-diastolic pressure, by application of the modified Bernoulli equation to the end-diastolic velocity of the pulmonary regurgitation Doppler signal. Mean PAP is PA systolic pressure + (2PADP)/3. Mean PA pressure can also be estimated from PW Doppler of the RVOT (**B**). Acceleration time is measured from the onset of ejection to peak ejection (*white lines* in **B**). Mean PAP = 79 – (0.45 × acceleration time); in patients with acceleration times less than 120 ms, mean PAP = 90 – (0.62 × acceleration time).

TABLE 1-5 ASSESSMENT OF RIGHT ATRIAL PRESSURE		
IVC Diameter	**Collapsibility Index**	**Estimated RA Pressure**
≤2.1 cm (normal)	>50% (normal)	3 mm Hg (normal)
>2.1 cm (dilated)	>50% (normal)	8 mm Hg (mildly elevated)
>2.1 cm	<50%	15 mm Hg
>2.1 cm	None	>15 mm Hg

Indicators of Elevated RA Pressure

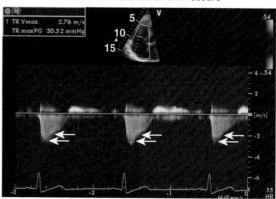

Figure 1-34. RV dilatation, often associated with systolic heart failure, may be associated with significant functional TR and elevated right atrial pressure. A cutoff sign ("V" sign) on the upstroke of the TR envelope (*white arrows*) indicates equalization of right ventricular and right atrial pressure in early systole as a result of elevation of right atrial pressure.

RA systolic pressure is estimated from the size and respiratory variability of the inferior vena cava (IVC) (Table 1-5).

Limitation
- Peak TR velocity may not be visible in the presence of trace TR.

Assessment of Right Ventricular End-Diastolic Pressure

The RV–pulmonary artery (PA) end-diastolic pressure gradient can be calculated from the end pulmonary insufficiency (PI) velocity as $4V^2$ (Figure 1-33). RA pressure is then added to this gradient to obtain RV end-diastolic pressure.

RA pressure is estimated from the IVC (see Table 1-5; see also Figure 1-19) and TR jet shape (Figure 1-34).

Summary of Echocardiographic Findings

Echocardiographic findings in systolic and diastolic heart failure are summarized in Tables 1-6 and 1-7.

Infiltrative Cardiomyopathy

While abnormalities in systolic function can be detected by TDI and speckle tracking, infiltrative cardiomyopathy manifests as a pure form of diastolic dysfunction on a conventional

TABLE 1-6 TWO-DIMENSIONAL ECHOCARDIOGRAPHIC FINDINGS IN SYSTOLIC AND DIASTOLIC HEART FAILURE

Echo Parameter	Systolic Heart Failure	Diastolic Heart Failure
LV size	Dilated	Normal
Wall thickness	Normal or increased	Usually increased
LV mass	Significantly increased	Normal to severely increased
LVEF	Moderate to severly reduced	Preserved
LV trabeculation	Often increased	Normal
LV thrombus	May be present	Absent
Atrial size	Usually enlarged	Enlarged disproportionate to LV size
Right ventricular size	Often enlarged	Normal to mildly enlarged
Right ventricular systolic function	Often reduced	Usually normal
Inferior vena cava	Normal to dilated	Dilated with reduced respiratory variation
Hepatic veins	Variable	Often dilated
Pleural effusion	Often present	Often absent
Pericardial effusion	Usually absent	Usually absent
Atrial fibrillation	May be present	Often present

TABLE 1-7 DOPPLER ECHOCARDIOGRAPHIC FINDINGS IN SYSTOLIC AND DIASTOLIC HEART FAILURE

Echo Parameter	Systolic Heart Failure	Diastolic Heart Failure
Mitral regurgitation	None to severe	None to moderate
Diastolic MR	May be present Often due to first-degree atrioventricular block (AVB)	May be present Often due to elevated LVEDP
MR peak velocity	Often reduced	Normal to elevated
MR dP/dt	Reduced	Often normal
Tricuspid regurgitation	None to severe Often due to first-degree AVB	None to moderate Often due to elevated LVEDP
Diastolic TR	May be present	May be present
Pulmonary artery pressure	Elevated proportionate to LV systolic dysfunction and/or MR	Elevated disproportionate to LV systolic dysfunction and/or MR
Mitral inflow	Grade I–IV diastolic dysfunction Grade often concordant to LV systolic function	Often grade II–IV diastolic dysfunction Grade often disconcordant to LV systolic function
Color M-mode	Propagation velocity (Vp) variable	Vp usually <45 cm/s and E/Vp > 1.5
Tricuspid inflow	Variable	Often restrictive filling
Pulmonary vein (PV) pattern	Grade I–IV May show systolic reversal with severe MR	Often grade III–IV Diastolic dominant pattern prominent atrial reversal with PV a_{dur} > mitral inflow a_{dur}
TDI E′	Often reduced	Often reduced

Continued

TABLE 1-7 DOPPLER ECHOCARDIOGRAPHIC FINDINGS IN SYSTOLIC AND DIASTOLIC HEART FAILURE—cont'd

Echo Parameter	Systolic Heart Failure	Diastolic Heart Failure
Septal annulus TDI S′	Markedly reduced	Mildly reduced
Mitral annulus	Dilated	Normal to moderately dilated
Tricuspid annulus	Dilated	Normal to moderately dilated
Tricuspid annulus TDI	S′ reduced	S′ often normal
Hepatic veins	Variable	S/D ratio <0.5, prominent atrial and ventricular reversal with inspiration and expiration

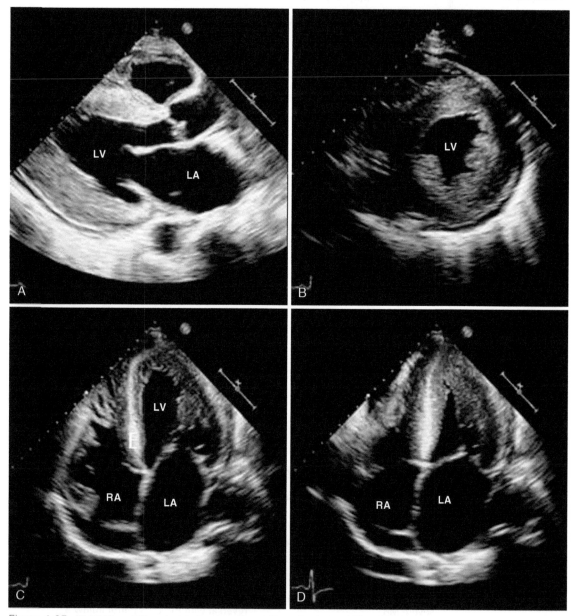

Figure 1-35. PLAX (**A** and **B**), apical 4-chamber (**C** and **D**), and subcostal (**E** and **F**) views in end-diastole and end-systole in a 45-year-old male with amyloid cardiomyopathy. Note a marked increase in LV and RV wall thickness, ground-glass appearance of LV and RV myocardium, normal to small LV end-systolic dimensions, marked left atrial enlargement, and small circumferential pericardial effusion, all hallmarks of restrictive cardiomyopathy from an infiltrative process.

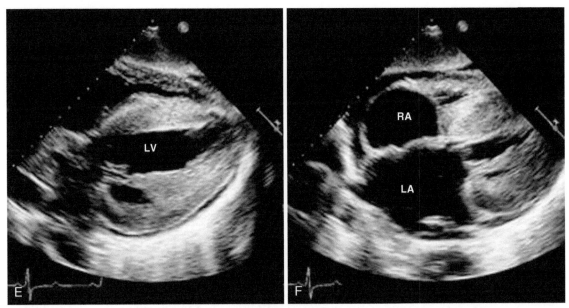

Figure 1-35, cont'd

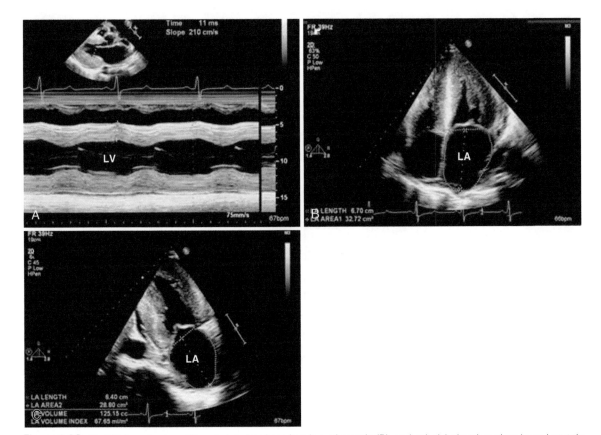

Figure 1-36. PLAX M-mode view (**A**), apical 4-chamber view in end-systole (**B**), and apical 2-chamber view in end-systole (**C**) in the same patient with infiltrative cardiomyopathy. Note again marked left ventricular hypertrophy on M-mode as well as ground-glass appearance of myocardium (**A**). Measurement of left atrial volume by area-length method revealed that the left atrial volume was severely increased at 68 mL/m².

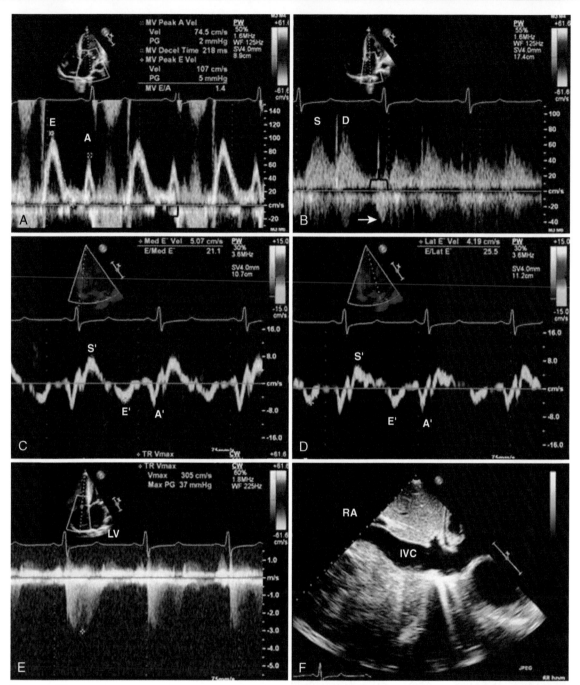

Figure 1-37. Mitral inflow (**A**), pulmonary vein inflow PW Doppler (**B**), TDI of medial (**C**) and lateral (**D**) mitral annulus, TR envelope (**E**), and subcostal view showing a dilated IVC (**F**) in the same patient with infiltrative cardiomyopathy. Note a pseudonormal-appearing mitral inflow with a DT of 213 ms. However, the pulmonary vein shows S/D ratio reversal with a ratio of 0.8. In addition, pulmonary vein atrial duration (*white arrow* in **B**) is greater than mitral inflow a duration in **A** (*black braces* in **A** and **B**) and E/E' is 21 and 25 at the medial and lateral annulus, respectively. These findings suggest grade III LV diastolic dysfunction and elevated left atrial pressure. IVC is dilated with reduced respiratory variation, suggesting RA pressure is approximately 15 mm Hg. This gives a PAP of 37 + 15 mm Hg = 52 mm Hg. Pulmonary hypertension in this patient is secondary to diastolic heart failure.

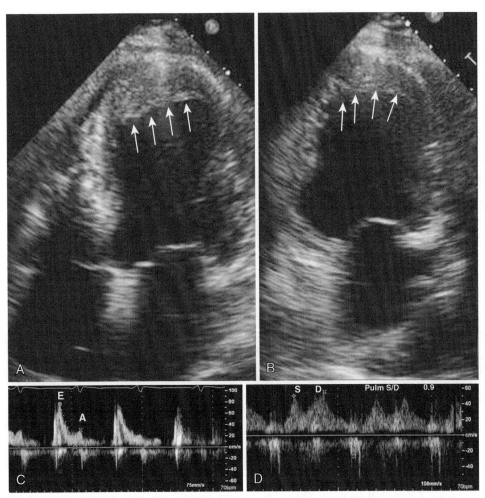

Figure 1-38. Apical 4-chamber (**A**) and 2-chamber (**B**) views in a 58-year-old male with a large recent left anterior descending coronary artery (LAD) territory infarct causing aneurysm formation of distal LV segments and a large apical thrombus (*white arrows* **A** and **B**). Mitral inflow (**C**) and pulmonary vein PW Doppler (**D**) show a restrictive filling pattern with increased E/A ratio and decreased S/D ratio.

Continued

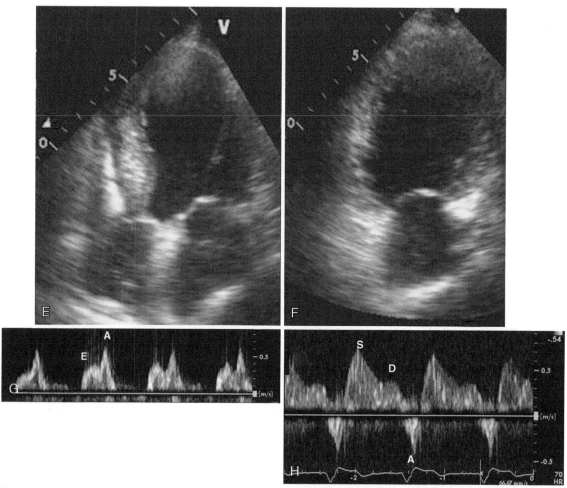

Figure 1-38, cont'd E through H are views obtained in the same patient 1 year later. Infarcted segments are still dyskinetic; however, LV size is smaller in apical 4-chamber (E) and 2-chamber (F) views and noninfarcted segments show better contractility. In addition, LV apical thrombus has resolved. A more significant improvement is noted in mitral inflow (G) that shows an E/A ratio less than 1 and pulmonary vein Doppler (H) that is S dominant. Prominent atrial reversal suggests elevated LVEDP.

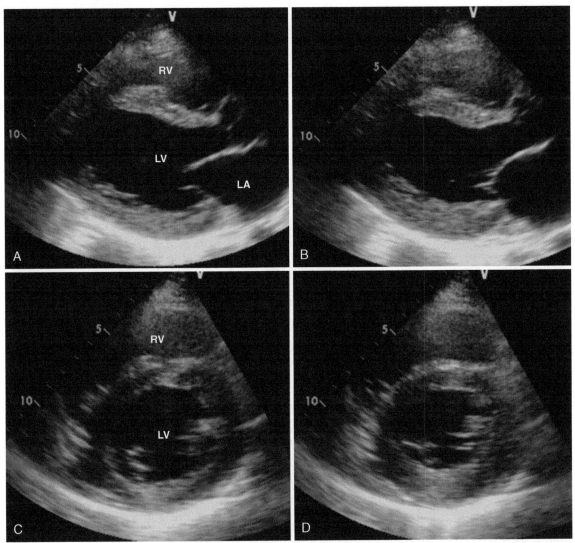

Figure 1-39. Two-dimensional echocardiographic views in PLAX at diastole (**A**) and systole (**B**), parasternal mid-LV SAX at diastole (**C**), and apical 4-chamber at diastole (**D**) in a 45-year-old Hispanic female with end-stage renal disease, on hemodialysis. Left ventricular concentric hypertrophy and reduced LV systolic function are evident by increased wall thickness and increased end-systolic diameter in the PLAX view (**B**).

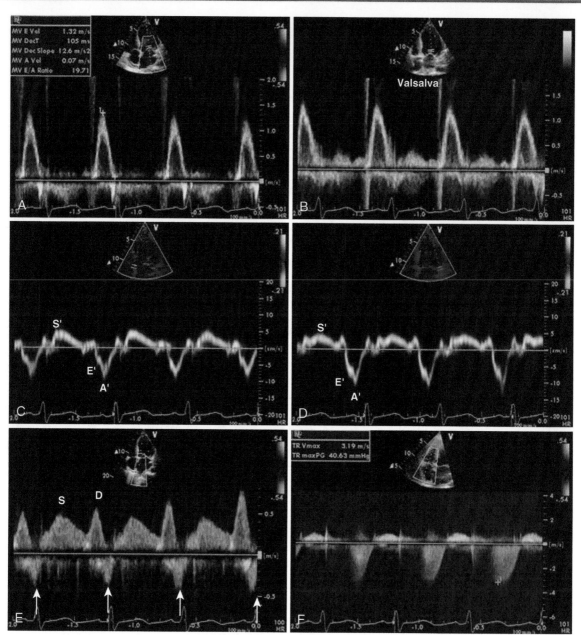

Figure 1-40. PW Doppler mitral inflow before (**A**) and after (**B**) Valsalva maneuver, TDI of medial (**C**) and lateral (**D**) mitral annulus, pulmonary vein inflow Doppler (**E**), and CW Doppler of TR (**F**) in same patient with end-stage renal disease on hemodialysis. Note E and A fusion on mitral inflow as well as TDI images due to sinus tachycardia in this patient that may make evaluation of diastolic function difficult. Pulmonary vein shows S/D reversal and prominent atrial reversal (*white arrows* in **E**), suggesting grade III diastolic dysfunction with elevation of LVEDP. Also note elevated RV-RA gradient of 41 mm Hg in **F**, suggesting pulmonary hypertension.

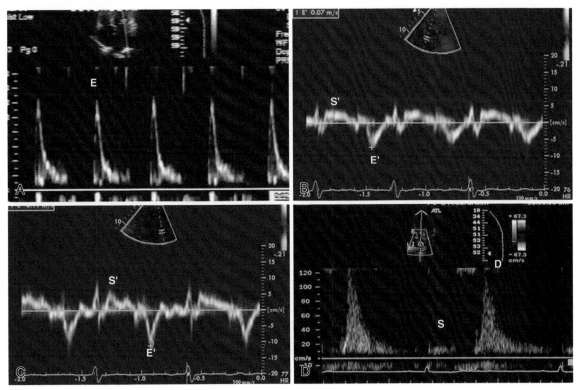

Figure 1-41. Mitral inflow (**A**), TDI of medial (**B**) and lateral (**C**) mitral annulus, and pulmonary vein PW Doppler (**D**) in a patient with atrial fibrillation. Lack of A wave does not allow evaluation of mitral inflow E/A ratio. However, E wave (160 cm/s), E-wave DT (120 ms), E/E' (17.7 for E' averaged over septal and lateral annulus), and pulmonary vein D-wave DT (130 ms) help in assessing diastolic function and left atrial filling pressures, which are elevated in this patient. E-wave height is more regular in patients with elevated LVEDP.

echocardiogram and initially presents as isolated diastolic heart failure (Figures 1-35 through 1-37).

Concomitant Systolic and Diastolic Dysfunction

In systolic heart failure, diastolic dysfunction is present parallel to the grade of systolic dysfunction. Figure 1-38 illustrates a patient with a large anterior acute MI complicated by LV aneurysm formation along with LV thrombus. Following bypass surgery, LV systolic function improved after a year. This was associated with an improvement in diastolic function grade.

Challenges in Assessment of Diastolic Function

Tachycardia makes evaluation of diastolic function difficult. Pulmonary vein flow may be most

helpful in this setting (Figures 1-39 and 1-40). In the presence of a prosthetic mitral valve, mitral stenosis, or significant mitral annular calcification, pulmonary vein flow is most reliable in assessing diastolic function.

Atrial fibrillation is another common condition that makes assessment of diastolic function difficult due to a loss of mechanical atrial function and highly variable cycle length. In chronic atrial fibrillation, it is difficult to separate the effects of the progression of diastolic dysfunction from further atrial remodeling related to atrial fibrillation itself. Pulmonary vein flow shows S-wave blunting and hence the S/D ratio is not very helpful. Mitral inflow E-wave DT, E/E', and pulmonary wave DT assist with evaluation of diastolic function and left atrial pressure (Figure 1-41).

Significant mitral regurgitation causes S-wave blunting. In addition, increased forward flow increases the E wave. Hence assessment of diastolic function in the presence of significant MR remains challenging.

Suggested Readings

1. Lang RM, Bierig M, Devereux RB, et al. Recommendations for chamber quantification: A report from the American Society of Echocardiography's Guidelines and Standards Committee and the Chamber Quantification Writing Group, developed in conjunction with the European Association of Echocardiography. *J Am Soc Echocardiogr.* 2005;18: 1440-1463.

2. Rudski LG, Lai WW, Afilalo J, et al. Guidelines for the echocardiographic assessment of the right heart in adults: A report from the American Society of Echocardiography. *J Am Soc Echocardiogr.* 2010;23:685-713.

3. Quinones MA, Otto CM, Stoddard M, Waggoner A, Zoghbi WA. Recommendations for quantification of Doppler echocardiography: A report from the Doppler Quantification Task Force of the Nomenclature and Standards Committee of the American Society of Echocardiography. *J Am Soc Echocardiogr.* 2002;15:167-184.

4. Nagueh SF, Appleton CP, Gillebert TG, et al. Recommendations for the evaluation of left ventricular diastolic function by echocardiography. *J Am Soc Echocardiogr.* 2009;22: 107-133.

Echocardiographic Assessment of Patients with Systolic Heart Failure

2

Sorin Pislaru and Maurice Enriquez-Sarano

Definition, Staging, and Etiology of Systolic Heart Failure

- Heart failure (HF): abnormality of cardiac function responsible for inability of the heart to provide blood flow at rates commensurate with tissue requirement, or to do so only at increased filling pressures.
- HF stages[1]
  Stage A: risk factors for HF, but normal ventricular function, no symptoms
  Stage B: ventricular dysfunction (systolic/diastolic), but no symptoms
  Stage C: ventricular dysfunction and mild symptoms
  Stage D: ventricular dysfunction and severe symptoms
- Systolic heart failure
  - Implies impairment of systolic ventricular function.
  - It is a common end stage for a variety of cardiac diseases.
  - It can be left ventricular, right ventricular, or biventricular.
- Various etiologies[2]
  - Coronary artery disease—approximately 60% to 70% of systolic HF
  - Dilated cardiomyopathy
    - Idiopathic
    - Infectious (viral, HIV, Chagas' disease, Lyme disease)
    - Toxic (alcohol, cocaine, anthracyclines)
    - Metabolic (thiamine and selenium deficiencies, thyroid disorders, hemochromatosis)
    - Genetic
  - Valvular disease
  - Other (peripartum, tachycardia-induced, autoimmune, familial, sarcoidosis, obstructive sleep apnea, etc.)
- The single most useful diagnostic test in the evaluation of patients with HF is the comprehensive two-dimensional (2D) echocardiogram coupled with Doppler flow studies.[1] The goals of echocardiography in systolic HF are:
  - Define etiology and in particular determine if systolic HF is due to a primary myocardial disease (including consequences of coronary disease) or a primary valve disease.
  - Define the degree of systolic ventricular dysfunction and remodeling (Table 2-1).
  - Define the degree of diastolic ventricular dysfunction (addressed in Chapter 3).
  - Define the presence and severity of functional mitral regurgitation (MR) and/or tricuspid regurgitation.
  - Define the hemodynamic consequences (cardiac output, pulmonary and atrial pressures).

Echocardiographic Methods for Assessment of Left Ventricular Systolic Function

Image Acquisition and Interpretation
- Various imaging modalities can be used for assessment of left ventricular systolic function (see Table 2-1).
- Classical indexes of left ventricular function are derived from linear and volumetric data.[3]
- Image optimization is a key step in obtaining accurate measurements. Always adjust focus depth, sector size, and lateral gains to optimize axial and temporal resolution.
- Harmonic imaging increases wall thickness and decreases internal dimensions slightly.
- Color B-mode maps and/or intravenous contrast may be needed for wall motion analysis.
- Assessment by Doppler echocardiography is always comprehensive, integrating all methods available (e.g., ejection fraction [EF] is judged visually and compounded with calculated EF from M-mode or 2D diameters or LV volumes).

TABLE 2-1 LEFT VENTRICULAR QUANTIFICATION METHODS: USE, ADVANTAGES, AND LIMITATIONS

Dimension/Volumes	Use/Advantages	Limitations
Linear		
M-mode	Reproducible High frame rates	Beam frequently off-axis Single dimension not representative in distorted ventricles
2D-guided	Assures orientation perpendicular to LV axis	Lower frame rates than in M-mode Single dimension only
Volumetric		
Biplane Simpson's method	Corrects for shape distortions Minimizes mathematic assumptions	Apex frequently foreshortened Endocardial dropout Relies on only two planes
Area-length method	Partial correction for shape distortion	Based on mathematic assumptions
3D echocardiography	Best correlation with MRI Further enhanced by contrast use	Endocardial definition

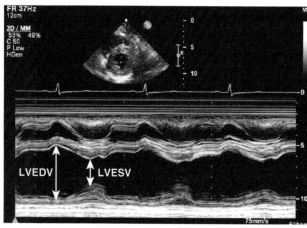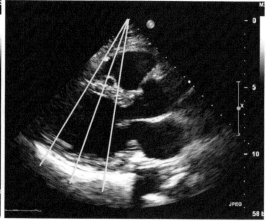

Figure 2-1. Left, M-mode measurement of left ventricular end-diastolic (LVEDD) and end-systolic (LVESD) dimensions. EF can be then calculated based on Teichholz or Quiñones formulas. **Right,** Note that only the M-mode obtained along the center line is perpendicular to the LV long axis. M-mode images obtained on the outer lines would overestimate left ventricular size, a common problem in M-mode measurements.

Indexes of Global Left Ventricular Systolic Function

- Left ventricular size
  - LV size is measured by the diameter at the mitral leaflet tips; calculation is simple but not linearly related to LV volumes.
  - Left ventricular volumes can be calculated from 2D imaging (area-length or method of disks) and from three-dimensional (3D) imaging with specific software. End-systolic volume index is an important index of LV remodeling and function.
- EF by visual assessment
  - This value is an estimation based on appreciation of ventricular area change in systole from multiple views.

- Calculation is simple but underestimates EF in the very low range (an area change of 10% equals an EF of 19%).
  - It serves as a background check for calculation methods.
- EF by linear measurements (Figure 2-1)
  - Calculation is based on the LV internal diameter at end-diastole and end-systole.
  - Electrocardiography (ECG) serves only as a guidance; valve and wall motion should also be considered in selecting end-diastolic and end-systolic frames.[3]
  - EF calculations are based on Teichholz or Quiñones methods.
  - Linear measurements (M-mode, 2D) have several disadvantages (see Table 2-1).

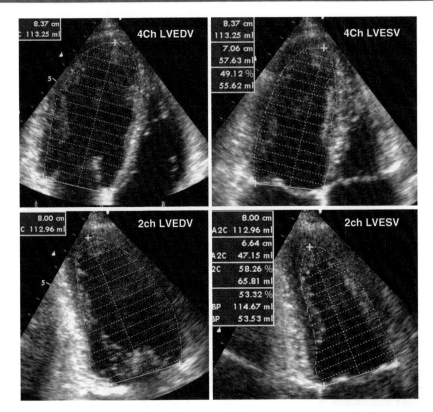

Figure 2-2. EF measurement based on the method of disks. End-systolic and end-diastolic frames are used to trace the endocardial border on standard apical 4-chamber (*top panel*, left ventricle on the left side) and 2-chamber (*bottom panel*) views.

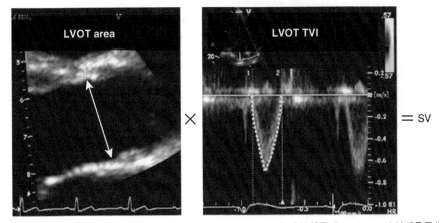

Figure 2-3. Stroke volume (SV) calculations are based on measurement of LVOT diameter and LVOT TVI. The LVOT is assumed to be circular and the area is calculated by the formula: $A = \pi \times d^2/4 = 0.785 \times d^2$. The cardiac output is then calculated by multiplying the SV and the heart rate at the time of acquisition.

- EF by volumetric measurements (Figure 2-2)
  - Calculation does not have geometric assumptions.
  - LV apical foreshortening and lateral resolution on 2D images can be significant limitations (see Table 2-1).
  - 3D contrast-enhanced echocardiography has the best correlation with magnetic resonance imaging (MRI) in terms of assessment of LV and RV volumes.

- Stroke volume and cardiac output (Figure 2-3)
  - These values are based on 2D (LV outflow tract [LVOT] dimension and calculated area) and Doppler (blood velocity) measurements, with calculation of stroke volume as the product of LVOT area by time-velocity integral (TVI).
  - LVOT diameter measurement can be underestimated, and small errors in LVOT measurements are squared in area calculation.

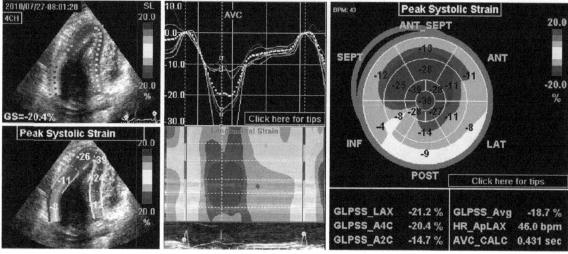

Figure 2-4. Measurement of left ventricular peak longitudinal systolic strain in a patient with hypertrophic cardiomyopathy. The software automatically tracks the area of interest and calculates left ventricular strain based on speckle tracking (*left panel*—example of tracking in 4-chamber view). The average peak negative systolic strain can be then calculated from measurements performed on each of the 17 segments, and can be displayed as a bull's-eye diagram (*right panel*); this can also serve for assessment of regional left ventricular function. The peak negative longitudinal systolic strain has gained importance in assessment of early changes in systolic function in patients with infiltrative and hypertrophic cardiomyopathies.

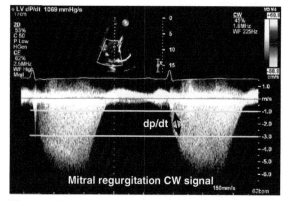

Figure 2-5. Measurement of left ventricular systolic *dP/dt* is based on the mitral regurgitant signal. Since in the very early phase of systole the MR does not significantly increase the atrial pressure, it can be assumed that the increase in MR regurgitant velocity directly reflects changes in intraventricular pressure. By measuring the time needed for the MR velocity to increase from 1 to 3 m/s, *dP/dt* can be calculated according to the formula: $dP/dt = (4 \times 3^2 - 4 \times 1^2)/\text{time} = 32/\text{time}$.

Careful zoomed imaging with decreased gain, and learning curve with calculation of cardiac index, are essential in accuracy.
- Other parameters used in assessment of global LV systolic function
  - Mitral annular systolic velocity (tissue Doppler imaging [TDI])
  - Global left ventricular peak systolic strain (Figure 2-4)
  - Estimated left ventricular *dP/dt* (Figure 2-5)
  - LV mass is measurable using wall thickness and LV size and is particularly important in

hypertensive patients. LV mass is always increased with LV dilatation, but prognosis is more based on quality than on quantity of muscle.

Assessment of Regional Left Ventricular Function
- Assessment of regional wall motion abnormalities (RWMAs)
  - The American Society of Electrocardiography (ASE) recommends a 17-segment LV model (Figure 2-6).
  - Motion of each segment is evaluated on a semiquantitative scale (1 = normal or hyperkinesis; 2 = hypokinesis; 3 = akinesis or negligible thickening; 4 = dyskinesis/paradoxical systolic motion; 5 = aneurysmal).
- RWMA due to ischemia does not occur at rest until epicardial coronary artery stenosis is greater than 85%.
- Echocardiography overestimates the area of ischemic or infarcted myocardium as adjacent regions are affected by tethering, regional loading conditions, and stunning.
- The presence of regional left ventricular dysfunction not respecting coronary distribution can be seen in various diseases, such as post–coronary artery bypass grafting, infiltrative cardiomyopathies (sarcoidosis), cardiac tumors, myocarditis, etc.
- Other tools are gaining momentum in assessing regional wall motion, particularly segmental left ventricular strain or strain rate (see Figure 2-4).

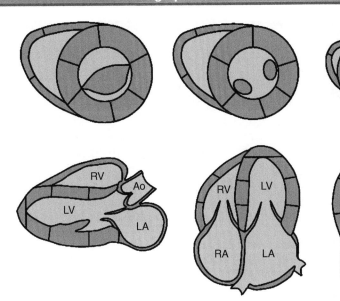

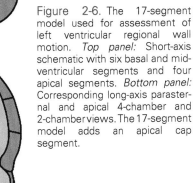

Figure 2-6. The 17-segment model used for assessment of left ventricular regional wall motion. *Top panel:* Short-axis schematic with six basal and mid-ventricular segments and four apical segments. *Bottom panel:* Corresponding long-axis parasternal and apical 4-chamber and 2-chamber views. The 17-segment model adds an apical cap segment.

Assessment of LV Diastolic Function

- LV relaxation is always slowed when systolic function is reduced.
- Diastolic dysfunction analysis is based on the combination of mitral and pulmonary venous flows and TDI.
- Simple relaxation abnormality (stage I) is benign, while restrictive filling (stage III/IV) indicates elevated filling pressures.

Assessment of Functional Regurgitation (Mitral, Tricuspid)

- Assess structural normalcy of valves.
- Estimate or, better, quantify regurgitation.

Assessment of Hemodynamic Consequences

- Estimate right atrial pressure using inferior vena cava size and variation, and right ventricular pressure using tricuspid regurgitation velocity.
- Calculate cardiac index.

KEY POINTS

- Left ventricular internal diameter and EF are key parameters in the diagnosis and follow-up assessment of systolic dysfunction.
- Several guidelines include LV size and EF in decision making.
- The ASE recommends use of biplane method of disks (modified Simpson's method) for EF calculations.
- Erroneous LVOT measurements can introduce large errors in estimation of cardiac output and severity of valvular disease.
- RWMAs at rest can occur both with ischemic and nonischemic cardiomyopathies.
- Assessment of LV strain and strain rate are increasingly used.

Echocardiographic Assessment of Specific Causes of Systolic Heart Failure

Ischemic LV Dysfunction

- Ischemic LV dysfunction is the most common cause of systolic HF.
- The presence of resting RWMAs in a coronary artery distribution pattern and/or evidence of old myocardial infarction (thinned, scarred myocardial wall; LV aneurysm) are key echocardiographic findings.
- Resting RWMAs can also be seen with stunned/hibernating myocardium and occasionally in non-ischemic disease.
- Intravenous contrast should be used whenever endocardial border definition is suboptimal in two or more contiguous segments.
- Stress echocardiography is an established method of assessment of myocardial ischemia.
  - Exercise (treadmill or stationary bike) is the preferred stress method. It can be combined with oxygen consumption for better quantification of exercise ability. Dobutamine is the most commonly used pharmacologic stress agent.
  - Interpretation is based on regional wall motion analysis and global response to stress (change in left ventricular dimension and EF with stress).
- With stress, RWMAs can occur with epicardial coronary stenoses as low as 50%.
- A biphasic response to dobutamine in at least two segments with resting RWMAs (improvement at low dose followed by worsening at high dose) is suggestive of viable myocardium and epicardial coronary artery disease (hibernating myocardium).

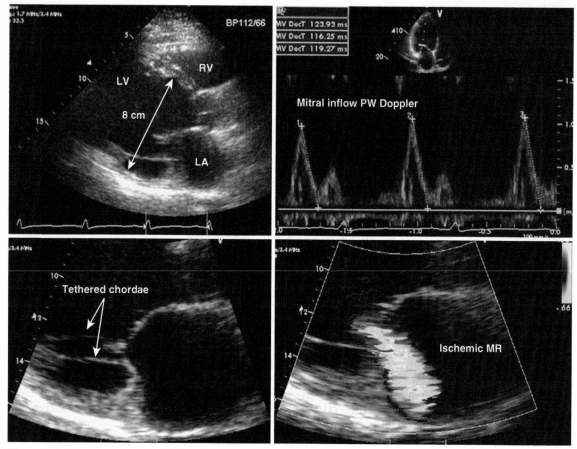

Figure 2-7. Typical appearance of ischemic MR in a patient with severe left ventricular dysfunction. Note extreme LV dilatation with thinned inferolateral wall (*top left*) and restrictive filling pattern on the mitral inflow (*top right*). Both mitral leaflets are tethered in systole, the posterior leaflet more than the anterior (*bottom left*). This results in incomplete coaptation and override of the anterior leaflet, with a posteriorly directed jet of MR (*bottom right*).

• MR can be associated with ischemic left ventricular dysfunction, and is most commonly due to tethering of the posterior mitral leaflet (Figure 2-7); an effective regurgitant orifice (ERO) greater than 0.20 cm² and a regurgitant volume greater than 30 mL are associated with poor prognosis.

• Always assess for intraventricular thrombus in patients with low EF and aneurysmal changes (Figure 2-8). This is best done by administration of intravenous contrast.

KEY POINTS

• RWMAs can be seen in a variety of conditions, but their most common cause is myocardial ischemia.
• The preferred stress modality is treadmill exercise.
• A biphasic response to dobutamine is suggestive of myocardial viability.

• Mitral regurgitation can be associated with ischemic left ventricular dysfunction.
• Intravenous contrast administration is helpful for accurate assessment of RWMAs and intracardiac thrombus.

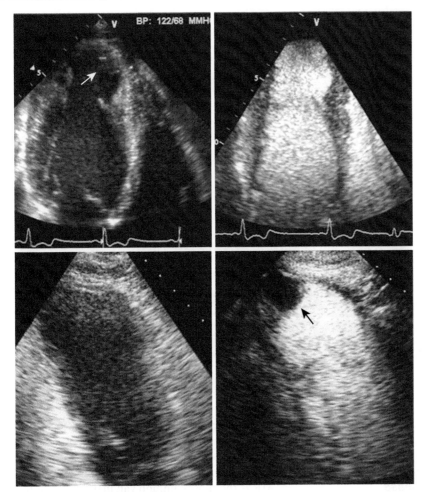

Figure 2-8. Intravenous contrast for assessment of intracardiac thrombus. *Top row:* Apical infarct with aneurysm formation in a patient with history of apical cardiomyopathy. *Left panel* shows wall thinning and intracavitary haziness at the apex (*arrow*), suspicious for apical thrombus. This is effectively ruled out on the contrast image (*right panel*). *Bottom row:* Apical aneurysm formation after LAD infarction. Note the inconspicuous appearance on standard 2D echocardiography (*left panel*). Since the endocardial definition was suboptimal, intravenous contrast was administered. This clearly shows the presence of an apical thrombus (*arrow*) but also apical LV wall thinning consistent with an old infarction (*right panel*).

Dilated Cardiomyopathy

- Idiopathic (~50%) and secondary dilated cardiomyopathies have similar echocardiographic findings.
- Diagnosis requires presence of an enlarged ventricle with reduced EF (<40%) or reduced fractional shortening (<25%).
- Generalized left ventricular hypokinesis is usually present, although some of the basal segments can be relatively spared.
- Valvular disease (functional MR and tricuspid regurgitation) is often present and may further worsen ventricular dysfunction.
- Treatment and prognosis vary depending on the etiology.
- Heart transplantation and/or left ventricular assist devices (LVAD) are frequently considered.
- Implanted continuous-flow LVADs have unique echocardiographic findings (Figure 2-9):
  - Lack of (or minimal) systolic opening of the aortic valve
  - Continuous aortic regurgitation (when present)
  - Left ventricular apical inflow cannula is usually well seen

- Continuous flow in the ascending aorta
- The outflow cannula is more difficult to visualize by the transthoracic approach (high position in the ascending aorta). Right parasternal imaging can help.
- Critical echocardiographic evaluations in LVAD patients are:
  - Assessment of valvular competency (especially aortic and tricuspid)
  - Assessment of possible inflow/outflow cannula obstruction by color Doppler and continuous wave (CW)/pulsed wave (PW) Doppler
  - Cardiac output can be estimated from careful assessment of the RV outflow tract (RVOT) diameter and RVOT TVI (similar to the left heart assessment).

KEY POINTS

- Idiopathic and secondary causes of dilated cardiomyopathy have similar echocardiographic features.
- Functional valvular regurgitation is often present.
- LVAD assessment has unique echocardiographic features.

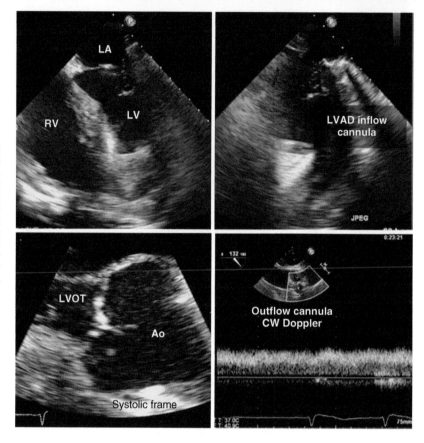

Figure 2-9. Typical appearance of an LVAD (HeartMate II) implanted as destination therapy. Orthogonal plane imaging from midesophageal position showing normal position of the apical inflow cannula (*top panels*). The aortic valve remains closed during systole (note position of the ECG marker; *bottom left*). CW Doppler in the ascending aorta at the tip of the outflow cannula shows continuous flow (*bottom right*).

Left Ventricular Dysfunction Resulting from Valvular Disease

- Long-standing severe aortic valve disease (both stenosis and regurgitation) and MR are associated with left ventricular dysfunction.
- Isolated mitral stenosis *is not* associated with left ventricular systolic dysfunction.
- Echocardiography is the cornerstone of evaluating valvular disease.
  - It establishes the etiology and responsible mechanism.
  - It allows reproducible quantification of disease severity.
  - Echocardiography-derived parameters have prognostic implications and are used in determining the need for surgical correction.
- Assessment of valvular disease severity is based on integrating data from several echocardiographic imaging modalities (Table 2-2).
- Formal volumetric quantification of valvular disease severity is based on the continuity-of-flow principle.
- Proximal isovelocity surface area (PISA) method (also based on continuity of flow) has become the preferred modality for evaluating regurgitant lesions (Figure 2-10).

Mitral Regurgitation

- MR is the most common valvular disease in the United States.[4]
- It is the result of the loss of normal systolic coaptation between the anterior and posterior leaflets.
- Echocardiography is uniquely positioned for comprehensive assessment of normal mitral valve anatomy (Figure 2-11).
  - The anterior and posterior mitral leaflets are further subdivided into three scallops (A1 through A3, P1 through P3).
  - The mitral annulus has a saddle shape as a result of which mitral valve prolapse is diagnosed based on the long-axis parasternal view (valve more than 2 mm below the annular plane).
- Echocardiographic approach to systematic evaluation of mitral regurgitation:
  - Step 1: establish the mechanism (Table 2-3).
    - "Organic" MR when the valve is structurally abnormal (Figure 2-12).
    - "Functional" MR when regurgitation is due to ventricular remodeling disturbing normal valvular anatomy.
    - Can be further classified according to leaflet mobility (Carpentier classification).

TABLE 2-2 ECHOCARDIOGRAPHIC CLASSIFICATION OF THE SEVERITY OF VALVULAR DISEASE IN ADULTS

Indicator	*Aortic Stenosis*		
	Mild	**Moderate**	**Severe**
Jet velocity (m/s)	<3.0	3.0–4.0	>4.0
Mean gradient (mm Hg)	<25	25–40	>40
Valve area (cm²)	>1.5	1.0–1.5	<1.0
Valve area index (cm²/m²)			<0.6

	Mitral Stenosis		
	Mild	**Moderate**	**Severe**
Mean gradient (mm Hg)	<5	5–10	>10
Pulmonary artery systolic pressure (mm Hg)	<30	30–50	>50
Valve area (cm²)	>1.5	1.0–1.5	<1.0

	Aortic Regurgitation		
	Mild	**Moderate**	**Severe**
Qualitative Color Doppler jet width	Central jet < 25% LVOT	Greater than mild but no signs of severe AR	Central jet > 65% LVOT
Doppler vena contracta (cm)	<0.3	0.3–0.6	≥0.6
Quantitative Regurgitant volume (mL per beat)	<30	30–59	≥60
Regurgitant fraction (%)	<30	30–49	≥50
Regurgitant orifice area (cm²)	<0.10	0.10–0.29	≥0.30
Additional Essential Criteria Left ventricular size			Enlarged

	Mitral Regurgitation		
	Mild	**Moderate**	**Severe**
Qualitative Color Doppler jet area	Small, central jet < 4 cm² or < 20% LA area		Large central jet > 40% of LA area Wall-impinging jet of any size, swirling in LA
Doppler vena contracta (cm)	<0.3	0.3–0.69	≥0.70
Quantitative Regurgitant volume (mL per beat)	<30	30–59	≥60
Regurgitant fraction (%)	<30	30–49	≥50
Regurgitant orifice area (cm²)	<0.20	0.20–0.39	≥0.40
Additional Essential Criteria Left atrial size			Enlarged
Left ventricular size			Enlarged

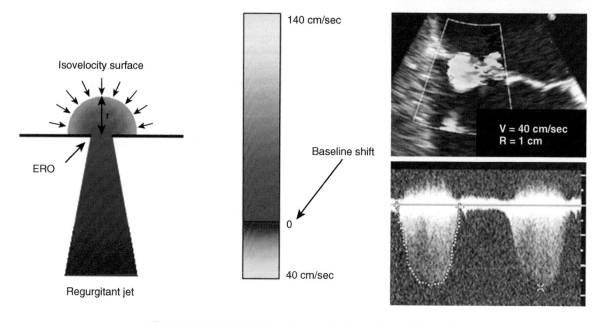

Flow at proximal isovelocity surface = flow through regurgitant orifice

$$2\pi r^2 \times \text{aliasing velocity} = \text{ERO} \times \text{regurgitant velocity}$$

$$\text{ERO} = (2\pi r^2 \times \text{aliasing velocity}) / \text{regurgitant velocity}$$

$$\text{Regurgitant volume} = \text{ERO} \times \text{regurgitant TVI}$$

Figure 2-10. PISA quantification method is based on the flow convergence concept. Blood flow progressively accelerates as it approaches the regurgitant orifice, forming hemispheric surfaces of equal velocity (isovelocity surfaces). Identification of such a surface is facilitated by shifting the 0 velocity line in the direction of the regurgitant jet. In this way, the velocity range in the direction of flow is significantly reduced, with aliasing occurring at lower velocity (hence further away from the orifice and easier to measure). The radius r is measured from the aliasing front line (sudden color change on color Doppler) to the narrowest point of the regurgitant jet (regurgitant orifice). Assuming the flow through the isovelocity surface area is equal with the flow through the regurgitant orifice, one can calculate the ERO and regurgitant volume according to the formulas outlined in the figure. *Right panels* show an example of PISA estimation of the ERO and RV in a patient with severe mitral regurgitation.

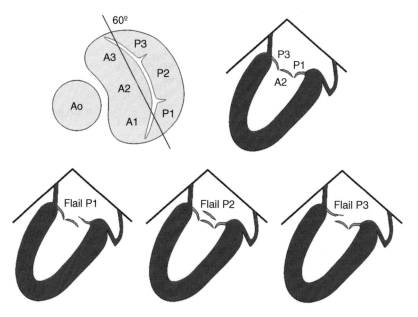

Figure 2-11. Schematic representation of the mitral valve scallops (*top*) and the typical appearance of flail posterior scallops on the TEE commissural view (*bottom*).

TABLE 2-3 CAUSES OF MITRAL REGURGITATION

	Organic			Functional
	Normal Leaflet Mobility (Type I)	**Increased Leaflet Mobility (Type II)**	**Reduced Leaflet Mobility (Type III)**	**Type I/Type III**
Nonischemic	Endocarditis (perforation) Degenerative (calcification) Congenital (cleft)	Degenerative (flail leaflets) Endocarditis (ruptured chords) Traumatic (ruptured chord/ papillary muscle) Rheumatic (acute)	Rheumatic (chronic) Radiation Drugs Inflammatory (lupus, hypereosinophilic syndrome, endomyocardial fibrosis)	Dilated cardiomyopathy Left ventricular dysfunction of any cause
Ischemic	—	Ruptured papillary muscle	—	Functional ischemic

- Step 2: evaluate disease severity.
  - Perform a quantitative analysis of the regurgitant lesion (effective regurgitant orifice, regurgitant volume).
  - Evaluate the hemodynamic consequences (left ventricle size and function, pulmonary pressures, etc.).
- Step 3: look for secondary clues to establish the etiology.
  - Ischemic
  - Non-ischemic
- Estimating disease severity based on color Doppler imaging alone is fraught with errors.
  - Severity can be overestimated as a result of low aliasing velocity limits on the color Doppler scale or of entraining left atrial stagnant blood by the high-velocity MR jet. These make the jet look worse than it actually is.
  - Eccentric, wall-hugging jets dissipate energy by contact with the atrial wall (Coanda effect); their color Doppler appearance can be underwhelming.
  - In patients with very high left atrial filling pressures, MR can be nearly silent Xon color Doppler alone (acute MR due to papillary rupture, functional ischemic MR).
- Left atrial volume reflects volume overload from MR and has prognostic value.

- Degenerative disease is the most common cause of MR in the western world (60% to 70% of cases).
- Surgical correction of MR is dependent on both cause and mechanism, which affect repairability. Therefore, comprehensive evaluation is of paramount importance in the decision for and planning of surgical intervention.
- Intraoperative real-time 3D transesophageal echocardiography (TEE) is particularly useful for assessment of the mitral valve.
- Echocardiography-derived indications for surgery in asymptomatic patients with severe MR:
  - Class I: left ventricular dysfunction (EF < 60% or left ventricular end-systolic dimension > 40 mm)
  - Class IIa: pulmonary artery pressure greater than 50 mm Hg at rest or 60 mm Hg with exercise[5]
- Indications for serial echocardiographic evaluation:
  - Every 6 to 12 months for patients with asymptomatic severe mitral regurgitation
  - Whenever change in symptoms is suspected to be secondary to MR
  - Contraindicated for routine follow-up of patients with mild MR

KEY POINTS

- MR results from lack of mitral coaptation due to organic or functional mechanisms.
- Color Doppler can over/underestimate disease severity. It should never be used as a sole assessment of disease severity.
- Systematic assessment of MR should include establishing the cause and mechanism, formal quantification of disease severity, and assessment of associated pathology.
- Success of surgical repair depends on both the etiology and the mechanism of MR.
- Serial echocardiograms are recommended in patients with severe asymptomatic MR.

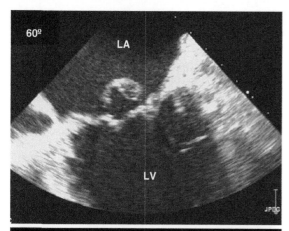

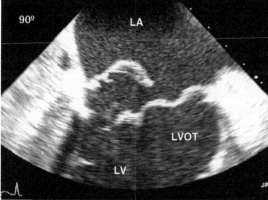

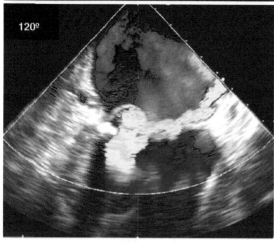

Figure 2-12. TEE images obtained from a patient with severe organic MR due to a flail P2 scallop of the mitral valve (*top*, commissural view; *middle*, long-axis midesophageal view). Note the very eccentric, anteriorly directed jet of MR. Compare with the functional MR shown in Figure 2-7.

Aortic Stenosis

- Left ventricular systolic dysfunction is a late manifestation of severe aortic stenosis (AS).
- Systematic echocardiographic evaluation of patients with AS:
  - Step 1: establish the location of the obstruction and native valve morphology.
    - Valvular/subvalvular/supravalvular

- Tricuspid/unicuspid/bicuspid/quadricuspid (Figure 2-13)
  - Step 2: evaluate severity of disease (see Table 2-2).
    - Estimate aortic valve gradient by systematic CW Doppler interrogation (all available windows, use of non-imaging CW Doppler probe).
    - Valve area calculation is based on continuity equation.
    - LVOT measurement can be difficult due to acoustic shadowing from calcification, which is prone to induce errors. Always perform on zoomed-up view.
    - Dimensionless indexes (aortic/LVOT TVI and velocity ratio) are helpful, especially when LVOT measurement is difficult.
    - Calculation of valve area by planimetry is unreliable on transthoracic echocardiography; TEE measurements correlate with calculated valve area at hemodynamic catheterization.
  - Step 3: evaluate for associated conditions.
    - Enlargement of ascending aorta, coarctation
- Serial echocardiographic evaluation:
  - Recommended every year for patients with asymptomatic severe aortic stenosis
  - Every 3 to 5 years for mild AS
- Left ventricular dysfunction (EF < 50%) is a class II indication for surgery in asymptomatic patients with severe AS.[5]
- Low-gradient, low-output aortic stenosis
  - Always consider this possibility in patients who have left ventricular dysfunction, severely reduced aortic leaflet mobility, but only a low aortic valve gradient (<30 mm Hg).
  - Use low-dose dobutamine stress echocardiography to determine severity.
  - Increase in stroke volume with increase in valve area greater than 0.2 cm² indicates that AS is unlikely to be severe.
  - Increase in stroke volume with unchanged valve area and an increase in gradient are suggestive of severe AS.
  - Lack of contractile reserve (<20% increase in stroke volume) is associated with a poor prognosis with either medical or surgical therapy.

KEY POINTS

- Assess location, native valve morphology, and associated aortic disease.
- LVOT measurement can be challenging; errors are amplified in valve area calculations.
- Use all available windows and non-guided Doppler for gradient assessment.
- A dimensionless index can be helpful.
- Low-gradient, low-output AS is best assessed with low-dose dobutamine stress.

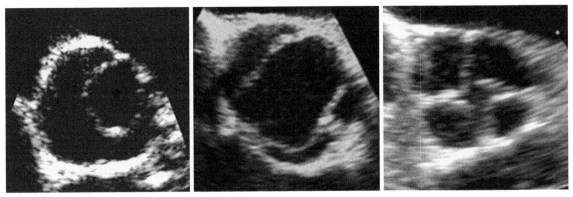

Figure 2-13. Typical appearance of unicuspid (*left*), bicuspid (*center*), and quadricuspid (*right*) aortic valve.

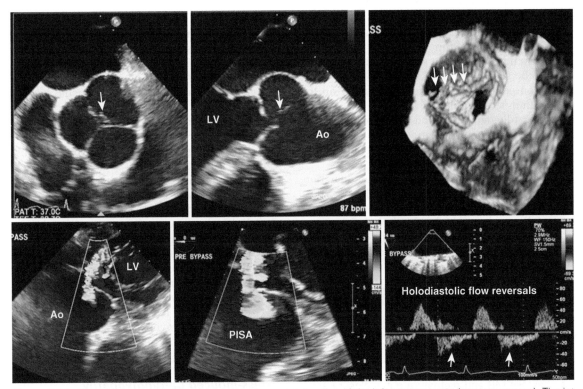

Figure 2-14. Severe AR resulting from a tear along the coaptation line of the left coronary cusp (*top row, arrows*). The jet is very eccentric (*bottom, left panel*), but excellent quantification by PISA method was possible from the deep transgastric view (*bottom, middle panel*). Also note prominent holodiastolic flow reversals in the descending thoracic aorta (*bottom right, arrows*). The patient underwent successful aortic valve repair.

Aortic Regurgitation

- Aortic regurgitation (AR) is a disease characterized by volume overload of the left ventricle, resulting in progressive dilatation of the LV with typically preserved EF for a long duration of time.
- The systematic echocardiographic approach is similar to that for MR:

- Step 1: establish mechanism.
  - Determine native valvular anatomy: tricuspid versus uni/bi/quadricuspid valve (see Figure 2-13).
  - Determine mechanism: degenerative, cusp prolapse/tear/perforation, annular enlargement, vegetations, etc. (Figure 2-14).

- Step 2: Evaluate disease severity.
  - Perform quantitative analysis of regurgitant lesion (see Table 2-2).
  - Evaluate hemodynamic consequences.
- Step 3: establish etiology and assess for associated conditions.
  - Degenerative/infectious/traumatic
  - Assessment of associated conditions (aortic enlargement, coarctation, multivalvular disease)
- Eccentric jets of AR are difficult to quantify. The presence of large holodiastolic flow reversals in the thoracic and abdominal aorta is highly suggestive of severe AR (see Figure 2-14).
- Assess for signs of impending hemodynamic compromise in acute severe AR (early diastolic closure of the mitral valve, diastolic MR).
- Serial echocardiographic evaluation
  - Recommended every 12 months for patients with asymptomatic severe AR and no evidence of LV dysfunction
  - Whenever change in symptoms is suspected to be secondary to AR
  - Contraindicated for routine follow-up of patients with mild AR
- Echocardiography-derived indications for surgery in asymptomatic patients with severe AR[5]
  - Class I: left ventricular dysfunction (EF < 50%)
  - Class IIb: severe left ventricular dilatation (end-diastolic dimension > 70 mm, end-systolic dimension > 50 mm)
  - Adjustment to body size is helpful, especially in women (less likely to develop left ventricular enlargement to that degree).

KEY POINTS

- Assess location of the obstruction, native valve morphology, and associated aortic disease (especially in bicuspid aortic valves).
- Large holodiastolic aortic flow reversals are consistent with severe AR.
- Diastolic MR and premature mitral closure are signs of impending hemodynamic compromise in patients with acute severe AR.
- Serial echocardiography is recommended in all patients with asymptomatic severe AR.
- Adjustment to body size is helpful, especially in women.

Peripartum Cardiomyopathy

- Four criteria have to be met for a diagnosis of peripartum cardiomyopathy[6]:
  - Development of HF in the last month of pregnancy or within 5 months of delivery
  - Absence of identifiable cause of HF
  - No heart disease prior to last month of pregnancy
  - Evidence of systolic LV dysfunction with EF less than 45%
- Echocardiographic findings
  - EF less than 45%
  - Left ventricular enlargement
  - Wall motion abnormalities in noncoronary distribution
  - Functional mitral and tricuspid regurgitation
  - Small pericardial effusion
- Only approximately 50% of the patients recover to an EF greater than 50%.
- Cardiomyopathy during previous pregnancy is associated with increased risk for subsequent pregnancies even if LV function has normalized.

Myocarditis

- Viral infection is the most common cause of myocarditis. Non-infectious causes include toxic causes, hypersensitivity reactions, and systemic disorders.[7]
- Echocardiography is the most valuable method of assessment of LV dysfunction.
- Typical echocardiographic findings include:
  - Reduced left ventricular EF
  - Typically global hypokinesis, but RWMAs can also be present
  - Occasionally exercise-induced RWMAs are seen and probably result from microvascular dysfunction.
  - Fulminant myocarditis is associated with normal left ventricular diastolic dimensions, but increased septal thickness. If the patient survives, LV function frequently normalizes.
  - Acute myocarditis is associated with a dilated left ventricle, but normal septal thickness. It may progress to persistent dilated cardiomyopathy.
- Strain and strain rate assessment may be useful, but large clinical studies are currently lacking.

Stress-Induced Cardiomyopathy (Tako-Tsubo, Apical Ballooning Syndrome)

- Stress-induced cardiomyopathy is transient systolic dysfunction of the apical and/or mid-segments of the left ventricle that mimics myocardial infarction without evidence of obstructive coronary artery disease, usually occurring after emotional/physical stress or sometimes acute medical illness.[8]
- It is a diagnosis of exclusion, as infarction of a large left anterior descending coronary artery (LAD) that wraps around the apex can be associated with similar wall motion abnormalities.

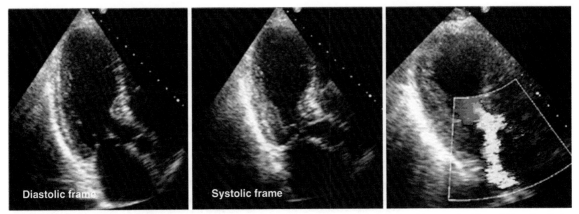

Figure 2-15. Apical long-axis views in a patient with stress-induced cardiomyopathy. Note typical hypo/akinesis of the apical and midventricular segments (*left,* end-diastolic frame; *middle,* end-systolic frame). In this patient who had pre-existing basal septal hypertrophy, hyperkinesis of the basal segments resulted in dynamic LVOT obstruction with severe systolic anterior motion of the mitral valve and severe posteriorly directed jet of MR (*right*).

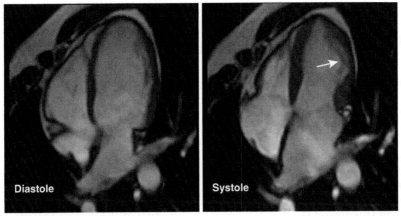

Figure 2-16. Stress-induced cardiomyopathy, atypical form (midventricular ballooning). Note significant thickening of all ventricular walls from diastole (*left frame*) to systole (*right frame*). The only area that is akinetic is located in the midventricular wall on this MRI 4-chamber view (*arrow*). Coronary angiography was normal in this patient; there was no evidence of delayed enhancement on MRI.

- Postulated mechanisms are catecholamine surge, vasospasm, and microvascular dysfunction.
- The typical form (apical ballooning) has hypo/akinesis of the apical and midventricular segments, with compensatory hyperkinesis of the basal segments (Figure 2-15).
- The atypical form (midventricular ballooning) can occur in up to 40% of cases and involves the midventricular segments exclusively (Figure 2-16).
- Hyperdynamic function at the base can result in dynamic LVOT obstruction and acute MR as a result of systolic anterior motion of the mitral valve (see Figure 2-15).
- Most patients survive and have rapid recovery of LV function.

KEY POINTS

- Stress-induced cardiomyopathy is a transient disease related to emotional stress.
- It is a diagnosis of exclusion.
- Apical and mid-ventricular forms have been described.
- Functional MR can result from dynamic LVOT obstruction.

Tachycardia-Mediated Cardiomyopathy

- Essentially all forms of chronic tachyarrhythmia can induce left ventricular dysfunction.
- It is difficult to make the distinction as to whether the arrhythmia is the cause or consequence of the left ventricular dysfunction.

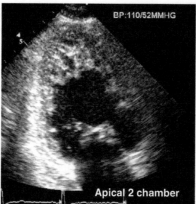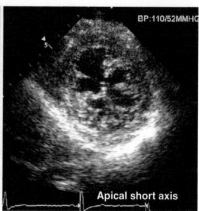

Figure 2-17. Noncompaction cardiomyopathy. Note prominent trabeculations of the distal third of the ventricle (*left:* apical 2-chamber view; *right:* short-axis para-apical view).

- A typical echocardiographic finding is the presence of left ventricular dysfunction (LV enlargement, reduced EF) in the context of tachyarrhythmia.
- Tachycardia-mediated cardiomyopathy is usually reversible with restoration of sinus rhythm or appropriate rate control.

KEY POINTS
• Non-compaction cardiomyopathy is a genetic form of LV dysfunction characterized by deep LV trabeculations.   • It occurs in isolation or associated with other congenital diseases.   • Intravenous contrast is helpful.

Genetic Causes of Left Ventricular Dysfunction
Non-compaction Cardiomyopathy
- Non-compaction cardiomyopathy is a form of genetic cardiomyopathy.
- It is possibly due to intrauterine arrest of fetal myocardial primordium compaction.
- It occurs in isolated form or in association with other disorders.
  - Isolated form (Figure 2-17)
    - Prominent trabeculations resulting in thickened myocardium with two layered appearance (trabeculated and compacted; see Figure 2-17).
    - Various criteria have been proposed. The most common one is a ratio of noncompacted to compacted myocardium greater than 2:1 at end-systole in the parasternal short-axis view.
  - Non-compaction associated with other disorders
    - Congenital disease (Ebstein's anomaly, ventricular septal defect [VSD], bicuspid aortic valve)
    - Neuromuscular disorders, genetic syndromes (Charcot-Marie-Tooth disease, nail-patella syndrome)
- Other echocardiographic features:
  - LV enlargement and decreased EF
  - Intracardiac thrombi
  - Abnormal papillary muscle structure
- Intravenous contrast is helpful for diagnosis and assessment of intracardiac thrombi.

Neuromuscular Disorders
- Duchenne muscular dystrophy
  - In Duchenne muscular dystrophy, there is extensive fibrosis of the posterobasal LV wall, but this can extend to the free lateral wall with disease progression.
  - There is frequently associated functional MR.
  - Female carriers can have cardiac manifestation of the disease (Figure 2-18).
- Becker muscular dystrophy
  - Cardiac involvement can be more severe than in Duchenne muscular dystrophy.
  - Early involvement of the right ventricular wall is frequently seen.
- Other neuromuscular disorders (myotonic dystrophy, Barth syndrome, Emery-Dreifuss muscular dystrophy and Friedreich's ataxia) are all associated with systolic LV dysfunction and conduction abnormalities.

Other Inherited Disorders
- Iron overload disorders
  - Iron overload disorders are caused by hemochromatosis or hereditary sideroblastic anemias and thalassemias.
  - Cardiac manifestation is part of a multi-organ disease, but can be the presenting feature.
  - Echocardiographic features are those of typical dilated cardiomyopathy.
- Fabry's disease
  - Lysosomal storage disease
  - Echocardiographic findings

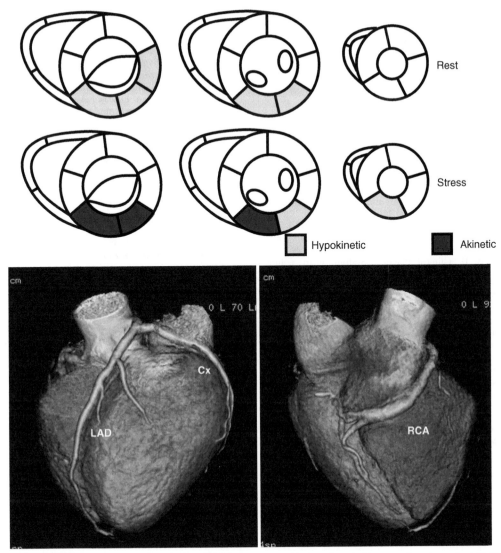

Figure 2-18. **Top,** Regional wall motion abnormalities seen at rest (*top row*) and after exercise stress test (*bottom row*) in a female carrier of Duchenne muscular dystrophy. **Bottom,** Note the normal computed tomography appearance of the coronary arteries (*left,* LAD and circumflex; *right,* right coronary artery with posterior descending and posterolateral branches). Mild persistent creatine kinase elevation was noted.

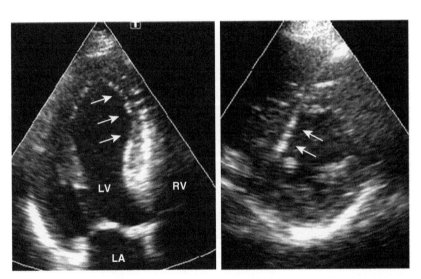

Figure 2-19. Typical appearance of Fabry's cardiomyopathy. There is mild left ventricular hypertrophy (septum measures 14 mm). Note the hyperechogenic endocardial stripe (*arrows*) seen both from the long-axis apical view (*left panel*) and the parasternal short-axis view (*right*). Left ventricular EF was still preserved in this patient.

- Left ventricular hypertrophy and LV dysfunction
- Presence of a hyper-echogenic endocardial stripe due to intracellular glycosphingolipid deposition in the endocardium (Figure 2-19)

References

1. Hunt SA, Abraham WT, Chin MH, et al. 2009 focused update incorporated into the ACC/AHA 2005 Guidelines for the Diagnosis and Management of Heart Failure in Adults: a report of the American College of Cardiology Foundation/American Heart Association Task Force on Practice Guidelines: developed in collaboration with the International Society for Heart and Lung Transplantation. *Circulation*. 2009;119:e391-e479.
   This is the reference document of the American College of Cardiology and American Heart Association for evaluation of heart failure. It is a "must read."
2. McMurray JJ. Clinical practice: Systolic heart failure. *N Engl J Med*. 2010;362:228-238.
   Part of the Clinical Practice series in the New England Journal of Medicine. The article starts with a clinical vignette, and briefly reviews systolic heart failure from a clinical perspective, including the role of imaging.
3. Lang RM, Bierig M, Devereux RB, et al. Recommendations for chamber quantification: A report from the American Society of Echocardiography's Guidelines and Standards Committee and the Chamber Quantification Writing Group, developed in conjunction with the European Association of Echocardiography, a branch of the European Society of Cardiology. *J Am Soc Echocardiogr*. 2005;18: 1440-1463.
   The reference text for echocardiographic chamber quantification. Note that echocardiography boards frequently test candidates on this topic.
4. Enriquez-Sarano M, Akins CW, Vahanian A. Mitral regurgitation. *Lancet*. 2009;373:1382-1394.
   A brief overview of the complex topic of MR, emphasizing the multiple types/mechanisms of this valvular disease. The reader will understand better what questions need to be answered when performing echocardiographic assessment of MR.
5. ACC/AHA 2006 Guidelines for the Management of Patients with Valvular Heart Disease: A report of the American College of Cardiology/American Heart Association Task Force on Practice Guidelines. *Circulation*. 2006;114: e84-e231.
   The reference document of the American College of Cardiology and American Heart Association for valvular heart disease. While lengthy, it is certainly the most comprehensive effort on valvular disease, including brief aspects of surgical management. Watch for an update soon.
6. Peripartum cardiomyopathy: National Heart, Lung, and Blood Institute and Office of Rare Diseases (National Institutes of Health) workshop recommendations and review. *JAMA*. 2000;283:1183-1188.
   Excellent review of this rare condition, with input from multiple disciplines (cardiovascular medicine, obstetrics, immunology, and pathology).
7. Cooper LT Jr. Myocarditis. *N Engl J Med*. 2009;360: 1526-1538.
   Part of the Review series in the New England Journal of Medicine, this article is an excellent summary of the topic. It includes an overview of echocardiographic findings, but also of competing imaging modalities (MRI).
8. Prasad A, Lerman A, Rihal CS. Apical ballooning syndrome (Tako-Tsubo or stress cardiomyopathy): A mimic of acute myocardial infarction. *Am Heart J*. 2008;155:408-417.
   A good review of stress-induced cardiomyopathy, including the role of imaging.

Evaluation of the Patient with Diastolic Dysfunction

Jacob Abraham, Kristian Eskesen, and Theodore Abraham

3

Identifying the Cause of Diastolic Dysfunction

Background
- Abnormal diastolic filling patterns in the presence of normal systolic function should alert the echocardiographer to the possibility of a cardiomyopathy (restrictive, hypertrophic) or constrictive pericarditis.

Restrictive Cardiomyopathy

Background
- Restrictive cardiomyopathies (RCMs) are rare disorders (Table 3-1) that cause abnormal stiffening of cardiac chambers, often associated with increased wall thickness (Figure 3-1). Contractile function is normal except in late stages of disease. Elevation of ventricular filling pressures and inability to augment stroke volume with exercise result in heart failure symptoms. Right heart failure often dominates the clinical picture.
- RCM and constrictive pericarditis (CP) have similar clinical presentations and echocardiographic findings. Differentiating RCM from CP is imperative as CP can be cured with pericardiectomy. The distinction is often difficult to make with echocardiography alone and requires integrating physiologic data from multiple investigations (Tables 3-2 and 3-3).

Echocardiographic Approach
General characteristic findings in RCM include (Figures 3-2 through 3-5):
- Nondilated left ventricle, often with increased wall thickness
- Normal LV systolic function
- Abnormal LV diastolic function
  - Mitral inflow: mitral inflow early-to-late diastolic velocity ratio (E/A) greater than 1.5, deceleration time (DT) less than 150 ms, isovolumic relaxation time (IVRT) < 60 ms

- Pulmonary venous inflow pattern
  - Systolic/diastolic ratio of pulmonary venous forward flow less than 0.4
  - Atrial reversal wave greater than 35 cm/s
- Hepatic venous flow
  - Blunted systolic forward wave
  - Prominant A-wave reversal
- Right ventricular free wall thickening
- Marked bi-atrial enlargement
- Dilated inferior vena cava
- Pulmonary hypertension

Specific Diagnoses
- **Cardiac amyloidosis:** increased RV/LV wall thickness, thickening of the interatrial septum and atrioventricular valves, presence of a small-to-moderate pericardial effusion, and "speckled" or "granular" myocardium (Figures 3-6 and 3-7).
- **Cardiac sarcoidosis:** Idiopathic, inflammatory multisystem granulomatous disease that commonly involves the lungs, skin, kidneys, eyes, and heart. Echocardiographic findings include both normal and dilated ventricular chambers; increased wall thickness and wall thinning, depending on stage and treatment, and aneurysm formation; segmental wall motion abnormalities not conforming to a coronary vascular distribution; and akinetic/dyskinetic wall segments adjacent to normokinetic wall segments.
- **Glycogen storage disease:** Unexplained left ventricular hypertrophy should prompt consideration of hypertrophic cardiomyopathy (HCM; see below) and the following glycogen storage disorders:
  - **Fabry's disease:** X-linked autosomal recessive disorder caused by lack of α-galactosidase A, leading to intracellular accumulation of ceramide trihexoside. The echocardiographic appearance is similar to HCM (see below). A specific finding for Fabry's disease is a binary appearance of the LV endocardial border, reflecting the endocardial and

subendocardial compartmentalization of gly-cosphingolipid material.

- **Danon's disease:** X-linked disorder typically affecting young men (<20 years old) caused by deficient lysosomal-associated membrane protein 2 (LAMP2). Phenotype of marked concentric HCM (wall thickness 20 to 60 mm) with severe LV systolic dysfunction, often associated with ventricular preexcitation. Extracardiac clinical features include skeletal myopathy, mental retardation, and hepatic disease, but systemic features may be absent or minimal.
- **PRKAG2 cardiomyopathy:** Autosomal dominant mutation in regulatory subunit of AMP-activated receptor kinase. Electrocardiographic (ECG) findings include preexcitation. Differentiated from Danon's disease clinically by absence of systemic disease.

Physiologic Data
- M-mode through the interventricular septum and inferior wall can reveal a square root sign.
- Diastolic mitral regurgitation (MR) may be present if left ventricular diastolic pressure is markedly elevated.

TABLE 3-1 CLASSIFICATION OF RCMS	
Site of Involvement	**Classification**
Myocardium	**Noninfiltrative** • Idiopathic cardiomyopathy • Familial cardiomyopathy • Hypertrophic cardiomyopathy • Scleroderma • Pseudoxanthoma elasticum • Diabetic cardiomyopathy
	Infiltrative • Amyloidosis • Sarcoidosis • Gaucher's disease • Hurler's syndrome • Fatty infiltration
	Storage • Hemochromatosis • Fabry's disease • Glycogen storage disease
Endomyocardium	• Endomyocardial fibrosis • Hypereosinophilic syndrome • Carcinoid heart disease • Metastatic cancers • Radiation • Toxic effect of anthracycline • Drugs (serotonin, methysergide, ergotamine, mercurial agents, busulfan)

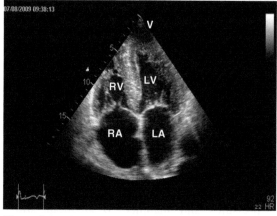

Figure 3-1. 2D 4-chamber view showing common findings in RCM, including nondilated hypertrophied left and right ventricles and enlarged left and right atria.

TABLE 3-2 OVERALL ECHOCARDIOGRAPHIC APPROACH FOR ASSESSING DIASTOLIC DYSFUNCTION		
Modality	**View/Technique**	**Findings**
2D	Apical, parasternal, subcostal	• Nondilated LV • Often increased LV wall thickness • RV free wall thickening • Bi-atrial enlargement • Dilated inferior vena cava
Pulsed wave Doppler	**4-chamber:** Ultrasound beam aimed at an angle of 20 degrees laterally to apex, and the sample volume between the tips of the mitral valve leaflets **Suprasternal short-axis** **Subcostal**	• Varying E, A, E/A, IVRT patterns (see text for details) • Pulmonary hypertension • Systolic:diastolic ratio of pulmonary forward flow ≤0.4 • Atrial reversal wave ≥35 cm/s • Blunted systolic forward flow • Prominant a-wave reversal
Tissue Doppler imaging	**4-Chamber:** 2-mm sample volume at the medial mitral annulus with the Doppler beam parallel to the longitudinal movement. Gain settings and wall filters should be low and velocity scale expanded.	Varying E, E/E patterns (see text for details)

TABLE 3-3 APPROACHES AND FINDINGS IN RCM

Modality	General Findings	Specific Findings
Chest radiograph	Normal-sized heart. Dilated atria. Signs of pulmonary congestion or interstitial edema. Pleural effusion may occur.	Mediastinal lymphadenopathy; pulmonary parenchymal disease in sarcoidosis.
Electrocardiogram	Nonspecific ST- and T-wave abnormalities. Conduction abnormalities. Same chamber and wall dimensions and functions as in echocardiography.	Low voltage in precordial leads is seen in ~50% of patients with amyloidosis with cardiac involvement. Pseudo-infarct pattern (QS wave in consecutive leads) is seen in ~50% of patients with cardiac amyloidosis. Fibrosis caused by cardiac sarcoidosis can be detected with late gadolinium enhancement. Trilaminar appearance (normal myocardium, thickened fibrotic endocardium, and overlying thrombus) may be detectable in endomyocardial diseases. Global reduction in T2* cardiac tissue is commonly seen in hemochromatosis.
CT	Same chamber and wall dimensions and functions as in echocardiography.	
Biposy	In most cases nonspecific.	Apple-green birefringence, electron microscopy findings in amyloidosis.
Radionuclide imaging	Mainly nonspecific findings in RCM.	With increased cardiac involvement in amyloidosis, Tc-99m labeled tracers are detectable.
Cardiac catheterization	Nonspecific findings of diastolic dysfunction (increased diastolic pressures, right-sided square root sign, and often LVEDP ≥5 mm Hg greater than RVEDP).	

LVEDP, LV end-diastolic pressure; RVEDP, RV end-diastolic pressure; Tc-99m, [99-m]technetium.

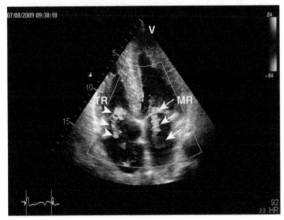

Figure 3-2. 2D 4-chamber view with color Doppler flow showing bilateral atrioventricular regurgitation. *Arrowheads* mark tricuspid regurgitation (TR) and mark mitral valve regurgitation (MR).

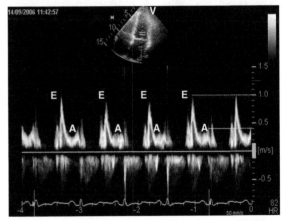

Figure 3-3. Pulsed wave Doppler over mitral valve showing typical signs of restrictive physiology with high (1 m/s) early (E) mitral inflow, increased E/A ratio (2.5), and decreased DT.

Anatomic Imaging (Acquisition/Analysis/Pitfalls)

- Abnormal diastolic filling patterns ranging from E/A reversal (grade I) to a restrictive filling pattern (grade IV) can be seen depending on the stage of disease and volume status.

- The term "restrictive pattern" is used to describe a high mitral E velocity seen in conditions of elevated atrial pressure and abbreviated early diastolic filling time (short DT). This pattern is not synonymous with RCM and can be observed in any cardiomyopathy

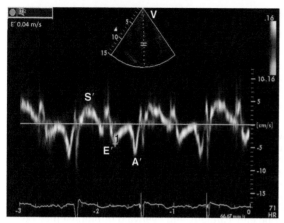

Figure 3-4. TDI of medial mitral annulus showing decreased systolic myocardial velocity (S') and early diastolic myocardial relaxation (E'). A', myocardial velocity associated with atrial contraction.

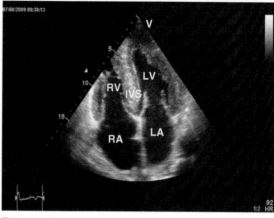

Figure 3-6. Four-chamber view of patient with amyloid. Enlarged walls and sparkling granular appearance are characteristic. IVS, interventricular septum.

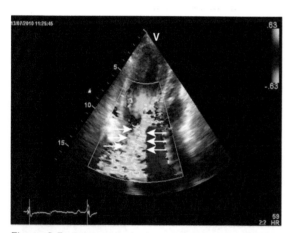

Figure 3-5. Severe mitral valve regurgitation due to RCM, indicated by *arrows*.

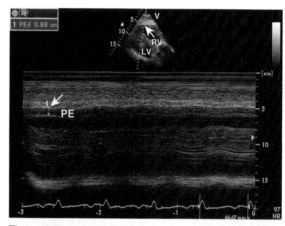

Figure 3-7. M-mode through right and left ventricles helps quantifying discrete pericardial effusion (PE), a typical finding in RCM.

leading to elevated ventricular filling pressures.

- Tissue Doppler imaging (TDI) myocardial velocity is recorded from the apical 4-chamber view. A small sample volume (2 mm) is positioned at the medial mitral annulus. The image should be optimized so that longitudinal deformation is parallel to the Doppler beam.
- Gain settings and wall filters should be low (i.e., <100 Hz) with an expanded velocity scale. A low early diastolic relaxation (E) (<8 cm/s) suggests RCM, whereas a high E (>12 cm/s) suggests CP. Caution is needed in interpreting Em in patients who may have confounding conditions (e.g., myocardial infarction, mitral annular calcification, right ventricular pressure overload) that can also impact septal TDI velocity.

Alternative Approaches
See Table 3-3.

Endomyocardial Fibrosis

- Endomyocardial fibrosis is a very rare form of RCM occurring in the hypereosinophilic syndrome, seen in Latin America, Africa, and Asia.

KEY POINTS
• The apex of the right or left ventricle is obliterated by thrombus, then fibrosis, in the absence of an underlying wall motion abnormality.
• Thrombus formation beneath the posterior papillary muscle and thickening of mitral valve leaflets with restricted motion can result in significant MR.
• Basal hypercontractility ("Merlon sign") is present.

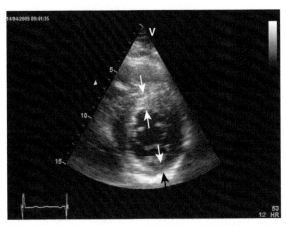

Figure 3-8. Short-axis view of LV in a patient with anterior HCM. *Upper white arrows* indicate severe thickening of anterior septal LV wall. *Lower white and black arrows* indicate less hypertrophy in posterior LV wall.

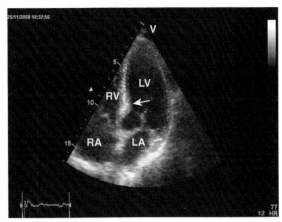

Figure 3-9. Patient with HCM mainly affecting the basal part of the septum. *Arrow* indicates a septal "knuckle."

Hypertrophic Cardioymopathy

- Autosomal dominant genetic myocardial disease with variable penetrance caused by mutations in genes encoding sarcomeric proteins and other genes.

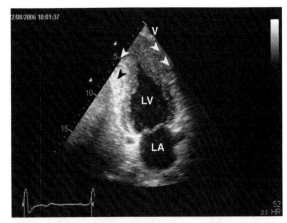

Figure 3-10. Two-chamber view of LV showing nondilated apical hypertrophy in patient with HCM. *Arrowheads* indicate apical hypertrophy.

KEY POINTS

- Patterns of left ventricular hypertrophy
  - Type 1: hypertrophy limited to anterior septum (Figures 3-8 and 3-9)
  - Type 2: hypertrophy involving the entire septum
  - Type 3: diffuse hypertrophy sparing the basal posterior wall
  - Type 4: apical hypertrophy (Figure 3-10)
- Echo contrast may be needed to define the endocardial border and demonstrate apical hypertrophy. Color or pulsed wave Doppler examination may also show absent blood flow. The ECG in apical hypertrophy often displays characteristic deep precordial T-wave inversions.
- The thickness of the basal posterior wall is usually normal.

Dynamic LV Outflow Tract (LVOT) Obstruction

- Narrowing of the outflow tract from hypertrophy
- Systolic anterior motion (SAM) of the mitral valve and submitral structures
- Hydrodynamic drag forces (Venturi effect)
- Midsystolic closure of the aortic valve due to early LV emptying

- Correlation between the extent and pattern of hypertrophy and the degree of obstruction
  - Resting obstruction common in patients with extensive septal hypertrophy
- Late-peaking, high-velocity flow in the outflow tract with typical "dagger" shape (Figure 3-11)
- Worsening of outflow obstruction with post–premature ventricular contraction beat, amyl nitrate, or Valsalva maneuver (Figure 3-12)

Mitral Regurgitation
- SAM of the mitral valve and submitral structures contributes to LVOT obstruction.
- Anterior displacement of the anterior mitral leaflet in systole causes posterior MR in mid- to late systole. Non-posterior MR suggests intrinsic mitral valve disease.
- Repeated contact between the mitral valve and septum can cause thickening of the anterior mitral leaflet and subaortic septal endocardial fibrosis.

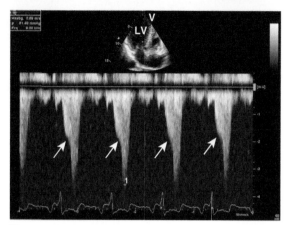

Figure 3-11. Pulsed wave Doppler through LVOT shows signs of obstruction revealing the characteristic "dagger"-shaped flow.

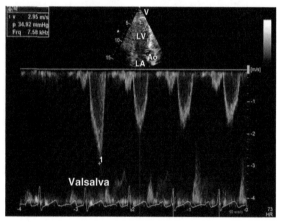

Figure 3-12. Pulsed wave Doppler of patient with HCM, showing difference in gradient with and without Valsalva maneuver.

Diastolic Filling Patterns

- Impaired relaxation is most common.
- No correlation exists between extent of hypertrophy and severity of diastolic filling abnormalities.[1]
- No correlation exists between mitral filling patterns and invasive hemodynamics. However, estimation of filling pressure using ratio of E/E or E/propagation velocity (Vp) correlates with hemodynamics at catheterization.[2]
- Screening of first-degree relatives older than 12 years is recommended when HCM is diagnosed. Abnormal TDI E has been described in genotype-positive subjects without left ventricular hypertrophy.[3,4] Because HCM may have late onset, screening is recommended every 5 years.

- Changes in early diastolic TDI velocity (E) correlate with improved diastolic function following alcohol ablation.[5]

Overview of Echocardiographic Approach
Acquisition
Wall Thickness

- M-mode placement should be guided by two-dimensional (2D) echo. The anatomic M-mode feature may be helpful to ensure measurement is perpendicular to the wall of interest.
- M-mode measurements are preferable to 2D because of inherently higher sampling rate, enabling more accurate visualization of the endocardial border.
- LV internal dimensions are measured from the parasternal region because the ultrasound beam is perpendicular to the blood-myocardium interface.
- A septal:inferior wall thickness ratio of at least 1.3:1 to 1.5:1 is suggestive of HCM.
- When hypertrophy is asymmetrical, measurements at specific sites should be reported.
- Care should be taken to avoid inclusion of RV trabeculation in measurement of septal thickness.

LVOT Obstruction

- M-mode of the mitral valve can accurately show SAM of the mitral valve and septal-anterior leaflet contact during systole.
- M-mode interrogation of the aortic valve can demonstrate early closure.
- Pulsed wave Doppler interrogation of the left ventricle is useful to localize the site of obstruction. High pulse repetition frequency Doppler should be used to localize the obstruction. The sample volume should be moved in small steps from the apex to the aortic valve.
- Dedicated continuous wave (CW) Doppler probes should be used to optimize the Doppler envelope for accurate quantification.
- The Doppler signal peaks in late systole (dagger-shaped CW Doppler profile; see Figure 3-11), in contrast to the mid-peaking signal seen in valvular disease.

Analysis/Pitfalls

A number of echocardiographic parameters (2D, M-mode, TDI, and strain) have been demonstrated to have diagnostic value in HCM.[6]

Differential Diagnosis

- **Pressure/volume loading:** Asymmetrical hypertrophy can also occur with right ventricular pressure overload (e.g., pulmonary hypertension, pulmonic stenosis, Eisenmenger's syndrome), left ventricular pressure overload (aortic stenosis, systemic hypertension), or glycogen storage disease (see above). Physiologic or pathologic causes of increased LV wall thickness/hypertrophy should be apparent from the history or during the remainder of the echocardiographic examination.

- **Elderly:** The presence of basal septal hypertrophy (septal "knuckle") can be a common finding in normal older individuals and arises because a tortuous aorta causes an acute angle between the basal septum and aortic root. However, resting and provokable gradients can be measured on occasion.
- **Athlete's heart:** An athlete's heart can be distinguished from HCM on the basis of a larger ventricular cavity (>55 mm), normal diastolic function, and clinical history. Left atrial enlargement can be seen in subjects who engage in endurance sports.
- **Hypertensive heart:** Hypertrophy in the patient with hypertension is usually due to hypertensive heart disease. Hypertensive hypertrophy causes concentric hypertrophy that includes the basal posterior wall. LVOT obstruction is midventricular, and SAM occurs at the chordal level.
- **Other causes of dynamic LVOT gradient:** Severe posterior mitral annular calcification; following anterior myocardial infarction with apical dysfunction and hyperdynamic basal contractility; after aortic valve replacement with hyperdynamic LV function and LV hypertrophy; following mitral valve repair.
- Technical factors
  - Improper angulation of the transducer can lead to underestimation of the outflow velocity.
  - Overestimation of the outflow gradient can occur if the Doppler measurement is contaminated by the flow signal from MR. Color Doppler should be used to optimally position the CW signal. The Doppler signal is characteristically "dagger" shaped in HCM (see Figure 3-11). The MR signal has an earlier onset, more rapid early acceleration, and higher peak velocity.
  - A peak velocity greater than 5.5 m/s is most likely secondary to MR rather than LVOT obstruction.
- Physiologic factors
  - The LVOT obstruction is load dependent and thus can vary from day to day. This variation is important to consider when evaluating the response to therapeutic interventions.

Alternative Approaches
- Cardiac magnetic resonance imaging (MRI) has emerged as a useful tool for diagnosing HCM by the magnitude and distribution of hypertrophy[7] and in prognosis (extent of delayed gadolinium enhancement, a radiographic surrogate for myocardial fibrosis, may predict sudden cardiac death).[8]

Estimating Clinical Prognosis

Echocardiographic Parameters
- Amyloidosis
  - LV wall thickness greater than 15 mm and RV wall thickness greater than 7 mm
  - RV dilatation
  - Mitral E-wave DT less than 150 ms
  - Increased myocardial performance index
- Idiopathic RCM
  - Left atrial dimension greater than 60 mm
- HCM: predictors of outcome[6]
  - Maximal wall or septal thickness greater than 30 mm
  - LVOT gradient (>30 mm Hg)
  - LV dysfunction (ejection fraction [EF] < 50%)
  - LA dilatation (>48 mm) or LA volume index greater than 34 mL/m^2
  - Intraventricular dyssynchrony (>45 ms), measured as the difference between the longest and shortest Q-Sm time intervals (beginning of Q wave in ECG to onset of systolic annular motion by TDI) among four different LV basal myocardial segments.

RCM versus Constrictive Pericarditis

- Because the rigid pericardium does not effectively transmit respiratory changes in intrathoracic pressure to the heart, the transmitral filling gradient decreases with inspiration and increases with expiration. Reciprocal respiratory changes occur in the right ventricular filling gradient. Consequently, ventricular interdependence is present and even enhanced in CP, but absent in RCM because of involvement of the ventricular septum. This provides the basis for the specific differences in M-mode, 2D, and Doppler findings between RCM and CP (Table 3-4).
- Diastolic dysfunction in CP is due to epicardial tethering and pericardial constraint, resulting in reduced circumferential deformation. In contrast, RCM is due to subendocardial dysfunction, resulting in reduced longitudinal

TABLE 3-4   RESTRICTIVE CARDIOMYOPATHIES VERSUS CONSTRICTIVE PERICARDITIS

	Modality	Findings in RCM	Findings in Constrictive Pericarditis
TTE	M-mode	Signs of ventricular interdependence rarely seen.	Net diastolic movement posteriorly of the posterior wall is <1 mm. Signs reflecting ventricular interdependence: abrupt septal movement in early diastole, septal movement toward LV in inspiration and toward RV in expiration.
	2D	Severe bi-atrial enlargement. Normal pericardial thickness.	Mild-moderate bi-atrial enlargement. Pericardium may be thickened. Reciprocal respiratory changes in LV and RV volumes.
	Speckle tracking	Reduced LV longitudinal strain, especially in the base.	Abnormal circumferential deformation, torsion, and untwisting velocity.
	Pulsed wave Doppler	Respiratory variation in mitral and tricuspid early diastolic flow velocity <15 mm Hg.	Respiratory variation in mitral and tricuspid early diastolic flow velocity >25 mm Hg (decrease in mitral flow velocity and increase in tricuspid flow velocity with inspiration).
	Tissue Doppler imaging	Reduced early diastolic mitral annulus velocity, septal <8 cm/s, lateral <11 cm/s.	Normal early diastolic mitral annulus velocity: septal >8 cm/s, lateral >11 cm/s.
BNP		High.	Moderate (depending on etiology).
MRI		Normal pericardium ($\approx$2 mm).	Global thickening of pericardium >4 mm. Late pericardial contrast enhancement.
CT		Bi-atrial enlargement; normal pericardium.	Local/global pericardial calcification.
Hemodynamic measurements		Respiratory concordance between RV and LV. End-diastolic pressure is more than one third of systolic pressure in most cases. Peak right ventricle systolic pressure is nearly always <60 mm Hg and often <40 mm Hg.	Respiratory discordance with increased systolic pressure in RV and decreased systolic pressure in LV during inspiration. Pressure equalization in all 4 chambers (around 20 mm Hg) within <5 mm Hg is seen in nearly all cases. Both RV and LV show dip and plateau (square root sign). End-diastolic pressure is often less than one third of systolic pressure. Peak right ventricle systolic pressure is frequently >40 mm Hg and occasionally >60 mm Hg.
Myocardial biopsy		Disease-specific findings.	Normal or nonspecific.

deformation. Speckle tracking imaging to assess strain can aid in differentiation of RCM and CP (see Table 3-4).

- Respiratory variation (>30%) in transmitral and trans-tricuspid inflow suggests CP. A respirometer is used to clearly identify inspiration and expiration. 2D and color flow images are used prior to Doppler measurement to ensure minimal respiratory variation in the angle between the ultrasound and direction of blood flow.
- Pulmonary artery pressure is typically normal in CP and elevated (secondary to elevated LV pressure) in RCM.

Approach
- Early diastolic filling is rapid with CP and reduced with RCM early in the disease course.
- Caveats
  - Respiratory changes in transmitral inflow may be absent in up to 20% of patients with CP because of a concurrent restrictive process or because of markedly elevated atrial pressures. In the latter circumstance, respiratory changes in left atrial pressure have relatively little effect on filling when the driving pressure (left atrial pressure − left ventricular pressure) is high. Reducing preload (by placing the patient in a sitting position or by

Valsalva maneuver) may unmask respiratory variation in E-wave velocity.

- Respiratory variation in diastolic filling is not specific for CP and may be seen in other conditions associated with exaggerated swings in intrathoracic pressure, such as asthma or chronic obstructive pulmonary disease. Measurement of flow velocity in the superior vena cava in pulmonary disease will show a marked increase in flow during inspiration because of the large negative intrathoracic pressure generated. No such changes are seen in CP or RCM.

Monitoring Effects of Treatment

Lusitropy

- The effect of interventions on diastolic function has recently become an endpoint in clinical trials. Tissue Doppler echocardiography has improved assessment of diastolic function by enabling distinction between normal and pseudonormal transmitral Doppler filling patterns.

Control of Blood Pressure (BP)
Mass

- BP potently influences LV mass. Antihypertensive drug classes have heterogeneous effects on LV mass for equivalent degrees of BP reduction.
- 2D targeted M-mode
  - In the parasternal short-axis view, a circular cross section at the level of the mitral leaflet tips is chosen. Eccentric cross sections should be excluded.
  - Choose beats with optimal definition of the posterior wall epicardial-pericardial interface.
  - Average beats from passive end-expiration during quiet respiration.
  - Measure left ventricular diastolic internal dimension (LVIDd), and septal thickness (STd), and posterior wall thickness (PWTd).
  - Mass = $0.8[1.04 (STd + LVIDd + PWTd)^3 - (LVIDd)^3]$ where 1.04 gm/mL is the specific gravity of myocardium and 0.8 is a correction factor (cube formula).
  - Assumes prolate ellipsoid geometry; thus it is invalid if regional wall motion abnormality or distorted chamber geometry is present.
- 2D echocardiography[9]
  - Cylindrical hemi-ellipsoid area-length method
    - The myocardial volume (V_{myo}) is approximated as total LV volume minus LV cavity volume ($V_{myo} = V_{total} - V_{cavity}$), where

volume is computed from the area-length formula, $V = 5/6\ A \times L$ (L = major axis length measured from apical view).
  - LV mass = $V_{myo} \times 1.04$ gm/mL.

- Three-dimensional echocardiography may improve the precision and accuracy of LV mass estimation.

Diastolic Function

- Systolic loading conditions, especially late systolic load and arterial compliance, are inversely related to E.[10]
- Reductions in systolic BP are associated with increased E.
- Antihypertensive drugs may have differential effects on diastolic function despite similar degrees of BP reduction. A recent substudy of the Anglo-Scandinavian Cardiac Outcomes Trial (ASCOT) showed that patients receiving an amlodipine-based regimen had higher E than patients receiving an atenolol-based regimen, independent of BP, heart rate, and other factors that may influence diastolic function.[11]

References

1. Nagueh SF, Lakkis NM, Middleton KJ, Spencer WH 3rd, Zoghbi WA, Quiñones MA. Doppler estimation of left ventricular filling pressures in patients with hypertrophic cardiomyopathy. *Circulation.* 1999;99:254-261.
   The first paper to identify Doppler parameters that accurately estimate filling pressures in HCM patients.
2. Nishimura RA, Appleton CP, Redfield MM, Ilstrup DM, Holmes DR Jr, Tajik AJ. Noninvasive Doppler echocardiographic evaluation of left ventricular filling pressures in patients with cardiomyopathies: A simultaneous Doppler echocardiographic and cardiac catheterization study. *J Am Coll Cardiol.* 1996;28:1226-1233.
   A definitive hemodynamic-echocardiographic correlation study demonstrating that E/A and DT are useful in predicting filling pressures in patients with systolic dysfunction, but not in patients with HCM.
3. Ho CY, Sweitzer NK, McDonough B, et al. Assessment of diastolic function with Doppler tissue imaging to predict genotype in preclinical hypertrophic cardiomyopathy. *Circulation.* 2002;105:2992-2997.
   A small study demonstrating the feasibility of detecting abnormal diastolic function in gene-positive but phenotypically normal subjects with a α-myosin heavy chain mutation.
4. Ho CY, Carlsen C, Thune JJ, et al. Echocardiographic strain imaging to assess early and late consequences of sarcomere mutations in hypertrophic cardiomyopathy. *Circ Cardiovasc Genet.* 2009;2:314-321.
   A comprehensive echocardiographic analysis of a large cohort of genotyped individuals with HCM. The authors validate that E, but not systolic strain or strain rate, is reduced in preclinical HCM, whereas individuals with overt hypertrophy have abnormal systolic mechanics as well as diastolic abnormalities, despite a normal EF.
5. Nagueh SF, Lakkis NM, Middleton KJ, et al. Changes in left ventricular diastolic function 6 months after nonsurgical septal reduction therapy for hypertrophic obstructive cardiomyopathy. *Circulation.* 1999;99:344-347.

This paper documents marked improvements in diastolic function following septal reduction in a small cohort of patients with hypertrophic obstructive cardiomyopathy.

6. Afonso LC, Bernal J, Bax JJ, Abraham TP. Echocardiography in hypertrophic cardiomyopathy: The role of conventional and emerging technologies. *JACC Cardiovasc Imaging.* 2008;1:787-800.
   A concise overview of echocardiographic findings in HCM with an emphasis on novel modalities such as strain imaging.

7. Rickers C, Wilke NM, Jerosch-Herold M, et al. Utility of cardiac magnetic resonance imaging in the diagnosis of hypertrophic cardiomyopathy. *Circulation.* 2005;112: 855-861.
   In a small minority of patients, cardiac MRI was able to detect regions of LV hypertrophy not readily detected by echocardiography. Echocardiography tends to underestimate the magnitude of hypertrophy, especially in the anterolateral free wall.

8. O'Hanlon R, Grasso A, Roughton M, et al. Prognostic significance of myocardial fibrosis in hypertrophic cardiomyopathy. *J Am Coll Cardiol.* 2010;56:867-874.
   One of several single-center studies showing that myocardial fibrosis measured by late gadolinium enhancement is an independent predictor of adverse cardiac outcomes. The study is limited by a small number of clinical events and relatively short follow-up.

9. Lang RM, Bierig M, Devereux RB, et al. Recommendations for chamber quantification: A report from the American Society of Echocardiography's Guidelines and Standards Committe and the Chamber Quantification Writing Group, developed in conjunction with the European Association of Echocardiography, a branch of the Europena Society of Cardiology. *J Am Soc Echocardiogr.* 2005;18:1440-1463.
   Extensive recommendations for echocardiographic measurement of heart chambers and aorta, with reference values.

10. Borlaug BA, Melenovsky V, Redfield MM, et al. Impact of arterial load and loading sequence on left ventricular tissue velocities in humans. *J Am Coll Cardiol.* 2007;50: 1570-1577.

This detailed and well-conducted study in human subjects convincingly demonstrates that late systolic loading and arterial compliance influence both systolic and diastolic tissue velocities.

11. Tapp RJ, Sharp A, Stanton AV, et al. Differential effects of antihypertensive treatment on left ventricular diastolic function: an ASCOT (Anglo-Scandinavian Cardiac Outcomes Trial) substudy. *J Am Coll Cardiol.* 2010;55: 1875-1881.
    This interesting ASCOT substudy shows a statistically significant improvement in E, E/E, and brain natriuretic peptide (BNP) with amlodipine versus atenolol, despite similar BP reductions. The clinical implications of these findings merit further investigation.

Suggested Readings

1. Dal-Bianco JP, Sengupta PP, Mookadam F, Chandrasekaran K, Tajik AJ, Khandheria BK. Role of echocardiography in the diagnosis of constrictive pericarditis. *J Am Soc Echocardiogr.* 2009;22:24-33.

2. Geske JB, Sorajja P, Nishimura R, Oomen SR. Evaluation of left ventricular filling pressures by Doppler echocardiography in patients with hyertrophic cardiomyopathy: Correlation with direct left atrial pressure measurement at catheterization. *Circulation.* 2007;116:2662-2665.

3. Ha JW, Ommen SR, Tajik AJ, et al. Differentiation of constrictive pericarditis from restrictive cardiomyopathy using mitral annular velocity by tissue Doppler echocardiography. *Am J Cardiol.* 2004;94:316-319.

4. Nagueh SF, Mahmarian JJ. Noninvasive cardiac imaging in patients with hypertrophic cardiomyopathy. *J Am Coll Cardiol.* 2006;48:2410-2422.

5. Nagueh SF, Appleton CP, Gillebert TC, et al. Recommendations for the evaluation of left ventricular diastolic function by echocardiography. *J Am Soc Echocardiogr.* 2009;22:107-133.

Echocardiographic Parameters Important for Decision Making

Robert L. McNamara

4

Background

Clinical decision making for patients with heart failure often requires obtaining a variety of important information in a timely fashion in a variety of locations, whether it is in a laboratory or at the bedside. Echocardiography is ideal for this task and is the most commonly used imaging modality to diagnose and follow patients with systolic heart failure. Left ventricular ejection fraction (LVEF) is instrumental in defining systolic heart failure. LVEF is an important prognostic indicator and identifies patients who likely will benefit from many evidence-based therapies. Echocardiography provides a wealth of information beyond the ejection fraction (EF).

Overview of Echocardiographic Approach

Not only is anatomic imaging essential for obtaining LVEF, but it provides valuable information on LV cavity size, right ventricular (RV) size and function, and left atrial (LA) size. Two-dimensional (2D) echocardiography is the major modality for obtaining anatomic information, but advances in three-dimensional (3D) echocardiography are proving increasingly valuable. Physiologic data are also critical for the assessment of patients with heart failure. LV diastolic function, mitral regurgitation (MR), and estimated pulmonary artery systolic pressure (PASP) are key components. The evidence base behind each of these anatomic and physiologic parameters is variable, but each is routinely used in clinical decision making.

Anatomic Imaging

LV Cavity Size and Systolic Function
Step 1: Determination of LV Cavity Size by 2D Echocardiography in Parasternal Long-Axis View
- LV cavity dimension can be measured by M-mode or by 2D.
- By convention, M-mode specifies that each point of the measurement be placed on the near edge (closest to the transducer) of the bright echo corresponding to the appropriate interface ("leading edge–to–leading edge" technique). For LV cavity measurements, these interfaces are located between the interventricular septum and the ventricular cavity and between the LV cavity and the posterior wall. While this technique has decades of data supporting its use, it gives information only along the lines that originate from the transducer. Unless the desired chamber size is exactly parallel to one of these lines, the measurements will overestimate the chamber sizes as compared with those obtained from 2D echocardiography. These differences are particularly notable in patients with "vertical" hearts (hearts with a more vertical axis in the parasternal long-axis view).
- 2D echocardiographic LV dimensions are measured at the interface between the bright myocardium and the echo-lucent cavity space. 2D imaging provides the flexibility of measuring along any line within the image plane. Improved image resolution and easier determination of precise timing during viewing have increased the use of 2D echocardiography for the determination of the same chamber measurements that can be obtained from M-mode. Measurements

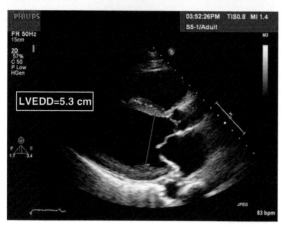

Figure 4-1. Parasternal long-axis view during diastole.

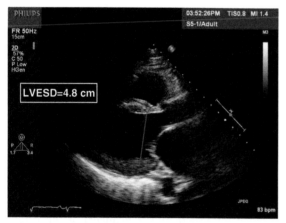

Figure 4-2. Parasternal long-axis view during systole.

made from 2D echocardiography provide an accurate representation of the chamber size.

- In the parasternal long-axis view in either M-mode or 2D, LV dimension is obtained at end-diastole (LVEDD) and end-systole (LVESD) (Figures 4-1 and 4-2 and Table 4-1)

Step 2: Estimation of LV Volumes and EF by 2D by Simpson's Method

- By making the geometric assumption that the LV is a stack of thin disks (Figure 4-3), LV volumes can be estimated. Outlines of endocardial walls in 4-chamber (4C) and 2-chamber views are combined with a linear measurement of the long axis to create a stack of individual volumes of multiple "disks" within the LV cavity.
- In the apical 4C view, obtain an image optimizing visualization of the endocardial borders of the LV, paying particular attention to include the true apex. Next trace an outline of the endocardial walls of the LV still frame images at end-diastole and end-systole (Figure 4-4).
- Repeat this procedure in the 2-chamber view.
- Estimates of the LV volumes are made by combining measurements in both views at end-diastole and at end-systole. Most modern echocardiography machines contain software that automatically combines these measurements. Stroke volume (SV; difference between the LV end-diastolic volume and the LV end-systolic volume) and EF (SV divided by the LV end-diastolic volume) are then estimated (Table 4-2).

Step 3: Determination of Estimated LV Volumes and EF by 3D

- With use of a pyramid-shaped ultrasound beam, accurate 3D data sets of the LV can be obtained.
- Images are obtained in the apical view. Current technology requires combining data from four cardiac cycles during a breath hold in order to obtain a full volume set.
- Although 3D echocardiography has been shown to estimate LV volume more accurately compared with MRI than does 2D echocardiography, care must still be taken to obtain images of the true apex for accurate volumes.
- In addition to estimated volume at end-diastole and end-systole only, volumes can be estimated at various points (typically 16 time points) throughout the cardiac cycle, enabling display of volume over time. The left ventricular cavity can be divided into 16 or 17 volumes corresponding the 16 or 17-wall-segment model and displayed over time (Figure 4-5).

TABLE 4-1 RECOMMENDATIONS FROM THE AMERICAN SOCIETY OF ECHOCARDIOGRAPHY FOR THE QUANTIFICATION OF LEFT VENTRICULAR SIZE AND VOLUME

	Women				Men			
	Reference Range	Mildly Abnormal	Moderately Abnormal	Severely Abnormal	Reference Range	Mildly Abnormal	Moderately Abnormal	Severely Abnormal
LV dimension								
LV end-diastolic diameter	3.9–5.3	5.4–5.7	5.8–6.1	≥6.2	4.2–5.9	6.0–6.3	6.4–6.8	≥6.9
LV diastolic diameter/BSA, cm/m²	2.4–3.2	3.3–3.4	3.5–3.7	≥3.8	2.2–3.1	3.2–3.4	3.5–3.6	≥3.7
LV end-diastolic diameter/height, cm/m	2.4–3.2	3.3–3.4	3.5–3.6	≥3.7	2.4–3.3	3.4–3.5	3.6–3.7	≥3.8
LV volume								
LV end-diastolic volume, mL	56–104	105–117	118–130	≥131	67–155	156–178	179–201	≥201
LV end-diastolic volume/BSA, mL/m²	*35–75*	*76–86*	*87–96*	*≥97*	*35–75*	*76–86*	*87–96*	*≥97*
LV end-systolic volume, mL	19–49	50–59	60–69	≥70	22–58	59–70	71–82	≥83
LV end-systolic volume/BSA, mL/m²	*12–30*	*31–36*	*37–42*	*≥43*	*12–30*	*31–36*	*37–42*	*≥43*

BSA, body surface area.

Bold italic values: Recommended and best validated.

Reprinted with permission from Lang RM, Bierig M, Devereux RB, et al. Recommendations for chamber quantification: A report from the American Society of Echocardiography's Guidelines and Standards Committee and the Chamber Quantification Writing Group, developed in conjunction with the European Association of Echocardiography, a branch of the European Society of Cardiology. *J Am Soc Echocardiogr.* 2005;18:1440-1463.

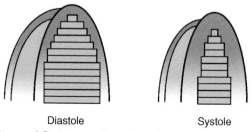

Figure 4-3. Cartoon illustrating Simpson's Method of Disks.

Diastole   Systole

Right Ventricle
Step 1: Determination of Right Ventricular Size by 2D

- Although a general sense of RV size can be obtained from the parasternal long- and short-axis views, because of the complex shape of the RV, neither definitive nor quantitative assessment of RV size is recommended in the parasternal view.
- The apical 4-chamber (4C) view provides a more complete and reliable perspective. Initially, a qualitative assessment is performed by noting RV apical location and overall size in comparison with the LV. The RV apex is normally closer to the base of the heart than the LV. With RV enlargement, the apex of the RV may be closer to or participate in forming part of the apex of the heart. Normally, the RV is approximately two-thirds the area of the LV in the 4C view. Qualitatively the degree of RV

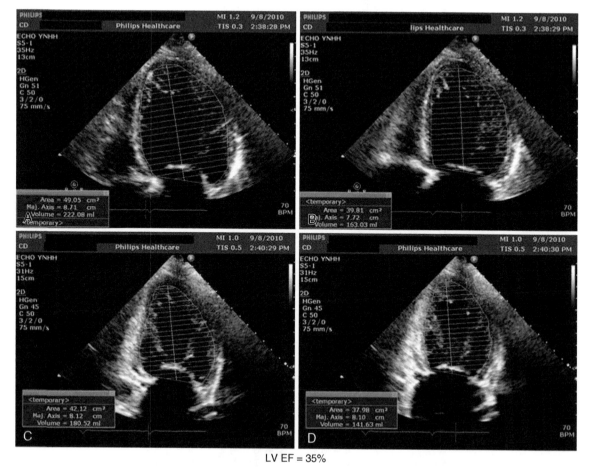

LV EF = 35%

Figure 4-4. Example of the use of Simpson's Method of Disks to estimate LVEF. From the 4C view, endocardial borders are traced at end-diastole (**A**) and end-systole (**B**). Similarly, in the 2-chamber view, endocardial borders are traced at end-diastole (**C**) and end-systole (**D**). Based upon these measurements, a computer algorithm calculates LVEF.

TABLE 4-2 RECOMMENDATIONS FROM THE AMERICAN SOCIETY OF ECHOCARDIOGRAPHY FOR THE QUANTIFICATION OF LEFT VENTRICULAR FUNCTION

	Women				Men			
	Reference Range	Mildly Abnormal	Moderately Abnormal	Severely Abnormal	Reference Range	Mildly Abnormal	Moderately Abnormal	Severely Abnormal
Linear method								
Endocardial fractional shortening, %	27–45	22–26	17–21	≤16	25–43	20–24	15–19	≤14
Midwall fractional shortening, %	15–23	13–14	11–12	≤10	14–22	12–13	10–11	≤10
2D method								
Ejection fraction, %	*≥55*	*45–54*	*30–44*	*<30*	*≥55*	*45–54*	*30–44*	*<30*

Bold italic values: Recommended and best validated.
Reprinted with permission from Lang RM, Bierig M, Devereux RB, et al. Recommendations for chamber quantification: A report from the American Society of Echocardiography's Guidelines and Standards Committee and the Chamber Quantification Writing Group, developed in conjunction with the European Association of Echocardiography, a branch of the European Society of Cardiology. *J Am Soc Echocardiogr.* 2005;18:1440-1463.

enlargement can be classified as: mild when the RV size is smaller than the LV but larger than three-fourths the size of the LV, moderate when the RV and LV are approximately equal in size, and severe when the RV is larger than the LV.

- A quantitative assessment can be obtained in the 4C view by measuring the minor axis at the tricuspid annulus, the minor axis at the midventricular level, and/or a longitudinal axis from the mid-tricuspid plane to the apex at end-diastole. In addition, the endocardial borders of the right ventricular cavity can be traced at end-diastole in the apical 4C view to obtain an RV diastolic area (Figure 4-6A and Table 4-3). Similar to LV measurements, it is important to avoid foreshortening, which may underestimate values.

KEY POINT

- Although somewhat less reliable, if the RV is not well visualized on the 4C view, similar qualitative and quantitative assessment can be performed in the subcostal view.

Step 2: Determination of RV Systolic Function

- Assessment of RV size and systolic function can be obtained from the parasternal and subcostal views. However, assessment of RV systolic function is optimally obtained in the 4C view.
- Qualitative judgment remains critically important in assessment of RV systolic function. Typical categorization includes hyperdynamic, normal, mildly decreased, moderately decreased, and severely decreased.
- Because of the complex geometry of the RV, estimates of volume by 2D are relatively unreliable. Thus, quantitative estimation of right ventricular ejection fraction (RVEF) is less common than LVEF. One means of quantitative assessment of RV systolic function is the change in fractional area in the 4C view, which can be obtained using Simpson's method as with the LV (see Figure 4-6B).
- A second quantitative assessment of RV systolic function can be obtained by measuring the

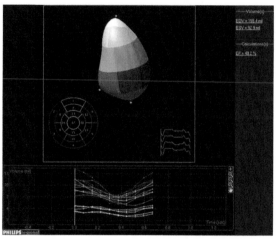

3D volume

Figure 4-5. The screen display of the results of a 3D analysis. In addition to left ventricular volumes and LVEF, shown in the upper right-hand corner, the main display shows a simulated cast of the left ventricular cavity, color-coded using the 17-segment model. In the lower section of the screen, segmental volumetric analysis of the cardiac cycle is demonstrated.

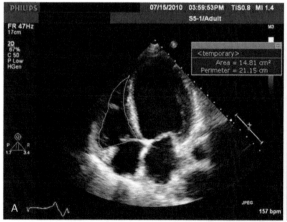
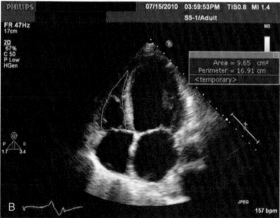

RV diastolic area = 14.81 cm²
RV systolic area = 9.85 cm²
Fractional area change = 33%

Figure 4-6. Example of the estimation of right ventricular fractional area change from endocardial tracing at end-diastole (**A**) and end-systole (**B**).

TABLE 4-3 RECOMMENDATIONS FROM THE AMERICAN SOCIETY OF ECHOCARDIOGRAPHY FOR THE QUANTIFICATION OF RIGHT VENTRICULAR SIZE AND SYSTOLIC FUNCTION

	Reference Range	Mildly Abnormal	Moderately Abnormal	Severely Abnormal
RV diastolic area, cm^2	11–28	29–32	33–37	≥38
RV systolic area, cm^2	7.5–16	17–19	20–22	≥23
RV fractional area change, %	32–60	25–31	18–24	≥17

Data from Weyman.[80]
Reprinted with permission from Lang RM, Bierig M, Devereux RB, et al. Recommendations for chamber quantification: A report from the American Society of Echocardiography's Guidelines and Standards Committee and the Chamber Quantification Writing Group, developed in conjunction with the European Association of Echocardiography, a branch of the European Society of Cardiology. *J Am Soc Echocardiogr.* 2005;18:1440-1463.

excursion of the tricuspid annulus during the cardiac cycle. A sample volume is obtained from the lateral tricuspid annulus by tissue Doppler imaging (TDI) in the apical 4C view. Normal tricuspid annular plane systolic excursion (TAPSE) is greater than 2.0 cm. Of note, TAPSE has been shown to be decreased in patients with normal RV systolic function but decreased LV systolic function.

KEY POINTS

- 3D echocardiography provides a more complete and reliable assessment of RV size. Quantitative assessment of RV size and RVEF by 3D has been shown to correlate better than that by 2D with other modalities, such as MRI.
- Assessment of RV diastolic function has not been validated to the degree that it has in determination of LV diastolic dysfunction. However, assessment of tricuspid inflow and diastolic parameters of TDI may become increasingly useful, particularly with improvements in 3D speckle tracking, which allows measurement of motion in all directions, not just in the direction of the probe.

LA Volume (LAV)
Step 1: Obtaining 2D Images
- LAV is best obtained in the apical 4C and 2-chamber views using the area-length method. In the final frame before mitral valve (MV) opening, approximating end-systole, endocardial borders of the left atrium are traced. Of note, the pulmonary veins and left atrial appendage should be carefully *excluded*, and a straight line should be drawn from one mitral annulus to the other (excluding the area immediately under the MV leaflets).

- The length of the left atrium is measured from the midpoint of the line connecting the two sides of the mitral annulus to the base of the atrium, again carefully *excluding* the pulmonary vein (Figure 4-7).

Step 2: Calculating LAV
- LAV is then calculated using the formula:

$$LAV = (8 * A_1 * A_2)/(3 * \Pi * L) \cong 0.85 * A_1 * A_2/L$$

  where A_1 is the area in the 4C view, A_2 is the area in the 2-chamber view, and L is the *shorter* of the major axes obtained (Table 4-4).
- Alternatively, LAV can be estimated using Simpson's method. The LA is divided into a "stack of disks," each with a set height and an area calculated from diameters obtained in the apical 4C and 2-chamber views.

KEY POINTS

- Care should be taken to avoid foreshortening.
- Avoid overgaining, which will result in underestimation of LAV.
- LAVs indexed to body surface area over 35 mL/m^2 have been correlated with worse prognosis.

Physiologic Data

LV Diastolic Function
Because LV myocardial relaxation and left atrial contraction during ventricular systole are heavily influenced by loading conditions, assessment of global LV diastolic function is a complex process requiring integration of multiple parameters.

Step 1: LV Inflow
- A spectral Doppler tracing is obtained with the sample volume placed at the MV leaflet tips.

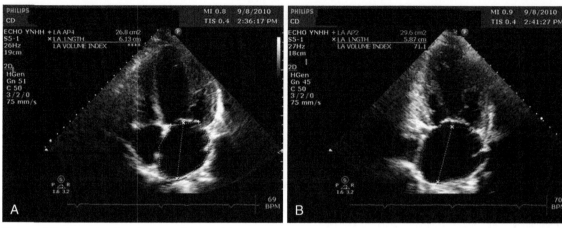

Figure 4-7. Example of estimation of left atrial volume by the area-length method, tracing left atrial borders at atrial end-diastole (**A**) and atrial end-systole (**B**).

- Normal LV inflow during diastole consists of a predominant early diastolic wave ("E wave"), caused by ventricular relaxation, and a smaller late diastolic wave ("A wave"), caused by atrial contraction. Thus, measurement of the peak velocity of each of these waves yields an E/A ratio greater than 1. Note that normal E/A ratios in adolescents and young adults can exceed 2. Normal E/A ratios in adults older than 40 years typically are in the 1 to 2 range.
- With abnormal LV relaxation, the early diastolic E wave decreases in velocity. To compensate, atrial contraction increases, yielding a higher velocity A wave. Once the E/A ratio decreases below 1.0, assessment is generally considered mild diastolic dysfunction (grade I). Note that, in people over the age of 65, the E/A ratio is frequently less than 1.0 and many echocardiographers do not consider it true diastolic dysfunction (Figure 4-8).
- As LV diastolic dysfunction progresses, left atrial pressure will increase to compensate, causing increase in the early diastolic E wave. Diastolic dysfunction can be considered moderate (grade II) once the E/A ratio increases above 1.0.
- As the LV becomes more restricted, left atrial pressure rises and left atrial contraction diminishes, resulting in further increases in the E/A ratio. Diastolic dysfunction can be considered severe when the E/A ratio exceeds 2.0. Typically, a decrease in preload will cause the E/A ratio to decrease below 1.0. If the E/A ratio reverses below 1.0 with the Valsalva maneuver, then the restriction is considered reversible (grade III). If it does not, it is considered irreversible (grade IV).

KEY POINTS

- While this system of diastolic function assessment can occur regardless of LV function, clinical application of diastolic function should be viewed in terms of coexisting reduced or preserved LVEF. In particular, given that the E/A ratio is greater than 1.0 in both normal and moderate diastolic dysfunction, relying solely on LV spectral Doppler flow velocities and pattern can be misleading.
  - Nonetheless, in patients with significantly abnormal systolic dysfunction, some degree of diastolic dysfunction is likely to be present. Thus, in patients with reduced EF, prognosis has been shown to be lower for patients with E/A ratios greater than 1.0.
  - For patients with preserved systolic function, typically determined by an EF greater than 50%, the LV inflow pattern may possess diagnostic value. The differential diagnosis of patients with preserved systolic function presenting with dyspnea is wide. An abnormal LV inflow pattern increases the likelihood of diastolic heart failure.

Step 2: Deceleration Time (DT) of Early Diastolic Filling

- In addition to the peak velocity, the DT of the E wave can yield valuable information. The DT is measured from the peak E wave to the baseline (see Figure 4-8).
- Normal values range from 140 to 200 ms. Values greater than 200 ms suggest mild diastolic dysfunction. As the LV diastolic dysfunction worsens, the E-wave DT will decrease into the normal range ("pseudonormal") and eventually below the normal range, consistent with restrictive physiology.

TABLE 4-4 RECOMMENDATIONS FROM THE AMERICAN SOCIETY OF ECHOCARDIOGRAPHY FOR THE QUANTIFICATION OF LEFT ATRIAL DIMENSIONS

	Women				Men			
	Reference Range	Mildly Abnormal	Moderately Abnormal	Severely Abnormal	Reference Range	Mildly Abnormal	Moderately Abnormal	Severely Abnormal
Atrial dimensions								
LA diameter, cm	2.7–3.8	3.9–4.2	4.3–4.6	≥4.7	3.0–4.0	4.1–4.6	4.7–5.2	≥5.2
LA diameter/BSA, cm/m²	1.5–2.3	2.4–2.6	2.7–2.9	≥3.0	1.5–2.3	2.4–2.6	2.7–2.9	≥3.0
RV minor-axis dimension, cm	2.9–4.5	4.6–4.9	5.0–5.4	≥5.5	2.9–4.5	4.6–4.9	5.0–5.4	≥5.5
RV minor-axis dimension/BSA, cm/m²	1.7–2.5	2.6–2.8	2.9–3.1	≥3.2	1.7–2.5	2.6–2.8	2.9–3.1	≥3.2
Atrial area								
LA area, cm²	≤20	20–30	30–40	>40	≤20	20–30	30–40	>40
Atrial volumes								
LA volume, mL	22–52	53–62	63–72	≥73	18–58	59–68	69–78	≥79
LA volume/BSA, mL/m²	*22 ± 6*	*29–33*	*34–39*	*≥40*	*22 ± 6*	*29–33*	*34–39*	*≥40*

Bold italic values: Recommended and best validated.

Reprinted with permission from Lang RM, Bierig M, Devereux RB, et al. Recommendations for chamber quantification: A report from the American Society of Echocardiography's Guidelines and Standards Committee and the Chamber Quantification Writing Group, developed in conjunction with the European Association of Echocardiography, a branch of the European Society of Cardiology. *J Am Soc Echocardiogr.* 2005;18:1440-1463.

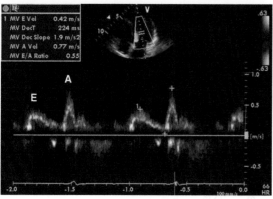

E/A = 0.71   Deceleration time = 224 ms

Figure 4-8. Pulsed wave Doppler of LV inflow with measurement of early diastolic (E) and late diastolic (A) wave ratio and DT.

KEY POINTS

- Deceleration time has been associated with mortality for patients with decreased LVEF.
- However, given the increase in DT with mild diastolic dysfunction, values need to be interpreted in the context of the individual patient.

Step 3: Isovolumic Relaxation Time (IVRT) and Myocardial Performance Index (MPI)

- The sample volume of the pulsed wave spectral Doppler determination is placed within the LV cavity to include both LV inflow during diastole and LV outflow during systole. The time between the end of outflow and the beginning of inflow represents the IVRT (Figure 4-9). The MPI incorporates the isovolumic contraction time (IVCT), the IVRT, and the LV systolic ejection time (LVET) into one assessment with the formula:

$$MPI = (IVCT + IVRT)/LVET$$

- IVRT has a normal range (60 to 100 ms), increases with mild diastolic dysfunction, decreases into the normal range with moderate dysfunction (pseudonormal), and decreases further below the normal range with severe dysfunction.

KEY POINT

- Accurate measurement of IVRT and IVCT is technically difficult and requires considerable training and practice.

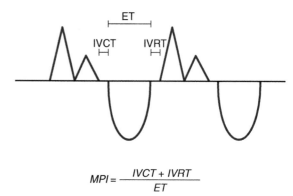

$$MPI = \frac{IVCT + IVRT}{ET}$$

Figure 4-9. Cartoon depicting measurement of IVCT, ET, IVRT, and MPI.

Step 4: Color Doppler M-Mode of LV Inflow to Obtain Propagation Velocity (Vp)

- In the apical 4C view, align the M-mode cursor in the center of the mitral annulus, as parallel as possible to the LV inflow.
- Obtain color Doppler images flow-superimposed upon M-mode with the color sector as narrow as possible. The Nyquist limit should be set at approximately 75% of the peak E-wave velocity. Sweep speed should be 150 mm/s to optimize measurements (Figure 4-10).
- The Vp is the slope of the change in color (at the first aliasing velocity) of the mitral inflow from the mitral annulus to 4 cm into the LV cavity. Normal values are greater than 50 cm/s.

KEY POINTS

- Obtaining a reliable color Doppler in M-mode that extends 4 cm from the mitral annulus is technically difficult and requires significant initial training and frequent use.
- While a color change of the first aliasing velocity (e.g., red to blue) is often recommended, change in other velocities (e.g., yellow to red) may provide a better image and a more reliable slope measurement.

Step 5: Spectral Doppler of Pulmonary Veins

- The superior right pulmonary vein from the apical 4C view provides the most reliable assessment of flow into the left atrium. The sample volume is obtained approximately 1 cm within the pulmonary vein. Flow consists of a forward systolic wave (S), corresponding to LV contraction and atrial relaxation; a second forward diastolic wave (D), corresponding to early mitral inflow; and a reverse late diastolic wave (A), corresponding to atrial contraction (Figure 4-11).

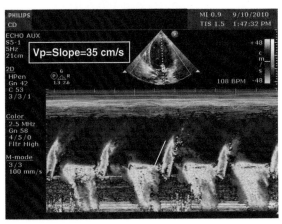

Figure 4-10. Example of measurement of Vp.

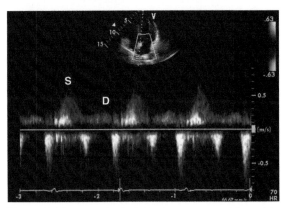

Figure 4-11. Example depicting flow measured from right upper pulmonary vein. D, flow during ventricular diastole; S, flow during ventricular systole.

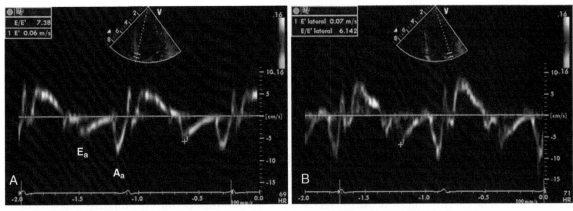

Figure 4-12. TDI in the apical 4C view of the septal (**A**) and lateral (**B**) mitral annulus.

KEY POINT

- In young patients, the D wave can significantly exceed the S wave. In normal middle-aged adults, the S and D waves have similar peak velocities. With mild diastolic dysfunction, the D wave decreases in velocity, similar to the decrease in the mitral inflow E wave. With more advanced diastolic dysfunction, ventricular compliance worsens allowing less complete atrial emptying, the velocity of the S wave decreases and that of the D wave increases.

Step 6: TDI of Mitral Annulus

- TDI is obtained in the apical views by placing the sample volume on the mitral annulus.
- Assessments can be obtained at the annulus of each wall in the three apical views (4-, 2-, and 3-chamber).
- In patients with normal diastolic function, the early diastolic TDI velocity (E_a) is higher than the late diastolic TDI velocity (A_a). Similar to mitral inflow, with mild diastolic dysfunction

the early diastolic flow decreases below the late diastolic flow (i.e., E_a/A_a becomes less than 1.0). However, in contrast to mitral inflow, with worsening diastolic dysfunction E continues to decrease. Thus, the pseudonormal mitral inflow E/A ratio of moderate diastolic dysfunction can be distinguished from normal diastolic function by a low E_a (typically below 8 or 9 cm/s) (Figure 4-12).

KEY POINTS

- Values can be averaged for all six segments; however, frequently the average of the septal and lateral walls in the 4C view is used.
- E_a has been shown to be correlated with mortality in patients with systolic dysfunction.
- A ratio of early diastolic flow velocities from mitral inflow and TDI (E/E_a) above 10 to 15 has been used to identify patients with elevated pulmonary capillary wedge pressures above 18 to 20 mm Hg. However, other studies have found no clinically significant correlation.

Step 7: Overall Assessment of LV Diastolic Function

- From the information obtained from the LV inflow, pulmonary veins, and TDI, an overall assessment of diastolic function can be made.
- Because all patients with significant systolic dysfunction have diastolic dysfunction, the major value of assessing degree of diastolic dysfunction in these patients is to identify those with moderate or severe dysfunction, or restrictive filling pattern (RFP).
- RFP has been shown to correlate with increased mortality.

Mitral Regurgitation

Step 1: Overall Assessment of Etiology

- Assessment of MR in patients with systolic heart failure begins with characterization of the anatomy of all components of the MV apparatus. Careful evaluation of the annulus, leaflets, chordae tendinae, and papillary muscle provides insight into the etiology and mechanism of MR, which will be critical toward determining optimal therapeutic intervention.
- The initial assessment in all patients with significant MR involves categorization into primary, due to abnormalities of the mitral apparatus, or functional, due to LV dilatation.
- Perhaps the most dramatic example of primary MR is a ruptured papillary muscle. While this scenario can be catastrophic, it is usually recognized acutely and, if addressed appropriately with timely surgical intervention, will not lead to chronic systolic dysfunction. Primary leaflet abnormalities, such as MV prolapse, can lead to systolic dysfunction. Patients with MV prolapse and significant MR should be evaluated clinically and echocardiographically serially for MV repair or replacement.
- Functional regurgitation frequently occurs in patients with significant LV dilatation. Myocardial infarction leading to regional wall remodeling can cause outward displacement of the papillary muscles. The chordae are stretched and tether the mitral leaflets, causing poor coaptation (Figure 4-13). An additional mechanism of functional MR is annular dilatation from regional or global LV dilatation. Functional MR can be addressed by decreasing afterload or limiting LV dilatation and assessment for mitral annular ring placement or MV replacement.

Step 2: Measurement of LV Diastolic and Systolic Size and Left Atrial Size (see above)

- See Anatomic Imaging section above.

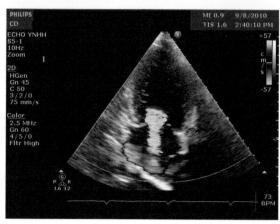

Figure 4-13. Two-chamber view of central MR due to annular dilatation resulting in poor leaflet coaptation.

Step 3: Color Doppler Evaluation

- Color Doppler evaluation of MR remains the foundation for assessment of severity and can also give clues toward etiology.
- Assessment includes estimation of the area of the jet as a proportion of the area of the left atrium in the 4C view, and estimation of the diameter of the vena contracta in the parasternal long-axis view. Severe MR has been defined as a jet area greater than 40% of the left atrium or a vena contracta greater than 7 mm.
- In addition to the quantitative assessment of these parameters, jet direction is an important factor. Severity of wall-impinging jets is significantly underestimated using jet area. Thus, MR may be severe with any wall-impinging jet. Direction of the jet also gives clues toward etiology. A posteriorly directed jet may be from a prolapsed anterior leaflet or a restricted posterior leaflet. Similarly, an anteriorly directed jet may be from a prolapsed posterior leaflet or a restricted anterior leaflet. Functional regurgitation is usually centrally directed.

KEY POINTS

- For color Doppler, the Nyquist limit should be set between 50 and 70 cm/s.
- Nyquist limits less than 50 cm/s can overestimate the degree of MR by including secondary movement of blood within the left atrium (i.e., blood displaced by the regurgitant jet) rather than the regurgitant jet only.
- Vena contracta is best measured in the parasternal view, where the direction of the jet is perpendicular to the ultrasound beam, because axial resolution is superior to lateral resolution.

Step 4: Spectral Doppler Evaluation

- The intensity of the spectral Doppler of the mitral jet is directly related to severity. Often a poorly characterized jet suggests a milder MR, but a very intense spectral Doppler signal suggests a more severe regurgitation.
- Assessment of pulmonary venous flow: a 1- to 2- mm sample volume is obtained in the right upper pulmonary vein (described above). Significant MR will blunt or reverse the systolic wave in the pulmonary vein.
- In addition, because of the relationship of velocity and pressure described in the Bernoulli equation, the rate of increase in velocity of the flow across the MV can estimate the change in pressure over time (*dP/dt*), which is an indicator of systolic function (Figure 4-14). A low *dP/dt* (<600 mm Hg/s) is an indicator of a poor prognostic, and may be helpful in determining management.

KEY POINT

- Although most modern echocardiography machines will automatically estimate a *dP/dt*, to manually estimate *dP/dt* on echocardiography, measure the time difference between when the mitral regurgitant jet is 1 m/s and 3 m/s. Because the change in pressure will be 32 mm Hg (36 mm Hg at 3 m/s – 4 mm Hg at 1 m/s), *dP/dt* = 32/Δ*t* (mm Hg/s).

Step 5: Integration

- While 2D, color Doppler, and spectral Doppler all are valuable independently, comprehensive quantitative assessment of MR severity requires a combination of all three.
- Flow-convergence analysis uses both color and spectral Doppler to estimate effective regurgitant orifice (ERO) area and regurgitant volume (RVo) by the proximal isovelocity surface area (PISA) method. The surface area of the jet approaching the MV is measured on color Doppler and the velocity and velocity-time integral (VTI) are measured on spectral Doppler (see Chapter 2 for further description of PISA). ERO above 40 mm^2 and RVo over 60 mL are considered severe mitral regurgitation.
- RVo can also be estimated by subtracting the SV across the aortic valve during systole from the volume across the MV during diastole. Stroke volume is estimated by measuring the diameter of the LV outflow tract and the VTI in the left ventricular outflow tract (LVOT). Diastolic flow across the MV is similarly estimated (assuming a circular cross section and obtaining 2D and spectral measurements at the level of the annulus).
- RVo can be estimated by subtracting SV from total change in volume of the LV cavity. SV is estimated as described above. LV volumes are typically estimated in 2D using Simpson's method.

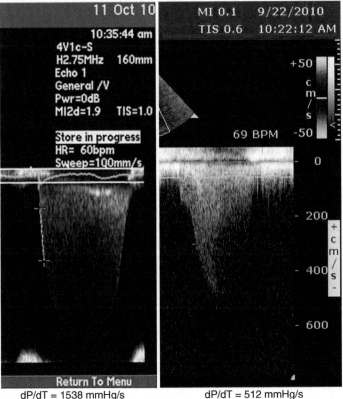

Figure 4-14. Example of measurement of the slope of the mitral regurgitant jet obtained by continuous wave across the MV in patients with normal (**A**) and abnormal (**B**) systolic function.

dP/dT = 1538 mmHg/s   dP/dT = 512 mmHg/s

- 3D echocardiography provides the promise to avoid some of the inaccuracies resulting from the geometric assumptions necessary for 2D quantitative analysis. 3D has been shown to provide more accurate assessments of LV volumes. LVOT and MV annular area assessment is likely improved with 3D. In addition, important advances are being developed to better render color Doppler 3D images of regurgitation.

Pulmonary Artery Systolic Pressure

Based on the law of conservation of energy, the pressure difference between two cardiac chambers can be estimated using the simplified Bernoulli equation: pressure equals four times the velocity squared ($P = 4v^2$). Thus, the peak velocity of the tricuspid regurgitant jet can be used to estimate the pressure difference between the right ventricle and atrium. With the assumption of no significant pulmonary stenosis and an estimation of the right atrial (RA) pressure, pulmonary artery systolic pressure can be estimated.

Step 1: Estimating the RV-to-RA Pressure Gradient

- The peak velocity of the tricuspid regurgitant Doppler envelope is measured in multiple views. The highest value from a regurgitant jet is used to estimate the systolic pressure gradient across the tricuspid valve with the use of the simplified Bernoulli equation ($P = 4v^2$) (Figure 4-15).

KEY POINTS

- While most patients have a sufficient tricuspid regurgitant jet for a reasonable measurement, a significant percentage do not. Care should be taken in using only those jets with a reasonable certainty that they represent the true peak velocity of blood across the tricuspid valve. Reporting that an estimation is not able to be accurately made is preferable to reporting a potentially inaccurate estimation.
- If a reasonable jet is obtained in multiple views, the jet with the highest velocity should be used (e.g., *not* an average of multiple views). The view with the jet with the highest velocity likely is the closest to parallel to the true jet. However, if within *one* view multiple different velocities are obtained (e.g., atrial fibrillation), an average of 3 to 5 beats is acceptable.

Step 2: Estimating the RA Pressure

- Right atrial pressure is estimated, usually based on evaluation of inferior vena cava size. A normal-sized inferior vena cava (<2.0 cm) and normal respiratory variation of this

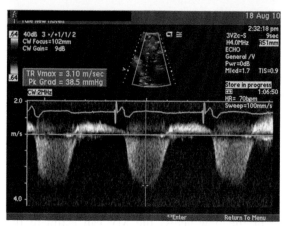

Figure 4-15. Pulsed wave Doppler across the tricuspid valve in the high parasternal view depicting a velocity of 3.1 m/s. By the modified Bernoulli equation, the gradient across the tricuspid valve is estimated to be 38 mm Hg (pressure = 4 times velocity squared). With an estimated right atrial pressure of 7 mm Hg (estimated from the size and reactivity of the inferior vena cava), pulmonary artery systolic pressure is estimated to be 45 mm Hg.

size with inspiration (e.g., "sniffing") (>50% decrease) signifies normal right atrial pressure (<10 mm Hg). Mildly increased size (2.0 to 2.5 cm) or decreased respiratory variation signifies mildly elevated right atrial pressure (10 to 15 mm Hg). A dilated inferior vena cava (>2.5 cm) and decreased respiratory variation signify elevated right atrial pressure (>15 mm Hg).

Step 3: Estimating PASP

- Assuming no significant pulmonary valvular stenosis, the PASP is estimated to be the sum of the estimated right atrial pressure and the estimated pressure gradient across the tricuspid valve. Often the values are reported in 5-mm Hg increments, as smaller increments suggest a higher precision than justified. Generally, values under 40 mm Hg are considered normal.

KEY POINTS

- Estimations of PASP on echocardiography have correlated well with invasive measurements. Not only can some patients avoid an invasive procedure, but the values can be followed more frequently to assist in decision making.
- PASP has been strongly correlated with prognosis in patients with systolic heart failure.

Alternate Approaches

While echocardiography is the foundation for providing the necessary cardiovascular imaging information to the clinician for the most appropriate clinical decision making both initially and in follow-up, other cardiovascular modalities certainly provide valuable additional imaging data.

MRI generally has higher spatial resolution and most frequently is used to provide additional anatomic information. MRI provides more accurate and precise left and right ventricular volumes as well as wall thicknesses. This precision can be particularly useful for following chamber volumes over time. The challenges presented to echocardiography as a result of the variable anatomy of the right heart, particularly in patients with dilated left ventricles, are largely overcome by MRI.

Most patients with systolic heart failure are evaluated for coronary artery disease. The noninvasive assessment of coronary perfusion by nuclear techniques, such as single-photon emission computed tomography (SPECT) with sestamibi (MIBI), provides additional physiologic data not obtained by conventional echocardiography and can give confirmation of left ventricular systolic function.

Right heart catheterization (RHC) measures cardiac pressures directly. Although right-sided pressures, such as PASP and RA pressure, are estimated by echocardiography, RHC has fewer assumptions and values are considered more accurate. Certainly the pulmonary capillary wedge pressure by RHC provides more accurate and precise estimations of left atrial pressures and left ventricular end-diastolic pressure than can be obtained by echocardiography.

Thus, many patients with systolic heart failure will benefit from a multimodality cardiovascular imaging approach. Echocardiography is generally the first-line imaging modality and can often direct the appropriate use of treatment and subsequent imaging when necessary.

Suggested Readings

1. Lang RM, Bierig M, Devereux RB, et al. Recommendations for chamber quantification: A report from the American Society of Echocardiography's Guidelines and Standards Committee and the Chamber Quantification Writing Group, developed in conjunction with the European Association of Echocardiography, a branch of the European Society of Cardiology. *J Am Soc Echocardiogr.* 2005;18:1440-1463.
   This document from the American Society of Echocardiography nicely describes the standards for measuring various chamber sizes, including the left ventricle, the right ventricle, and the left atrium.
2. Haddad F, Doyle R, Murphy AD, Hunt SA. Right ventricular function in cardiovascular disease, part II: Pathophysiology, clinical importance, and management of right ventricular failure. *Circulation.* 2008;117:1717-1731.
   This review outlines important physiologic principles of right ventricular function and provides a practical guide for placing these measurements in a clinical context.
3. Leung DY, Boyd A, Ng AA, Chi C, Thomas L. Echocardiographic evaluation of the left atrial size and function: Current understanding, pathophysiologic correlates, and prognostic implications. *Am Heart J.* 2008;156:1056-1064.
   This review summarizes the data and clinical importance of the relatively recent appreciation of the role of left atrial volume assessment in prognosis and clinical management.
4. Meta-Analysis Research Group in Echocardiography (MeRGE) AMI Collaborators, Møller JE, Whalley GA, Dini FL, et al. Independent prognostic importance of a restrictive left ventricular filling pattern after myocardial infarction: An individual patient meta-analysis. *Circulation.* 2008;117:2591-2598.
   This paper summarizes the results of a large effort to compile the evidence surrounding the prognostic significance of many echocardiographic parameters attempting to evaluate diastolic function in patients after myocardial infarction.

Hypertensive Heart Failure

Fay Y. Lin and Richard B. Devereux

5

Left Ventricular Hypertrophy

- Myocardial hypertrophy is a response to increased LV wall stress in accordance with Laplace's law.
  - Laplace's law describes the relationship of wall tension (T) to the transmural pressure difference (P), the radius (*r*) and thickness (*h*) of the LV (Figure 5-1).
  - High pressure stimulates compensatory increases in wall thickness. Increased volume dilates the cavity and causes higher wall tension for constant pressure, stimulating compensatory LV hypertrophy (LVH) (Figure 5-2).
- Both volume and pressure load influence LVH in hypertension.
- LVH and left ventricular mass (LVM) are strong, independent predictors of all-cause death, congestive heart failure, sudden cardiac death, and other cardiovascular events.

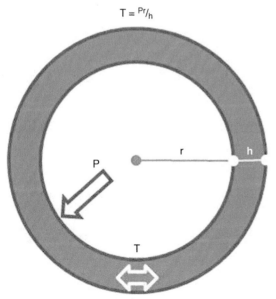

$$T = {}^{Pr}/_h$$

Figure 5-1. Laplace's law describes the relationship of wall tension and pressure to ventricular size and thickness.

How to Evaluate LV Mass

- LV mass may be evaluated using linear, two-dimensional (2D), or three-dimensional (3D) measurements. LV mass is measured by subtracting LV cavity volume from LV epicardial volume to obtain LV myocardial volume, and multiplication of volume by myocardial density to obtain LV mass.
- LVM quantitation requires adequate endocardial and epicardial definition, and on-axis imaging.

Linear Measurements

> **KEY POINTS**
>
> - Linear measurements of interventricular septal wall thickness (SWT), posterior wall thickness (PWT), and LV diastolic internal dimension (LVIDd) should be made from the parasternal long-axis window in end-diastole (Figure 5-3).
> - Measurements should be taken at the level of the LV minor axis, at the papillary muscle level.
> - Linear measurements can be made directly from 2D images or using 2D-targeted M-mode echocardiography. M-mode recordings aligned perpendicular to the LV long axis may facilitate exclusion of trabeculae and false tendons from the LV wall.
> - Linear measurements should be made from leading edge to leading edge.
> - To avoid inclusion of RV and LV trabeculae, measurements should be taken from the most rapidly moving myocardial interface.
> - Oblique imaging planes may overestimate cavity size and wall thickness (Figure 5-4).
> - LVM may be estimated by the following necropsy-validated formula (Figure 5-5):
>
>   LVM = 0.8 × {1.04[(LVIDd + PWTd + SWTd)³ − (LVIDd)³]} + 0.6 g
>
> - Relative wall thickness (RWT) may be estimated as:
>
>   RWT = (2 × PWTd)/LVIDd

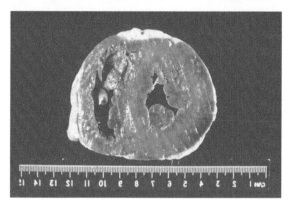

Figure 5-2. Gross pathology of LVH.

2D Measurement of LVM

KEY POINTS

- Epicardial and endocardial contours are traced in the 4-chamber and 2-chamber views at end-diastole.
- Traced contours are used to calculate LV volumes by the biplane Simpson method.
- Foreshortening of the LV apex can systematically underestimate LV cavity volumes, with variable impact on LVM measurement.

3D Measurement of LVM

KEY POINTS

- 3D measurement requires high-quality 3D LV volume acquisition with clear endocardial and epicardial interfaces.
- This may be unobtainable with atrial fibrillation or poor acoustic windows.
- Echocardiographic contrast may be useful for poor endocardial definition.
- Select anatomically correct 2- and 4-chamber views with the largest long-axis dimensions (Figure 5-6).
- Epicardial and endocardial contours are traced in the 4-chamber and 2-chamber views at end-diastole. Traced contours are used to calculate LV volumes by use of the biplane Simpson formula similar to 2D measurement of LVM.
- 3D measurement has lower interobserver variability than 2D measurement (Figure 5-7).

Definition of LVH and Abnormal LV Geometry

LV Hypertrophy

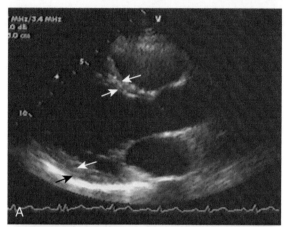

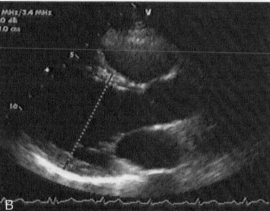

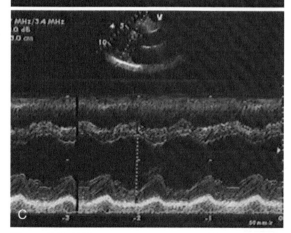

Figure 5-3. LV linear measurements. **A,** The endocardial interface (*arrows*) should be measured from the most rapidly moving myocardial interface to avoid inclusion of RV and LV trabeculae. **B,** Measurements should be taken at the level of the LV minor axis. **C,** 2D-directed M-mode measurements in the same patient using the most rapidly moving myocardial interface.

KEY POINTS

- LV mass is related to body size. LVM is higher among men than women (Table 5-1).
- LVM indexed to body surface area (BSA) is widely used to define LVH.
- Use of BSA may misclassify obesity-induced LVH as normal, so indexing LV mass to the allometric power of height ($h^{2.7}$) may be preferred.
- Small differences are observed between partition values for linear and 2D measurements.
- 95% confidence intervals are used for partition values to identify abnormality.

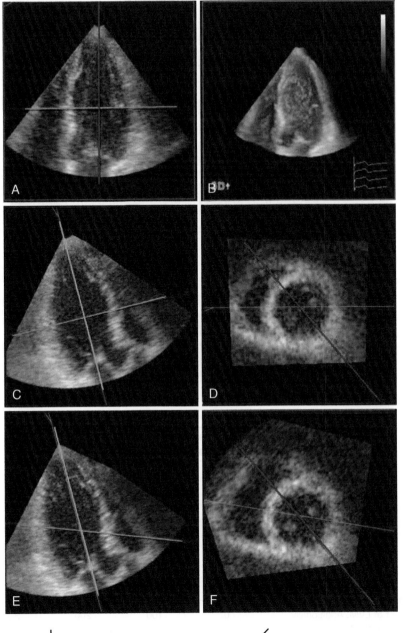

Figure 5-4. 3D echocardiography illustrates potential pitfalls in LV measurement due to off-axis imaging. The green, red, and blue lines represent the four-chamber (**A**), two-chamber, and short-axis planes, respectively, from the 3D volume (**B**). A correctly oriented LV minor axis plane (**C**) results in a short-axis image (**D**) with smaller diameter and thinner apparent wall thickness than an off-axis plane (**E** and **F**), without grossly visible differences in short axis.

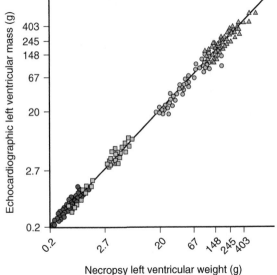

Figure 5-5. Echocardiographic LV mass has a high correlation ($r \geq 0.90$) versus necropsy in humans and experimental animals. *(Reproduced with permission from Devereux RB, Alonso DR, Lutas EM, et al. Echocardiographic assessment of left ventricular hypertrophy: Comparison to necropsy findings. Am J Cardiol. 1986;57:450-458.)*

Figure 5-6. Reorientation of planes using 3D echocardiography. The four-chamber (**A,** *green*), two-chamber (**B,** *red*), and short-axis (**C,** *blue*) planes are identified by corresponding lines in other projections (**D**). The short-axis plane is defined by positioning the blue line in both apical views (**A** and **B**) at the midpapillary muscle level perpendicular to the long axis of the ventricle. The apical views are iteratively selected by repositioning the red and green lines to pass through the midcavity to the apex, ensuring that the resulting views have the largest long-axis dimension. End-diastolic epicardial and endocardial contours are traced in 4-chamber and 2-chamber views to obtain myocardial volume and mass. *(Reproduced with permission from Mor-Avi V, Sugeng L, Weinert L, et al. Fast measurement of left ventricular mass with real-time three-dimensional echocardiography: Comparison with magnetic resonance imaging. Circulation. 2004;110:1814-1818.)*

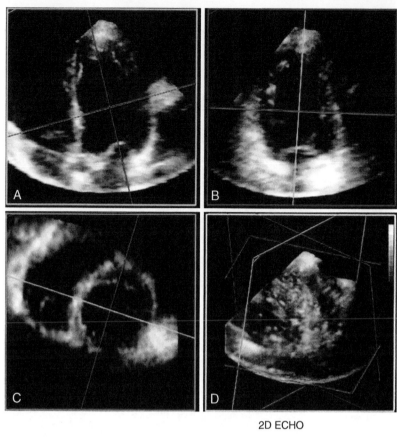

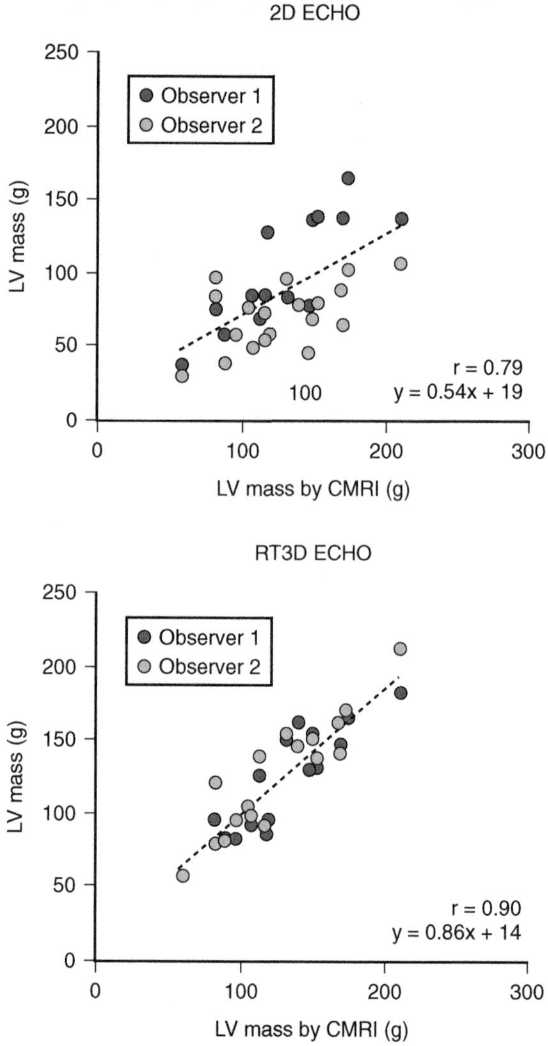

Figure 5-7. 3D measurement of LVM has lower interobserver variability than 2D measurement of LVM. Additionally, 3D measurement of LVM has high agreement with measurement by cardiac magnetic resonance imaging (CMRI). *(Reproduced with permission from Mor-Avi V, Sugeng L, Weinert L, et al. Fast measurement of left ventricular mass with real-time three-dimensional echocardiography: Comparison with magnetic resonance imaging. Circulation. 2004;110: 1814-1818.)*

TABLE 5-1 REFERENCE LIMITS AND PARTITION VALUES OF LEFT VENTRICULAR MASS AND GEOMETRY

	Women				Men			
	Reference Range	Mildly Abnormal	Moderately Abnormal	Severely Abnormal	Reference Range	Mildly Abnormal	Moderately Abnormal	Severely Abnormal
Linear Method								
LV mass, g	67–162	163–186	187–210	≥211	88–224	225–258	259–292	≥293
LV mass/BSA, g/m²	*43–95*	*96–108*	*109–121*	*≥122*	*49–115*	*116–131*	*132–148*	*≥149*
LV mass/height, g/m	41–99	100–115	116–128	≥129	52–126	127–144	145–162	≥163
LV mass/height$^{2.7}$, g/m$^{2.7}$	18–44	45–51	52–58	≥59	20–48	49–55	56–63	≥64
Relative wall thickness, cm	0.22–0.42	0.43–0.47	0.48–0.52	≥0.53	0.24–0.42	0.43–0.46	0.47–0.51	≥0.52
Septal thickness, cm	*0.6–0.9*	*1.0–1.2*	*1.3–1.5*	*≥1.6*	*0.6–1.0*	*1.1–1.3*	*1.4–1.6*	*≥1.7*
Posterior wall thickness, cm	*0.6–0.9*	*1.0–1.2*	*1.3–1.5*	*≥1.6*	*0.6–1.0*	*1.1–1.3*	*1.4–1.6*	*≥1.7*
2D Method								
LV mass, g	66–150	151–171	172–182	≥193	96–200	201–227	228–254	≥255
LV mass/BSA, g/m²	*44–88*	*89–100*	*101–112*	*≥113*	*50–102*	*103–116*	*117–130*	*≥131*

Bold italic values: Recommended and best validated.
Reproduced with permission from Lang RM, Bierig M, Devereux RB, et al. Recommendations for chamber quantification: A report from the American Society of Echocardiography's Guidelines and Standards Committee and the Chamber Quantification Writing Group, developed in conjunction with the European Association of Echocardiography, a branch of the European Society of Cardiology. *J Am Soc Echocardiogr.* 2005;18:1440-1463.

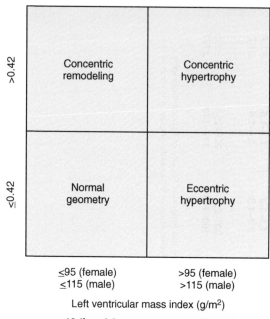

Concentric remodeling	Concentric hypertrophy	>0.42
Normal geometry	Eccentric hypertrophy	≤0.42

≤95 (female)   >95 (female)
≤115 (male)   >115 (male)

Left ventricular mass index (g/m²)

≤46 (female)   >46 (female)
≤49.2 (male)   >49.2 (male)

LVM/height²·⁷ (g/m²·⁷)

Figure 5-8. Definition of abnormal LV geometry.

LV Geometry (Figure 5-8)

<table>
<tr><td colspan="1" align="center">KEY POINTS</td></tr>
<tr><td>
<ul>
<li>LV geometry is defined by RWT and LV mass (Figure 5-9).
  <ul>
  <li>Normal LVM with normal or increased RWT is classified as normal LV geometry or concentric LV remodeling.</li>
  <li>LVH (increased LV mass) with normal or increased RWT is classified as eccentric or concentric hypertrophy.</li>
  <li>LV geometry has incremental value for prognostication of mortality (Figure 5-10) and to heart failure events, all-cause mortality, and composite cardiac events (Figures 5-11 and 5-12).</li>
  </ul>
</li>
</ul>
</td></tr>
</table>

Clinical Vignettes

Case 1

A 48-year-old diabetic, hypertensive man with unlimited exercise tolerance was referred to echocardiography to evaluate atypical chest pain. His blood pressure was 160/100 mm Hg on valsartan and hydrochlorothiazide. He was mildly overweight with a normal exam. The LV ejection fraction (LVEF) was normal with normal valvular function. On echocardiographic exam, LV geometry was normal (Figure 5-13A):

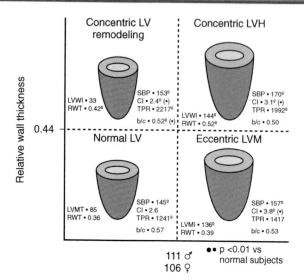

Figure 5-9. Hemodynamic and geometric profiles in hypertensive patients with four patterns of LV geometry. Compared with normal geometry, concentric LV remodeling is associated with lower cardiac output, as lower end-diastolic volume limits SV for the same EF. Concentric LVH is associated with higher systolic blood pressure. Eccentric LVH is associated with higher systolic blood pressure and cardiac output, as higher end-diastolic volumes increase SV for the same EF. (Reproduced with permission from Ganau A, Devereux RB, Roman MJ, et al. Patterns of left ventricular hypertrophy and geometric remodeling in essential hypertension. J Am Coll Cardiol. 1992;19:1550-1558.)

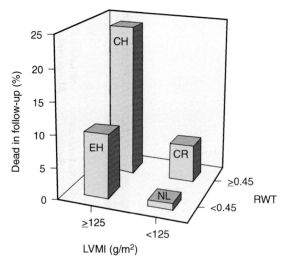

Figure 5-10. Relationship of LV geometry to mortality in patients with uncomplicated hypertension. Concentric hypertrophy (CH) carries the greatest risk, followed by eccentric hypertrophy (EH) and concentric remodeling (CR). NL, normal. (Adapted with permission from Koren MJ, Devereux RB, Casale PN, Savage DD, Laragh JH. Relation of left ventricular mass and geometry to morbidity and mortality in uncomplicated essential hypertension. Ann Intern Med. 1991;114:345-352.)

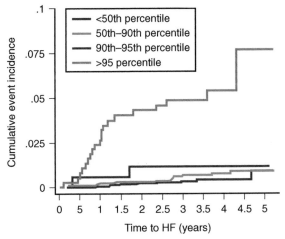

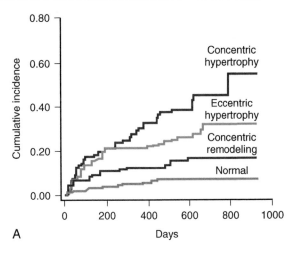

Figure 5-11. LVM and LVH raise the risk of incident heart failure events in the Multi-Ethnic Study of Atherosclerosis. *(Reprinted with permission from Bluemke DA, Kronmal RA, Lima JA, et al. The relationship of left ventricular mass and geometry to incident cardiovascular events: The MESA (Multi-Ethnic Study of Atherosclerosis) study. J Am Coll Cardiol. 2008;52:2148-2155.)*

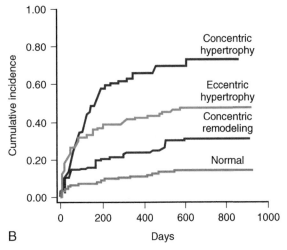

- SWT 1.0 cm, LVIDd 4.6 cm, PWT 1.0 cm
- LVM 136 gm, LVM index (LVMI) 69 gm/m^2 (normal)
- RWT 0.35% (normal)
- LVEF was normal without wall motion abnormalities. Left atrial (LA) size was normal with a diameter of 4.0 cm.
- Off-axis imaging increased the apparent cavity diameter and wall thickness.

The mitral filling pattern was also normal (Figure 5-13B):

- E/A 1.2, deceleration time 178 ms
- Isovolumic relaxation time (IVRT) 77 ms
- Septal E' 7 cm/s, E/E' 8
- Lateral E' 17 cm/s, E/E' 3

The patient went on to nuclear stress testing demonstrating normal exercise electrocardiogram (ECG) and perfusion imaging, but severe exercise-induced hypertension. Blood pressure medication was increased.

Case 2

A 60-year-old man with hypertension, myelofibrosis, and multiple falls underwent echocardiography during evaluation of presyncope. His blood pressure was 131/77 mm Hg on amlodipine and captopril. He was normal weight with a normal exam. His hemoglobin was 8.0 gm/dL. The LVEF was normal with normal valvular function (Figure 5-14A). On echocardiographic exam:

- SWT 0.8 cm, LVIDd 4.2 cm, PWT 0.8 cm
- LVM 136 gm, LVMI 69 gm/m^2 (normal)

Figure 5-12. Relationship of LV geometry to all-cause mortality and composite cardiac events (cardiovascular death, recurrent myocardial infarction, heart failure, stroke, and resuscitated sudden death) post myocardial infarction in the VALIANT study. Concentric hypertrophy has the highest risk, followed by eccentric hypertrophy and then concentric remodeling. *(Reproduced with permission from Verma A, Meris A, Skali H, et al. Prognostic implications of left ventricular mass and geometry following myocardial infarction: The VALIANT (VALsartan In Acute myocardial iNfarcTion) Echocardiographic Study. JACC Cardiovasc Imaging. 2008;1:582-591.)*

- RWT 0.38% (normal)
- LA diameter 4.0 cm (normal)

The mitral filling pattern was normal for age (Figure 5-14B):

- E/A 0.9, deceleration time 292 ms
- IVRT 103 ms
- Septal E' 8 cm/s, E/E' 8
- Lateral E' 9 cm/s, E/E' 7

Despite the E/A reversal and prolonged deceleration time and IVRT, tissue Doppler velocities were normal for age and there was no evidence of elevated LV filling pressures. The inferior

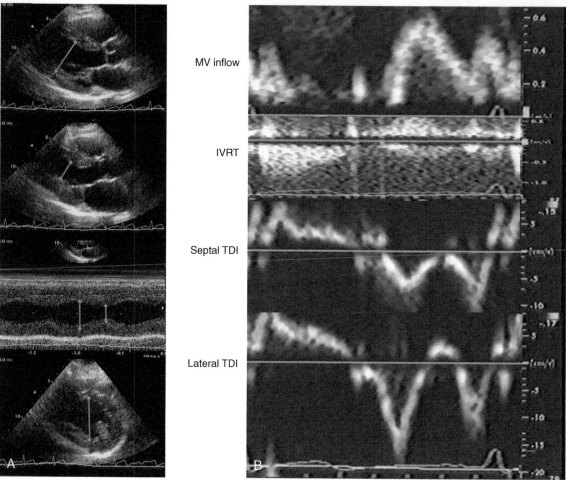

Figure 5-13. Normal LV geometry (**A**) and normal mitral filling pattern (**B**) in a diabetic, hypertensive man with atypical chest pain. MV, mitral valve; TDI, tissue Doppler imaging.

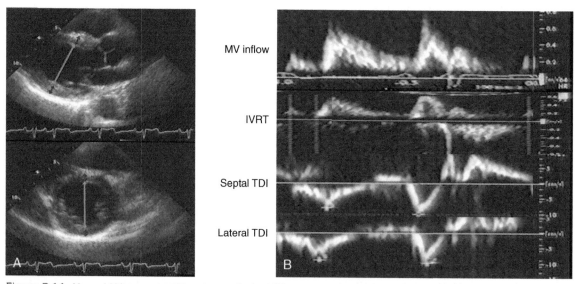

Figure 5-14. Normal LV geometry (**A**) and normal mitral filling pattern for age (**B**) in a 60-year-old hypertensive man with presyncope.

vena cava (IVC) had normal respiratory variation, consistent with right atrial (RA) pressures between 5 and 10 mm Hg. An E/E' ratio ≤ 8 was consistent with normal LV filling pressures. The patient was diagnosed with seizure by electroencephalography.

Case 3

A 75-year-old woman with hypertension underwent echocardiography during evaluation of palpitations. She had unlimited exercise tolerance with no other symptoms. Her blood pressure was 135/70 mm Hg on atenolol. She was normal weight with a I/VI systolic murmur at the left upper sternal border and trace lower extremity edema. The LVEF was normal with normal valvular function. There was mild mitral and aortic annular calcification. Estimated glomerular filtration rate (GFR) by MDRD was 57 mL/min (Figure 5-15A). On echocardiographic exam, LV geometry was consistent with borderline eccentric hypertrophy:

- SWT 1.0 cm, LVIDd 4.9 cm, PWT 0.9 cm
- LVM 164 gm, LVMI 98 gm/m^2 (LVM/$h^{2.7}$ of 46.2 gm/m^2 is borderline LVH)
- RWT 0.37% (normal)
- LA size was normal.

The filling pattern was normal for age (Figure 5-15B):

- E/A 0.9, deceleration time 243 ms
- IVRT 116 ms

- S-dominant pulmonary venous inflow, consistent with decreased ventricular compliance
- Septal E' 6 cm/s (normal for age); E/E' 13
- Lateral E' 7 cm/s (normal for age); E/E' 11[6]

The IVC was normal in size with normal respiratory collapse. She had an abnormal relaxation pattern with E/A reversal and prolonged deceleration time and IVRT, and S-dominant pulmonary venous flow, which may be consistent with normal aging (Figure 5-16).

Case 4

A 94-year-old woman with diabetes was referred to evaluate dyspnea on exertion. She had a ½ block exercise tolerance without other signs or symptoms of heart failure. Her blood pressure was 112/76 mm Hg on no antihypertensives. Her brain natriuretic peptide (BNP) was 23. An ECG demonstrated sinus tachycardia. The LVEF was normal with mild aortic stenosis. LA size was normal for age and body size (Figure 5-17A). On echocardiographic exam, the LV geometry was consistent with concentric remodeling:

- SWT 1.1 cm, LVIDd 4.0 cm, PWT 1.0 cm
- LVM 135 gm, LVMI 83 gm/m^2 (normal)
- RWT 0.50% (concentric)

The stroke volume (SV) was relatively low at 55 mL, with maintenance of a normal cardiac index of 3.4 L/min/m^2 with tachycardia.

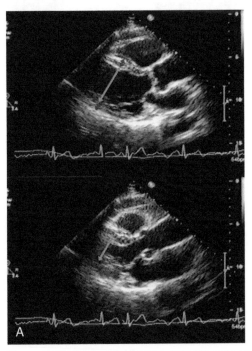
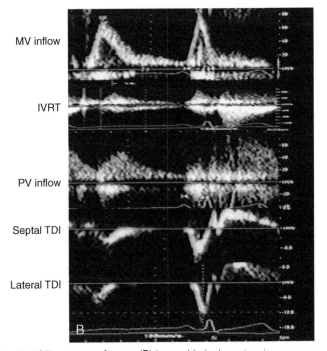

MV inflow

IVRT

PV inflow

Septal TDI

Lateral TDI

Figure 5-15. Borderline eccentric LVH (**A**) and normal mitral filling pattern for age (**B**) in an elderly, hypertensive woman with palpitations. PV, pulmonary valve.

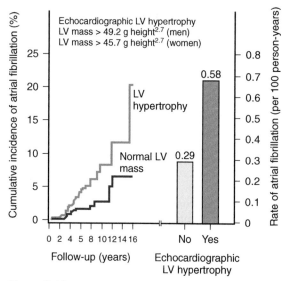

Figure 5-16. Echocardiographic LVH increases the risk of atrial fibrillation. *(Reprinted with permission from Verdecchia P, Reboldi G, Gattobigio R, et al. Atrial fibrillation in hypertension: Predictors and outcome. Hypertension. 2003;41:218-223.)*

There was evidence of elevated LV filling pressures (Figure 5-17B):

- E/A 0.7, deceleration time 242 ms, IVRT 129 ms
- S-dominant pulmonary vein flow
- Septal E′ 5 cm/s, E/E′ 20; lateral E′ 3 cm/s, E/E′ 33

LV filling parameters were suggestive of heart failure with a normal EF[7] (Figure 5-18).

Case 5

A 93-year-old woman with hypertension and a history of non-sustained ventricular tachycardia was referred to echocardiography for syncope. Her blood pressure was 94/56 mm Hg before and 115/70 mm Hg after hydration. The LVEF was hyperdynamic with moderate mitral and tricuspid regurgitation (Figure 5-19A). On echocardiographic exam, LV geometry was consistent with concentric remodeling:

- SWT 1.2 cm, LVIDd 4.0 cm, PWT 1.0 cm
- LVM 146 gm, LVMI 92 gm/m², RWT 0.5%

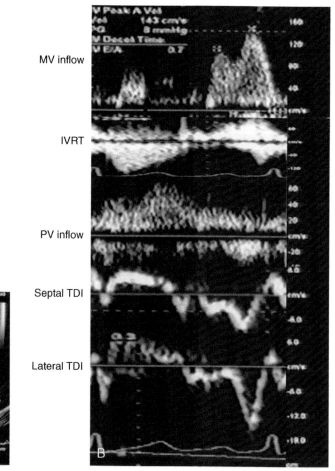

Figure 5-17. Concentric remodeling (**A**) and evidence of elevated LV filling pressures (**B**) in a woman of advanced age with dyspnea on exertion.

Filling parameters were consistent with abnormal relaxation and elevated LV filling pressures (Figure 5-19B):

- E/A 0.7, deceleration time 261 ms
- Septal E′ 3 cm/s, E/E′ 33; lateral E′ 3 cm/s, E/E′ 33
- Tricuspid regurgitation (TR) velocity 2.8 m/s, consistent with pulmonary artery (PA) systolic pressure of 37 to 41 mm Hg.

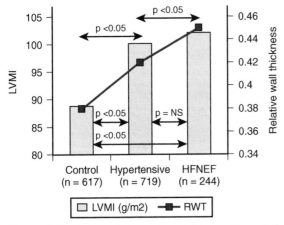

Figure 5-18. LV morphology of heart failure with normal ejection fraction (HFNEF). Relative wall thickness (RWT, *red line*) is significantly higher with HFNEF than in asymptomatic hypertensive or normal patients in the community. *(Adapted with permission from Borlaug BA, Melenovsky V, Redfield MM, et al. Impact of arterial load and loading sequence on left ventricular tissue velocities in humans. J Am Coll Cardiol. 2007;50:1570-1577.)*

The IVC was normal in size with normal respiratory variation, consistent with RA filling pressures of 5 to 10 mm Hg.

Case 6

A 41-year-old man with stage V chronic kidney disease secondary to hypertension was referred to echocardiography for an abnormal ECG. He had an unlimited exercise tolerance with no symptoms of heart failure. His blood pressure was 140/93 mm Hg on amlodipine, labetalol, furosemide, hydralazine, and isosorbide dinitrate. On exam, he had trace lower extremity edema without jugular venous distention or crackles. The LVEF was normal with normal valvular function. The LA was severely dilated by volume measurement (Figure 5-20A). On echocardiographic exam, LV geometry was consistent with concentric hypertrophy:

- SWT 1.3 cm, LVIDd 4.8 cm, PWT 1.3 cm
- LVM 245 gm, LVMI 142 gm/m², RWT 0.54%

LV filling parameters were consistent with pseudonormalization and mildly elevated LV filling pressures (Figure 5-20B):

- E/A 1.3, deceleration time 221 ms
- Septal E′ 4 cm/s, E/E′ 21; lateral E′ 6 cm/s, E/E′ 12
- Pulmonary venous inflow with mild systolic blunting, increased A reversal
- Peak pulmonic regurgitation (PR) velocity 1.0 m/s, consistent with PA diastolic pressure of 19 to 24

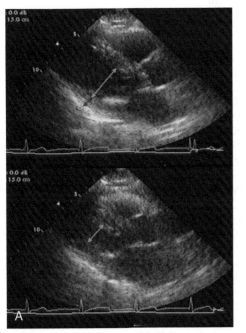

Figure 5-19. Concentric remodeling (**A**) evidence of elevated filling pressures (**B**) in a woman of advanced age with syncope.

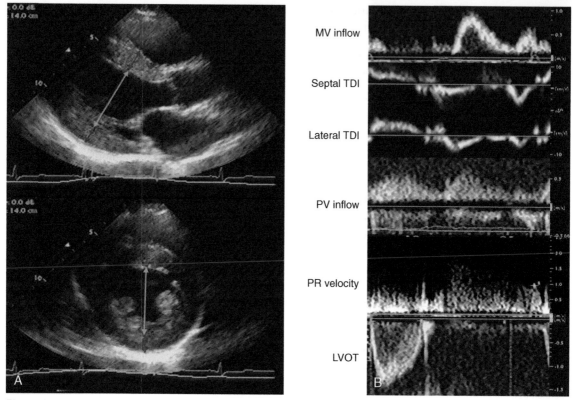

Figure 5-20. Concentric hypertrophy (**A**) and evidence of elevated filling pressures (**B**) in an asymptomatic hypertensive man with stage V chronic kidney disease.

- LV outflow tract (LVOT) velocity-time integral (VTI) 26 cm and SV 106 mL, consistent with volume overload

The IVC was dilated without respiratory variation, consistent with elevated RA filling pressures of 15 to 20 mm Hg.

Case 7

A 64-year-old man was referred for echocardiography to evaluate LV function after discharge from hospitalization for a hypertensive emergency. He had an unlimited exercise tolerance and no symptoms. His blood pressure was 144/66 mm Hg on carvedilol, losartan, amlodipine, and furosemide. His estimated GFR was 73 mL/min. LV function was normal with normal valvular function. The LA was dilated, with an LA volume index of 47 mL/m². Two years later, he had progression of renal insufficiency and was referred to echocardiography for lower extremity edema. Exercise tolerance was unlimited. The blood pressure was 160/88 mm Hg on carvedilol, amlodipine, furosemide, isosorbide dinitrate and hydralazine in lieu of losartan due to hyperkalemia (Figure 5-21A).

LV geometry in 2008 was consistent with concentric LVH:

- 2008 SWT 1.6 cm, LVIDd 5.8 cm, PWT 1.5 cm
- 2008 LVM 425 gm, LVMI 195 gm/m², RWT 0.52%

LV geometry in 2010 was consistent with less severe concentric LVH:

- 2010 SWT 1.6 cm, LVIDd 5.1 cm, PWT 1.5 cm
- 2010 LVM 349 gm, LVMI 156 gm/m², RWT 0.59%

LV filling in 2008 was consistent with pseudonormalization and possibly elevated LV filling pressures (Figure 5-21B):

- 2008 E/A 1.2, deceleration time 215 ms, IVRT 85 ms
- 2008 Septal E′ 3 cm/s, E/E′ 23; lateral E′ 5 cm/s, lateral E/E′ 14
- 2008 Pulmonary veins demonstrated very mild systolic blunting.

LV filling in 2010 was consistent with abnormal relaxation and normal LV filling pressures:

- 2010 E/A 0.8, deceleration time 341 ms, IVRT 95 ms
- 2010 Septal E′ 3 cm/s, E/E′ 17; lateral E′ 8 cm/s, lateral E/E′ 9
- 2010 Pulmonary veins were S dominant.

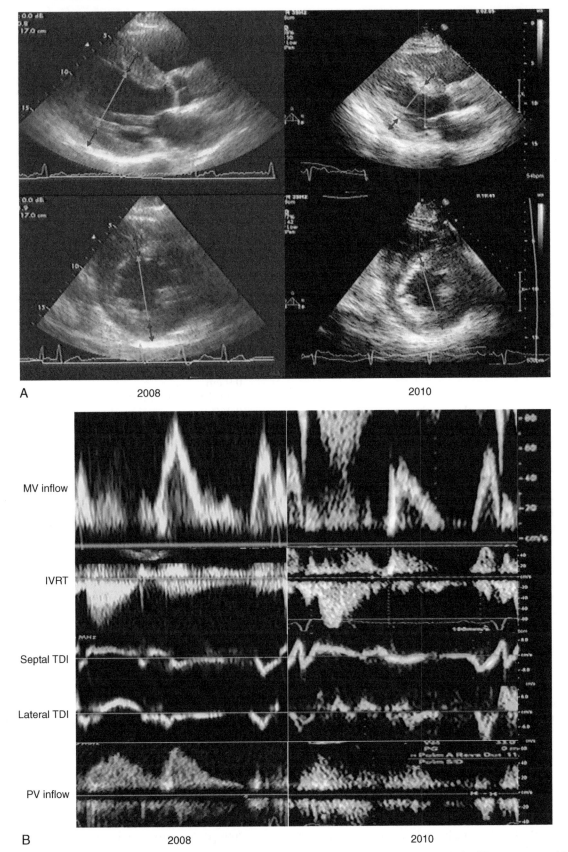

Figure 5-21. Concentric hypertrophy in a hypertensive emergency (**A**) and improved left ventricular filling pressure with medical therapy and LVH regression (**B**) in a hypertensive man.

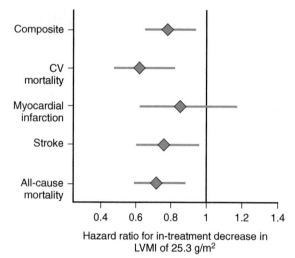

Figure 5-22. Association of in-treatment LV mass with risk of cardiovascular (CV) events in the LIFE trial: results of Cox multivariable proportional hazards analysis. Hazards are adjusted for baseline LVMI, treatment with atenolol or losartan, and blood pressure lowering. *(Adapted with permission from Devereux RB, Wachtell K, Gerdts E, et al. Prognostic significance of left ventricular mass change during treatment of hypertension. JAMA. 2004;292:2350-2356.)*

Figure 5-22 shows the association of in-treatment LV mass with risk of cardiovascular events.

Case 8

A 41-year-old man with stage III chronic kidney disease secondary to hypertension underwent echocardiography for dyspnea with exertion. His blood pressure was 134/75 mm Hg on amlodipine, labetalol, furosemide, hydralazine, and isosorbide dinitrate. On exam, he had jugular venous distention to the jaw and bibasilar crackles with mild pedal edema. His LVEF was normal with normal valvular function. The left atrium was mildly dilated (Figure 5-23A). On echocardiographic exam, LV geometry was consistent with concentric hypertrophy:

- SWT 1.3 cm, LVIDd 4.7 cm, PWT 1.3 cm
- LVM 237 gm, LVMI 116 gm/m², RWT 0.55%

Doppler parameters were consistent with pseudo-normalized filling, indeterminate LV filling pressures and high cardiac output (Figure 5-23B).

- E/A 1.1, deceleration time 129 ms
- Septal E' 7 cm/s, septal E/E' 16; lateral E' 10 cm/s, E/E' 11
- Pulmonary vein S/D 1
- PR end-diastolic velocity 1.7 m/s, consistent with PA diastolic pressures of 22 to 27 mm Hg
- Peak TR velocity 3.2 m/s, consistent with PA systolic pressures of 51 to 56 mm Hg

- LVOT VTI 31 cm, consistent with SV of 107 mL and cardiac index of 5.1 L/min/m²

The IVC was dilated with absence of respiratory variation consistent with RA filling pressures of 15 to 20 mm Hg. The clinical presentation was consistent with high-output heart failure.

Case 9

A 73-year-old man with diabetes and a history of kidney transplantation, congestive heart failure with preserved EF, and triple-vessel coronary artery disease (CAD) was referred for echocardiography in 2008 to evaluate postoperative dyspnea after coronary artery bypass grafting. His blood pressure was 144/70 mm Hg on carvedilol, lisinopril, amlodipine, and furosemide. His exam was notable for an intact arteriovenous (AV) fistula, trace lower extremity edema, and no other evidence of volume overload. His echocardiogram in 2008 demonstrated inferolateral hypokinesis with mildly reduced left ventricular function (LVEF 47%) and a left pleural effusion. LV geometry was normal:

- 2008 SWT 1.0 cm, LVIDd 5.0 cm, PWT 0.9 cm
- 2008 LVM 170 gm, LVMI 107 gm/m², RWT 0.36%

Two years later, he was referred for echocardiography to evaluate LV function in the setting of worsening renal insufficiency. His blood pressure was 156/62 mm Hg on higher doses of the same medications, with no edema or evidence of volume overload. The follow-up echocardiogram demonstrated normal LV function without wall motion abnormalities. The patient was diagnosed with chronic allograft rejection (Figure 5-24A). LV geometry in 2010 was consistent with eccentric LVH:

- 2010 SWT 1.2 cm, LVIDd 5.1 cm, PWT 1.0 cm
- 2010 LVM 214 gm, LVMI 134 gm/m², RWT 0.39%

Over 2 years, with poorly controlled hypertension and chronic allograft rejection, there were increased LV wall thicknesses and increased LVM, with progression of LV geometry from normal to eccentric LVH. With recovery of stunned myocardium post–bypass surgery as well as LV remodeling, LVEF improved.

Filling parameters were consistent with abnormal relaxation and elevated LV filling pressures (Figure 5-24B):

- 2008 E/A 1.0, deceleration time 205 ms
- 2008 Septal E' 3 cm/s, septal E/E' 32; lateral E' 5 cm/s, lateral E/E' 20
- 2008 Pulmonary venous S/D 1, with preserved S_1

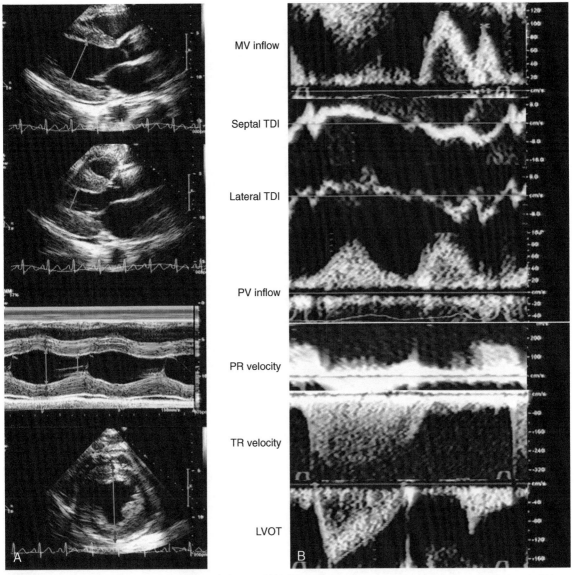

MV inflow

Septal TDI

Lateral TDI

PV inflow

PR velocity

TR velocity

LVOT

A

B

Figure 5-23. Concentric hypertrophy (**A**) and abnormal LV filling (**B**) in a hypertensive man with stage 3 chronic kidney disease and clinical heart failure symptoms.

- 2008 PR end-diastolic velocity 1.2 m/s, estimated PA diastolic pressure 11 to 16 mm Hg; TR velocity 2.2 m/s (not shown in Figure 5-24)

The IVC was normal in size with normal respiratory variation, consistent with RA filling pressures of 5 to 10 mm Hg.

Over 2 years, there was evidence of progressive diastolic dysfunction from abnormal relaxation to pseudo-normalization, with evidence of increasing LV filling pressures and PA pressures, in the setting of progressive LVH and eccentric LV remodeling:

- 2010 E/A 1.2, deceleration time 196 ms
- 2010 Septal E′ 3 cm/s, E/E′ 47; lateral E′ 5 cm/s, E/E′ 28

- 2010 Pulmonary venous systolic blunting and loss of S_1 was consistent with pseudonormalization. Atrial reversal velocity was not well visualized by transthoracic echocardiography.
- 2010 PR end-diastolic velocity 1.4 m/s, estimated PA diastolic pressure 13 to 18 mm Hg, estimated RV systolic pressure 36 to 41 mm Hg (not shown in Figure 5-24).

Case 10

A 36-year-old woman with poorly controlled type 1 diabetes and stage III chronic kidney disease was referred to echocardiography for evaluation of dyspnea with exertion and lower extremity edema.

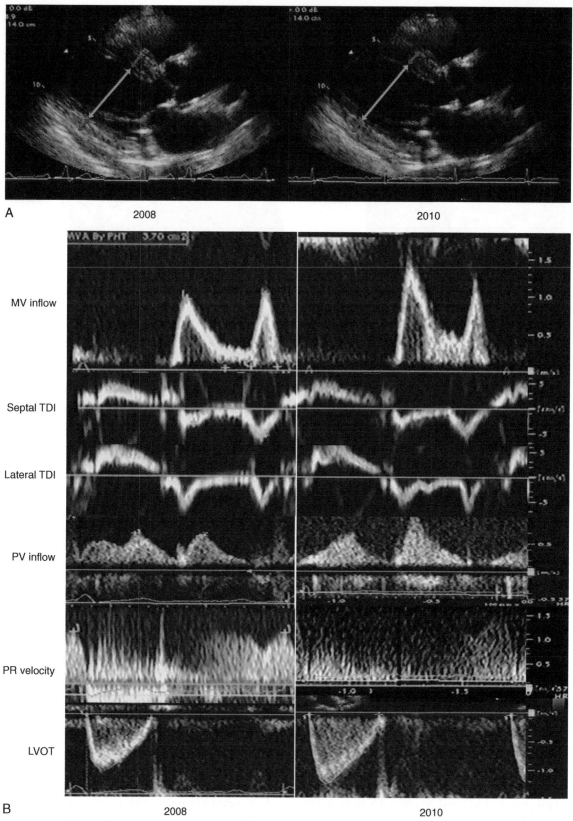

Figure 5-24. Worsening eccentric hypertrophy (**A**) and increasing LVM and progression of abnormal diastolic filling (**B**) in a hypertensive man with CAD, heart failure, and poorly controlled hypertension over 2 years.

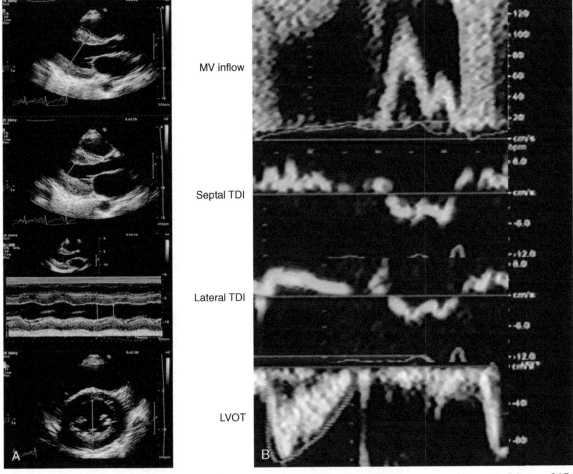

Figure 5-25. Concentric hypertrophy (**A**) and abnormal LV filling (**B**) in a hypertensive woman with type 1 diabetes, CAD, and mildly depressed LV function.

Her blood pressure was 176/90 mm Hg on labetalol and enalapril. Her exam was notable for a 2/6 holosystolic murmur, an S_4, and no evidence of volume overload. Her echocardiogram demonstrated diffuse mild hypokinesis with mildly reduced LV function (LVEF 53%), moderate to severe mitral regurgitation with a regurgitant fraction of 50%, and severe TR. She underwent cardiac catheterization and was diagnosed with three-vessel CAD. The LV end-diastolic pressure was 22 mm Hg (Figure 5-25A). On echocardiographic exam, LV geometry was consistent with concentric LVH:

- SWT 1.2 cm, LVIDd 4.7 cm, PWT 1.2 cm
- LVM 218 gm, LVMI 116 gm/m², RWT 0.50%

The LA size was normal by volumetric measurement (not shown in Figure 5-25).

Filling parameters were consistent with restrictive physiology and elevated LV filling pressures confirmed by cardiac catheterization (Figure 5-25B):

- E/A 2, deceleration time 127 ms
- Septal E′ 5 cm/s, septal E/E′ 22; lateral E′ 5 cm/s, lateral E/E′ 22
- LVOT VTI 18.6 cm, consistent with a mildly depressed SV of 47 mL despite only mildly depressed LV function with low end-diastolic volume. The cardiac index of 2.5 L/min/m² was maintained with elevated heart rate.
- Estimated PA systolic pressure 74 to 79 mm Hg, PA diastolic pressure 17 to 21 mm Hg (not shown in Figure 5-25)

The IVC was dilated with absence of respiratory variation, consistent with RA filling pressures of 15 to 20 mm Hg.

Case 11

A 50-year-old Native American diabetic woman had normal LVEF with normal valvular function at initial evaluation:

- 2004 SWT 0.7 cm, LVIDd 5.3 cm, PWT 0.6 cm; LVM 115 gm, LVMI 67 gm/m², RWT 0.22%

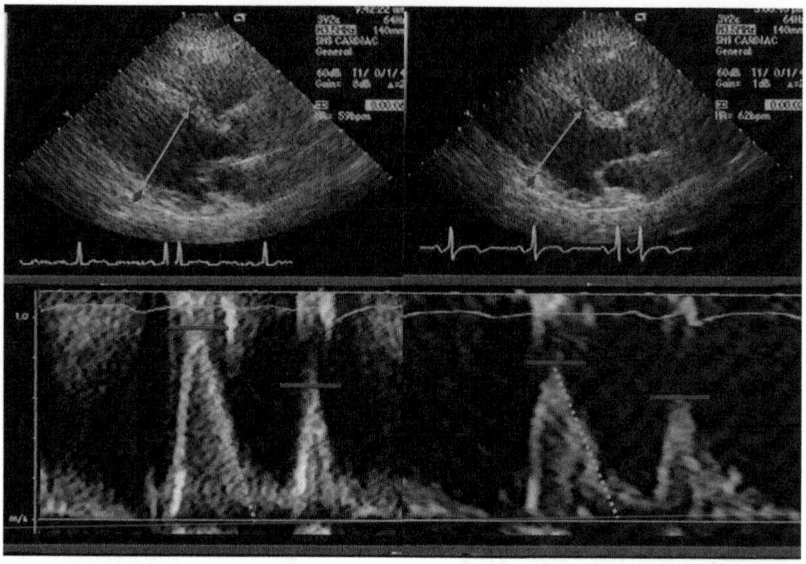

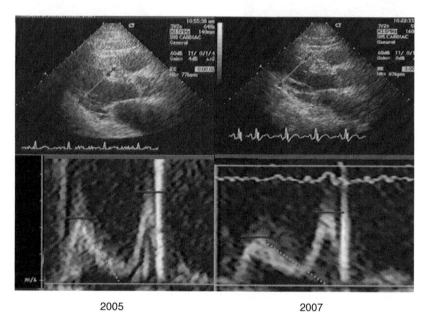

Figure 5-26. LVH regression and improved LV filling in a type 2 diabetic with blood pressure control and weight loss.

2004   2006

Figure 5-27. LVH regression with blood pressure control in a type 2 diabetic with systolic heart failure.

2005   2007

- 2004 E/A 1.5, deceleration time 241 ms, IVRT 75 ms

The LA diameter was normal at 3.6 cm (Figure 5-26).

During 2 years of aggressive blood pressure reduction, she also lost 27 pounds with lifestyle modification. The LA diameter also decreased to 3.4 cm. Evaluation was consistent with treatment-associated reduction of LV mass within the normal range and improvement of LV filling from pseudo-normalization to abnormal relaxation:

- 2006 SWT 0.7 cm, LVIDd 4.6 cm, PWT 0.6 cm; LVM 90 gm, LVMI 57 gm/m², RWT 0.26%

- 2006 E/A 1.4, deceleration time 211 ms, IVRT 100 ms. Deceleration time indexed to E, which outperforms deceleration time alone in predicting cardiovascular outcome, prolonged from 2.45 to 2.67.[9]

Case 12

A 78-year-old Native American diabetic man with a prior history of myocardial infarction had severely depressed LVEF (33%) with inferior and inferolateral akinesis at baseline (2005), and unchanged left ventricular function at follow-up in 2007 after reduction of blood pressure from 163/82 to 132/73 mm Hg (Figure 5-27):

- 2005 SWT 1.1 cm, LVIDd 5.2 cm, PWT 0.7 cm; LVM 169 gm, LVMI 89 gm/m^2, RWT 0.27%
- 2005 E/A 0.7, deceleration time 180 ms, IVRT 110 ms
- 2007 SWT 1.0 cm, LVIDd 4.8 cm, PWT 0.7 cm; LVM 154 gm, LVMI 81 gm/m^2, RWT 0.29%
- 2006 E/A 0.8, deceleration time 208 ms, IVRT 85 ms

Left atrial diameter was unchanged at follow-up. Evaluation is consistent with a mild decrease in LV mass with baseline normal LV geometry and no major changes in LV filling parameters and stable systolic heart failure.

References

1. Devereux RB, Alonso DR, Lutas EM, et al. Echocardiographic assessment of left ventricular hypertrophy: Comparison to necropsy findings. *Am J Cardiol.* 1986;57: 450-458.
   This paper established the echocardiographic validation of left ventricular mass and hypertrophy.
2. Mor-Avi V, Sugeng L, Weinert L, et al. Fast measurement of left ventricular mass with real-time three-dimensional echocardiography: Comparison with magnetic resonance imaging. *Circulation.* 2004;110:1814-1818.
   This paper validated the evaluation of left ventricular mass using three-dimensional echocardiography against cardiac magnetic resonance.
3. Ganau A, Devereux RB, Roman MJ, et al. Patterns of left ventricular hypertrophy and geometric remodeling in essential hypertension. *J Am Coll Cardiol.* 1992;19: 1550-1558.
   This study was the first to characterize differing patterns of ventricular hypertrophy and left ventricular geometry.
4. Koren MJ, Devereux RB, Casale PN, Savage DD, Laragh JH. Relation of left ventricular mass and geometry to morbidity and mortality in uncomplicated essential hypertension. *Ann Intern Med.* 1991;114:345-352.
   This paper was the first to demonstrate the independent prognostic value of left ventricular geometry for major adverse cardiac events.
5. Verma A, Meris A, Skali H, et al. Prognostic implications of left ventricular mass and geometry following myocardial infarction: The VALIANT (VALsartan In Acute myocardial iNfarcTion) Echocardiographic Study. *JACC Cardiovasc Imaging.* 2008;1:582-591.
   This paper validates the prognostic value of left ventricular hypertrophy and geometry in coronary artery disease for major adverse cardiac events.
6. Nagueh SF, Appleton CP, Gillebert TC, et al. Recommendations for the evaluation of left ventricular diastolic function by echocardiography. *J Am Soc Echocardiogr.* 2009;22:107-133.
   This consensus document establishes methodology for evaluation of left ventricular diastolic dysfunction.
7. Paulus WJ, Tschope C, Sanderson JE, et al. How to diagnose diastolic heart failure: A consensus statement on the diagnosis of heart failure with normal left ventricular ejection fraction by the Heart Failure and Echocardiography Associations of the European Society of Cardiology. *Eur Heart J.* 2007;28:2539-2550.
   This European consensus document establishes diagnostic workup for heart failure with normal left ventricular ejection fraction.
8. Devereux RB, Wachtell K, Gerdts E, et al. Prognostic significance of left ventricular mass change during treatment of hypertension. *JAMA.* 2004;292:2350-2356.
   This landmark study demonstrates the mortality benefit of left ventricular mass regression among treated hypertensives above and beyond blood pressure.
9. Mishra RK, Galloway JM, Lee ET, et al. The ratio of mitral deceleration time to E-wave velocity and mitral deceleration slope outperform deceleration time alone in predicting cardiovascular outcomes: The Strong Heart Study. *J Am Soc Echocardiogr.* 2007;20: 1300-1306.
   This paper refines evaluation of mitral inflow deceleration time for left ventricular diastolic evaluation.
10. Drazner MH, Rame JE, Marino EK, et al. Increased left ventricular mass is a risk factor for the development of a depressed left ventricular ejection fraction within five years: The Cardiovascular Health Study. *J Am Coll Cardiol.* 2004;43:2207-2215.
    This paper demonstrates the prognostic value of LVH for systolic dysfunction.
11. Fox ER, Taylor J, Taylor H, et al. Left ventricular geometric patterns in the Jackson cohort of the Atherosclerotic Risk in Communities (ARIC) Study: Clinical correlates and influences on systolic and diastolic dysfunction. *Am Heart J.* 2007;153:238-244.
    This paper demonstrates the association of LVH and LV geometry with systolic and diastolic dysfunction.
12. From AM, Scott CG, Chen HH. The development of heart failure in patients with diabetes mellitus and preclinical diastolic dysfunction a population-based study. *J Am Coll Cardiol.* 2010;55:300-305.
    This paper demonstrates the intermediate role of diastolic dysfunction in the development of heart failure among type 2 diabetics.
13. Lonn E, Shaikholeslami R, Yi Q, et al. Effects of ramipril on left ventricular mass and function in cardiovascular patients with controlled blood pressure and with preserved left ventricular ejection fraction: A substudy of the Heart Outcomes Prevention Evaluation (HOPE) Trial. *J Am Coll Cardiol.* 2004;43:2200-2206.
    This randomized controlled trial demonstrates that LVM and remodeling are modifiable with angiotensin receptor blocker therapy.
14. Howard BV, Roman MJ, Devereux RB, et al. Effect of lower targets for blood pressure and LDL cholesterol on atherosclerosis in diabetes: The SANDS randomized trial. *JAMA.* 2008;299:1678-1689.
    This randomized controlled trial demonstrated greater decrease in LVM with more aggressive blood pressure control among Native Americans with type 2 diabetes.
15. Devereux RB, Roman MJ, Liu JE, et al. Congestive heart failure despite normal left ventricular systolic function in a population-based sample: The Strong Heart Study. *Am J Cardiol.* 2000;86:1090-1096.
    This population-based study characterizes the clinical and echocardiographic findings of patients with CHF and normal LV function, with more impaired early diastolic LV relaxation and concentric LV geometry compared to those with no CHF.
16. Liao Y, Cooper RS, McGee DL, Mensah GA, Ghali JK. The relative effects of left ventricular hypertrophy, coronary artery disease, and ventricular dysfunction on survival among black adults. *JAMA.* 1995;273: 1592-1597.
    This landmark paper highlights the high prevalence and relative risk of LVH among African-American patients with heart disease. LVH is associated with a greater relative and attributable risk than CAD severity, highlighting the importance of risk factor control.

17. Liao Y, Cooper RS, Durazo-Arvizu R, Mensah GA, Ghali JK. Prediction of mortality risk by different methods of indexation for left ventricular mass. *J Am Coll Cardiol.* 1997;29:641-647.
    This paper establishes the optimal method of indexing left ventricular mass to body size in the clinical setting.

18. Bluemke DA, Kronmal RA, Lima JA, et al. The relationship of left ventricular mass and geometry to incident cardiovascular events: The MESA (Multi-Ethnic Study of Atherosclerosis) study. *J Am Coll Cardiol.* 2008;52: 2148-2155.
    This population-based study demonstrates in a large multi-ethnic registry the prognostic value of LVM for HF, stroke and CHD, and of LV geometry for stroke and CHD.

19. Verdecchia P, Reboldi G, Gattobigio R, et al. Atrial fibrillation in hypertension: Predictors and outcome. *Hypertension.* 2003;41:218-223.
    This paper demonstrates the excess risk of atrial fibrillation with increasing LVM. LA size predisposes to chronicity of atrial fibrillation but not to incidence.

20. Borlaug BA, Melenovsky V, Redfield MM, et al. Impact of arterial load and loading sequence on left ventricular tissue velocities in humans. *J Am Coll Cardiol.* 2007;50: 1570-1577.
    This careful study demonstrates the impact of arterial afterload, particularly late-systolic loads as often found in late-systolic vascular stiffening, on abnormal diastolic relaxation by tissue Doppler velocities.

21. Lang RM, Bierig M, Devereux RB, et al. Recommendations for chamber quantification: A report from the American Society of Echocardiography's Guidelines and Standards Committee and the Chamber Quantification Writing Group, developed in conjunction with the European Association of Echocardiography, a branch of the European Society of Cardiology. *J Am Soc Echocardiogr.* 2005;18:1440-1463.
    This consensus document establishes methodology for evaluation of cardiac chamber size and hypertrophy.

Echocardiographic Assessment of Heart Failure Resulting from Coronary Artery Disease

6

Martin St. John Sutton, Yan Wang, and Theodore J. Plappert

Acute and Chronic Ischemic Heart Failure

Basic Principles

- Heart failure (HF) is caused by coronary artery disease (CAD) in more than 65% of patients and may be acute or chronic. There are two major causes of acute post–myocardial infarction (MI) HF:
  - First, MI involving the loss of 25% to 35% of the LV precipitates acute HF because the remaining myocytes cannot sustain a normal cardiac output.
  - The second cause of acute HF post-MI is due to the onset of volume overload from mitral regurgitation (MR) or rupture of the ventricular septum producing a ventricular septal defect (VSD). These complications usually occur 3 to 5 days post-MI.
- Chronic HF results from progressive LV dilatation due to stretching of the infarct zone and expansion of the normal remote myocardium.
- LV dilatation increases wall stress that induces hypertrophy to normalize LV load and redistribute the elevated wall stress uniformly within the LV walls.
- Increased wall stress and neurohormonal activation drive the remodeling process, favoring LV dilatation and deterioration in function until a new equilibrium is reached between restraining forces exerted by the extracellular matrix and distending forces that promote LV dilatation.
- Myocardial repair involves collagen deposition and scar formation that provide an ideal substrate for re-entrant ventricular arrhythmias.
- Early diagnosis and treatment of HF is important because the prognosis of New York Heart Association (NYHA) class III/IV heart failure is poor (50% at 5 years).
- Doppler echocardiography provides a unique array of metrics for risk-stratifying patients with acute as well as chronic heart failure.

KEY POINTS

- The hallmark of HF due to CAD is regional wall motion abnormalities (RWMAs) (Figure 6-1).
- Knowledge of the distribution of coronary artery blood flow in the 17-segment model of the LV is important for identifying the culprit coronary artery and the likely location of the flow-limiting coronary stenosis (Figure 6-2). Subtle RWMA at rest can be amplified by exercise or pharmacologic stress.
- In ischemic cardiomyopathy with a dilated LV and an ejection fraction (EF) less than 20%, it may be difficult to rule out RWMA because endocardial excursion is severely reduced.
- LV regional wall thickness and systolic wall thickening are reduced in infarcted myocardium.
- Variation in the composition of the LV walls causes a heterogeneous acoustic signature from the myocardium, with increased brightness in infarcted regions due to the increased fibrosis (Figure 6-3).
- LV end-diastolic and end-systolic dimensions and volumes are both increased. The increase in end-systolic volume (ESV) is greater than the increase in end-diastolic volume (EDV), accounting for the fall in ejection fraction in acute HF.
- Percent fractional shortening:

([end-diastolic diameter – end-systolic diameter]/end-diastolic diameter) ×100%

is decreased in HF.
- The LV ejection fraction (LVEF) is usually less than 40%:

$$EF = ([EDV - ESV]/EDV) \times 100\%$$

- LV size as linear dimensions or LV volumes provides unique prognostic information for early risk stratification in HF. LV shortening and LVEF are both strong predictors of survival and adverse cardiovascular events.
- Meridional and circumferential wall stress can be calculated from echocardiographic measurements of wall thickness, cavity radius, cavity length, and LV pressure (Figure 6-4). Wall stress is a major determinant of hypertrophy and

Continued

structural and functional LV remodeling. Calculation of wall stress requires that two contingencies be met—that the LV behaves uniformly without regional abnormalities (RWMAs) and that the material properties of myocardium are constant. Neither of these contingencies is met in ischemic HF. However, longitudinal, radial, and circumferential myocardial strain can be measured and used as surrogates for wall stress.

- Early detection of complications of acute post-MI HF is essential. These include LV thrombus, MR, VSD, pericardial effusion, right ventricular (RV) infarction, increase in QRS duration, and LV dyssynchrony.

Quantification of LV Size and Function in HF

Basic Principles
Step 1
- M-mode echocardiography measurements of LV size in patients with CAD, RWMA, and abnormal LV shape may not be representative of the heart as a whole.

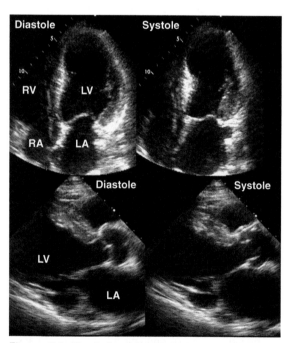

Figure 6-1. The hallmark of HF resulting from CAD is the presence of RWMAs. *Upper panels:* A 4-chamber view at end-diastole and at end-systole of a HF patient with an RWMA involving the mid- to apical anterior septum that exhibits contraction at the base and akinesis of the distal septum consistent with an anteroseptal infarction in the LAD territory. *Lower panels:* Abnormal regional LV function in parasternal long-axis views at end-diastole (*left panel*) and at end-systole (*right panel*) with a thin scarred inferior LV wall consistent with infarction in the right coronary artery territory.

- Use of systolic shortening or LVEF derived from linear dimensions should be avoided for similar reasons in ischemic HF.

Step 2
- LV size in HF due to CAD should be estimated as LV volumes.
- Paired images of the apical 4-chamber and 2-chamber views should be used to estimate LV volumes using Simpson's rule and indexed to body surface area (BSA) or height.
- LV cavity lengths should be similar in the two apical images to avoid foreshortening of the cavity, causing spuriously small volumes.
- Quantification of LV volumes at end-diastole and at end-systole (Figure 6-5) enables calculation of LVEF:

$$LVEF = (LVEDV - LVESV)/LVEDV$$
$$= \text{Stroke volume (SV)}/LVEDV$$

Step 3
- LVEF is often assessed visually by experienced echocardiographers, and correlates closely with LVEF calculated from digitized biplane images.
- The correlation above breaks down in large left ventricles with EF less than 30% and distorted LV cavity shape.
- The myocardial performance index (MPI) or Tei index has been used as an indicator of LV function that is determined as:

$$MPI = (IVCT + IVRT)/LVET$$

where IVRT is the isovolumic relaxation time, IVCT is the isovolumic contraction time, and LVET is the LV ejection time.
- Regional LV function is estimated visually using the 17-segment model during rest and stress. The overall wall motion score predicts cardiac outcome.
- Regional LV function can also be evaluated using tissue Doppler imaging (TDI), in which myocardial velocities are measured. In ischemic or infarcted regions, myocardial velocities are reduced to below normal (Figure 6-6).

Step 4
- Regional myocardial ischemia can be located by measuring regional strain using speckle tracking. Myocardial strain (S) is defined as the change in length (ΔL) at end systole as a function of resting length (L_0) and strain rate is the rate of change of strain with time:

$$\text{Strain (S)} = (\Delta L)/(L_0)$$

$$\text{Rate of change of strain: } dS/dt$$

- Strain can be measured from the apex to base as longitudinal strain. The echo-derived values

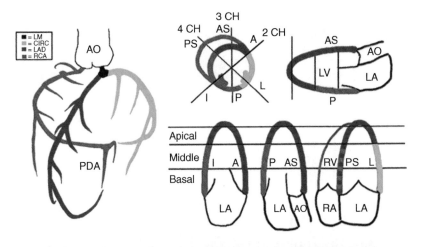

Figure 6-2. Color-coded schema of the coronary artery anatomy (**left**), and the 17-myocardial-segment model color-coded for the coronary artery perfusion of the segments (**right**).

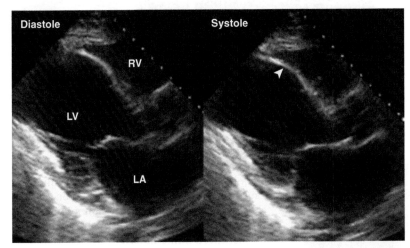

Figure 6-3. Left parasternal echocardiographic images of the LV long axis in diastole (*left panel*) and in systole (*right panel*) showing a thin and scarred distal septum (*arrowhead*). This occurs due to greater reflection of the ultrasound by the infarct than by the adjacent normal myocardium as a result of the greater content of fibrosis.

Left ventricular end-systolic meridional wall stress:

$$(S_m) = \frac{1.33 \times P \times A_c}{A_t - A_c}$$

Left ventricular end-systolic circumferential wall stress:

$$(S_c) = \frac{1.33 \times P \times \sqrt{A_c}}{\sqrt{A_t} - \sqrt{A_c}} \left(\frac{1 - \sqrt{A_c} \left(\frac{A_c}{(0.5L)^2} \right)}{\sqrt{A_t} + \sqrt{A_c}} \right)$$

Figure 6-4. Formulas for end-systolic meridional wall stress (Sm) and end-systolic circumferential wall stress (Sc). A_c, LV short axis cavity area; A_t, the total area of the LV short axis enclosed by the epicardium; L, LV cavity length; P, LV pressure.

for myocardial strain have been validated against magnetic resonance imaging and have correlated closely both in healthy normal subjects and in a number of disease entities. Ischemic or infarcted myocardial segments in HF associated with CAD can be identified by the depressed regional and global longitudinal strain values and by the different times to peak strain from the various myocardial regions in the infarcted/ischemic versus normal segments (Figure 6-7).

Echocardiographic Detection of Thrombus in HF

Basic Principles

- Thrombus usually occurs at the LV apex or adjacent to a region of LV wall that is severely hypokinetic or dyskinetic. The amplitude of endocardial motion in the infarct zone is low, such that there is slow adjacent intracavitary blood flow velocity that looks like "smoke" and is a precursor of thrombus formation.
- Left atrial (LA) dilatation is common in HF due to high filling pressures. LA thrombus is especially frequent in the LA and the LA appendage in patients with atrial fibrillation and atrial flutter. Thrombus in the left heart

Figure 6-5. Quantification of LV
end-diastolic volume (LVEDD) and
end-systolic volume (LVESD) from
paired biplane images of the LV
apical 4-chamber (A4C) and LV
apical 2-chamber (A2C) views as
recommended by the American
Society of Echocardiography.
*(Reprinted with permission from
Lang RM, Bierig M, Devereux RB,
et al. Recommendations for
chamber quantification: A Report
from the American Society of
Echocardiography's Guidelines
and Standards Committee and
the Chamber Quantification Writing Group, developed in conjunction with the European Association
of Echocardiography, a branch of
the European Society of Cardiology. J Am Soc Echocardiogr.
2005;18:1446.)*

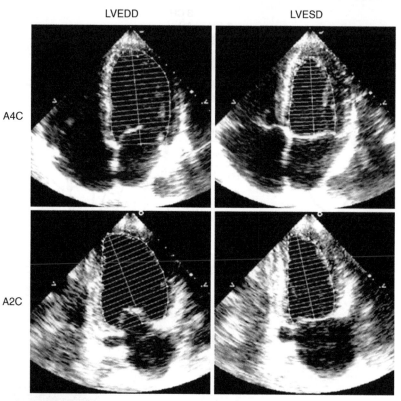

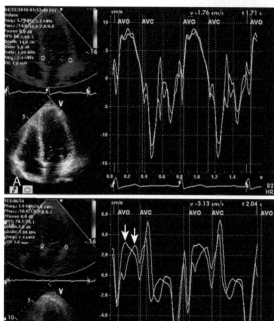

Figure 6-6. Graphic display of myocardial velocities from
the septal and lateral walls at the level of the MV annulus
throughout the cardiac cycle in a normal subject (**A**) and in
a patient with HF due to CAD (**B**). Note that, in the normal
subject, the two velocities track and peak simultaneously,
while in the patient with CAD, there is a delay in the time
to peak septal and peak lateral wall velocities (*arrows*).

chambers has the potential for cardioembolism,
causing stroke or loss of organ function. Detection of LV thrombus is of paramount importance because appropriate anticoagulation can
be instituted immediately.

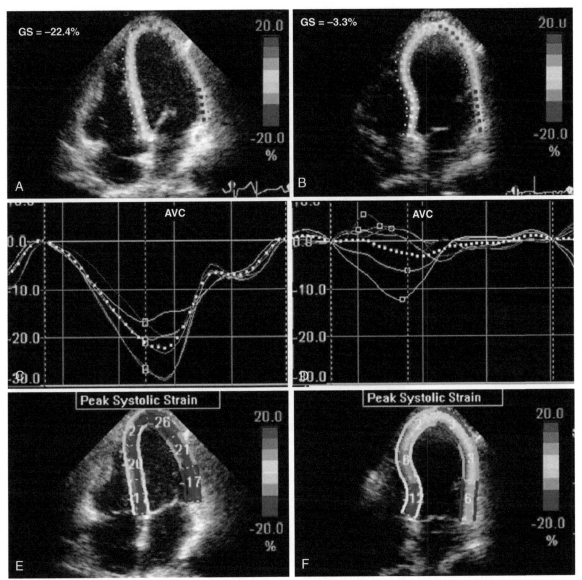

Figure 6-7. Graphic display of systolic strain in a normal subject (**A, C,** and **E**) and a patient with an antero-apical LV aneurysm (**B, D,** and **F**). Global strain (GS) and regional myocardial strain are both severely reduced (**B** and **D**) in the patient with CAD and HF, and the normal exquisite synchrony of the timing of peak strain is lost.

Postinfarction Ventricular Septal Defect

Basic Principles

• Persistent refractory acute HF or new-onset intractable HF several days post-MI should suggest severe LV volume overload due to MR (Figure 6-11) or rupture of the interventricular septum into the right ventricle (VSD) (Figure 6-12).

• Distinguishing the two mechanical lesions purely on the auscultatory features of a harsh holosystolic murmur is unreliable despite claims to the contrary.

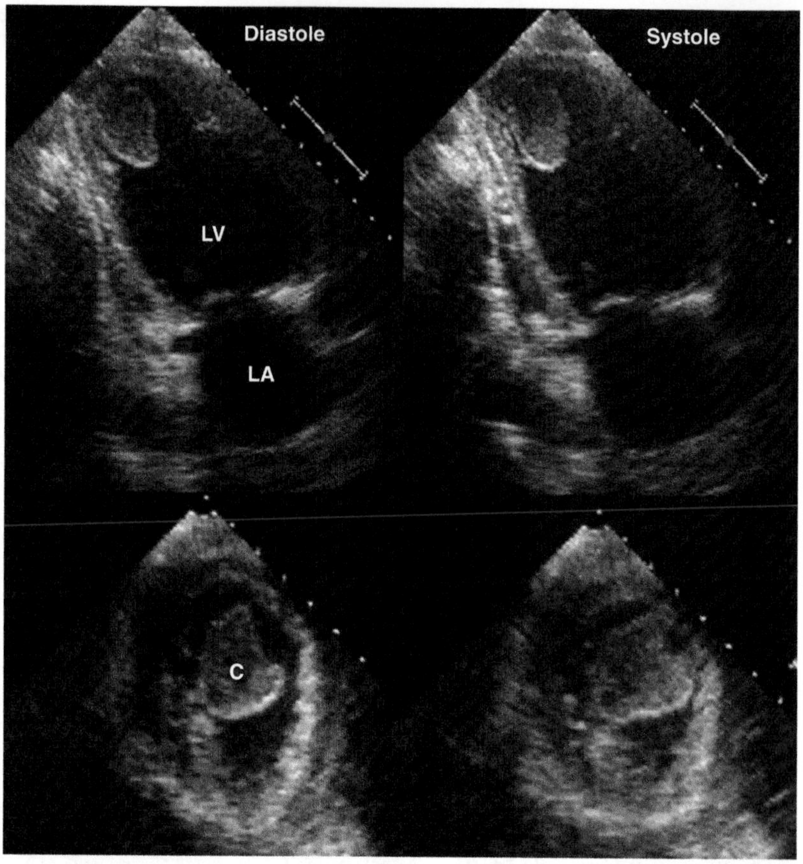

Figure 6-8. Left ventricular thrombus adherent at the apex of the cavity where there is an apical wall motion abnormality shown by the absence of endocardial motion from diastole (*upper left panel*) to systole (*upper right panel*). *Lower panels:* Short-axis images at the apex of the LV demonstrating a large clot (C).

- Doppler echocardiography removes the clinical doubt because color flow Doppler technology enables unequivocal localization of the VSD and at the same time can rule out MR (see Figure 6-12).

- The size of the defect in the ventricular septum can often be visualized directly and semiquantified by the maximal width of the color flow Doppler jet.

KEY POINTS

Step 1
- When an infarct-related VSD is suspected as the cause of new-onset refractory HF post-MI, it is important to obtain a complete assessment of the hemodynamics noninvasively.
- Cuff systolic blood pressure should be recorded with the two-dimensional (2D) echocardiogram. If the aortic valve is normal, cuff systolic pressure (CSP) can be substituted for LV peak pressure (LVPP).
- Measurement of the trans-septal gradient across the VSD allows the RV peak pressure to be estimated. Pulmonary artery peak systolic pressure (PASP) will be the same as RV peak systolic pressure if the pulmonary valve is normal:

$$CSP = LVPP$$

$$PASP = LVPP - \text{trans-VSD gradient}$$

Step 2
- The location of the VSD can be determined using color flow Doppler velocity mapping. Post-MI

VSDs usually occur in the anterior apical septum following a left anterior descending coronary artery (LAD) occlusion. Inferoposterior VSDs result from a right coronary artery occlusion or a dominant left circumflex artery occlusion.
- Color flow mapping should be used to direct the continuous wave Doppler beam to achieve an angle of incidence between the direction of transseptal flow and the insonating Doppler beam close to 0 degrees. This is frequently difficult with inferior VSDs that follow a serpiginous course through the posterior septum. The entrance of the jet in the septum and its exit are separated sometimes by several centimeters, which makes orientation of the Doppler beam difficult if not impossible.

Step 3
- Assessment of the magnitude of the shunt flow across the VSD should be achieved by quantifying blood flow in the pulmonary circulation (Qp) and the systemic circulation (Qs) using the

Doppler principle that volume flow can be calculated as the product of the velocity-time integral (VTI) and the cross-sectional area (CSA) of the flow stream.
- The main pulmonary artery is visualized in its long axis either from the left parasternal view of the short axis of the aortic valve (Figure 6-13) or from the corresponding view from the subcostal window to measure the diameter (d) of the main pulmonary artery. The pulmonary artery is assumed to be circular in CSA and equals $2\pi(d/2)^2$. The velocity signal in the main pulmonary artery is recorded from exactly the same location as the diameter is measured, so that pulmonary flow (Qp) is calculated as:

$$Qp = VTI \times CSA$$

$$Qp = VTI \times 2\pi(d/2)^2$$

- Aortic flow (Qs) is quantified in the same way from the left parasternal region and the apical long-axis view (see Figure 6-13):

$$Qs = VTI \times 2\pi(d/2)^2$$

- Shunt flow across the infarct VSD is expressed as the ratio Qp/Qs. In a normal subject without a VSD, the Qp/Qs = 1.0:1.0. In the presence of a VSD, the larger the shunt (Qp/Qs), the greater the pulmonary blood flow (Qp) and the greater the hemodynamic burden on the failing ventricles.

Postinfarction MR

Basic Principles
- MR occurs in almost two thirds of patients with acute and chronic HF, and results in an increase in LV load that often escalates the deterioration in an already dysfunctional LV, worsening the

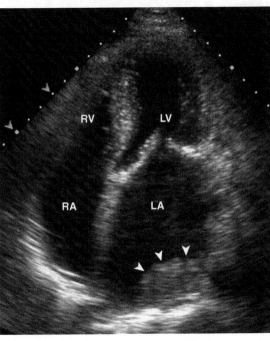

Figure 6-9. An apical 4-chamber view of the heart showing a dilated left atrium (LA) with a large sessile mural thrombus within it (*arrowheads*).

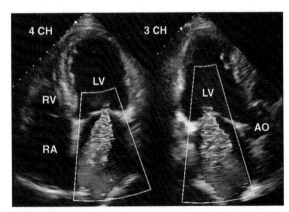

Figure 6-11. Color flow Doppler velocity mapping showing moderate MR with the regurgitant blood flow extending to the roof of the LA and penetrating the pulmonary veins in a patient with HF.

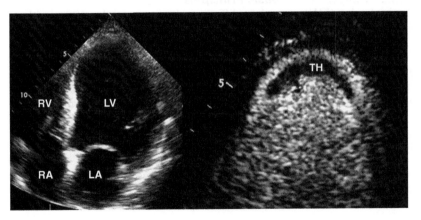

Figure 6-10. Laminated LV thrombus that required intravenous contrast (Definity) to enhance endocardial definition to establish the presence of thrombus (TH).

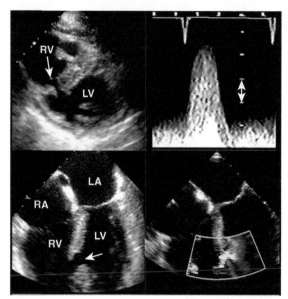

Figure 6-12. Transesophageal echocardiogram in a patient with the onset of HF 4 days post-MI showing a VSD (*bottom left panel, arrow*) and with color flow Doppler demonstrating left-to-right flow across the defect in the 4-chamber view obtained (*bottom right panel, arrow*). The VSD can be seen in the images of the LV short-axis view with RV enlargement from the shunt flow (*top left panel*). A Doppler velocity signal obtained from across the VSD shows that the VSD is restricted but nevertheless causes RV dilatation (*top right panel*).

risk for HF and death from complex ventricular arrhythmias.

- The mechanism of MR in chronic HF is usually progressive increase in LV chamber size and secondary mitral annular dilatation. The latter perturbs the geometry of the mitral subvalve apparatus, increases the tenting area, and prevents normal leaflet coaptation, causing MR (Figure 6-14).
- In acute HF, the mechanism of MR is different from that in chronic heart failure. Acute HF is most frequently due to ischemia that damages the papillary muscles, occasionally causing papillary muscle rupture and severe MR (Figure 6-15). More commonly, ischemia disrupts the temporal coordination of the mitral valve (MV) and subvalve apparatus during valve closure.
- In both acute and chronic HF, the MV leaflets are intrinsically normal.
- Color flow Doppler velocity mapping is exquisitely sensitive to MR such that even mild MR is easily detected as a turbulent regurgitant jet in the LA during systole.
- Since the onset of MR may have dire hemodynamic consequences and necessitate surgical repair of the MV in already high-risk patients, it is important to be able to quantify the severity of MR accurately and determine whether the valve is repairable.

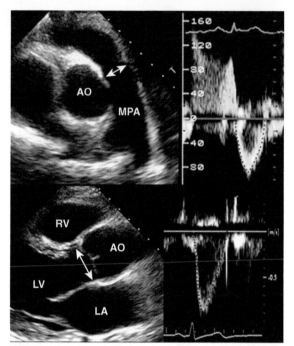

Figure 6-13. The *top panels* demonstrate the method for quantifying pulmonary blood flow as the product of the CSA of the flow stream and the pulmonary VTI. The diameter of the main pulmonary artery is measured to calculate CSA as $2\pi\,(d/2)^2$ and the VTI is digitized. *Bottom panels:* The diameter of the LV outflow tract (*bottom left panel, arrow*) and the digitized Doppler velocity signal (*bottom right panel*), both of which are required to calculate aortic blood flow. The velocity signals are obtained from the exact location at which the diameters are recorded.

- There are methods for quantifying the severity of MR that involve making a single measurement, and more labor-intensive methods that necessitate multiple measurements. In general, the more measurements made, the greater the likelihood of inclusion errors.

Mitral Regurgitant Volume

Basic Principles
- Any difference between total antegrade blood flow across the MV and antegrade blood flow across the aortic valves (AVs) represents the mitral regurgitant volume (MRV) flow, or backward flow into the LA during systole. Blood volume flow is computed as the product of the VTI and the CSA of the flow stream:

$$MRV = (MV\text{-}CSA \times MV\text{-}VTI) - (AV\text{-}CSA \times AV\text{-}VTI)$$

- When this method is used, whether with 2D or three-dimensional (3D) echo, several key points are important (Figure 6-16).

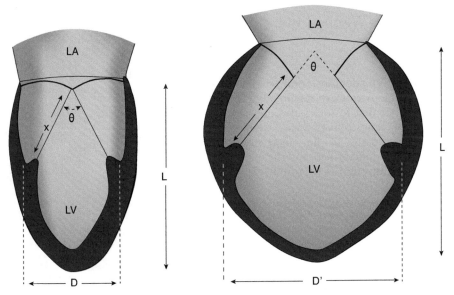

Figure 6-14. Schema showing a normal LV (**left**) and the extensive remodeling that occurs as the normal LV transitions to HF (**right**). This involves progressive LV dilatation and assumption of a spherical rather than an ellipsoidal shape, which disrupts the geometry of the mitral valve and subvalve apparatus. The papillary muscles are separated, and since there is no change in the length of the chordae or leaflets, failure of appropriate coaptation of the leaflets results in MR that ranges from mild to severe.

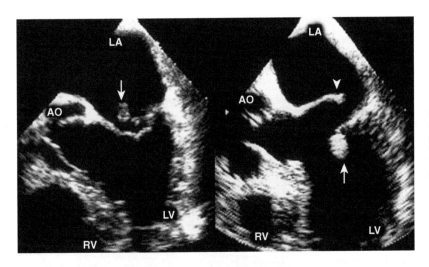

Figure 6-15. Transesophageal echocardiography showing the tip of the ruptured papillary muscle attached to the posterior mitral valve leaflet (*arrow*) prolapsing into the LA and subsequently appearing in the LV.

KEY POINTS

- Calculation of volume flow by this method requires attention to detail because volume computation is dependent upon accurate measurement of diameter of the LV inflow and outflow tracts for calculation of CSA. Even small errors in measurement of diameter are amplified by a square-power function and thus have a major effect on blood volume flow determination.
- The blood flow velocity signals across the LV inflow and outflow tracts must be recorded at the exact same site at which the diameter measurements are made.

- Doppler signals must be high quality and continuous. Of equal importance, they must be digitized very carefully in order to generate an accurate and meaningful VTI. This is particularly relevant with the LV inflow tract signal, and this is best achieved by ensuring that the baseline is downshifted to provide the velocity signal as a full-scale deflection. This large velocity signal enables accurate digitization and a more fiducial VTI.
- Occasionally, both the MV and AV are regurgitant, in which case the pulmonary valve diameter and VTI can be substituted for the AV to estimate forward volume flow.

Measurement of the Width of the Vena Contracta

Basic Principles

- The vena contracta (VC) demonstrated by color flow Doppler is the narrowest region of the mitral regurgitant jet that resides between the proximal zone of flow convergence, where the jet velocity increases as the blood flow approaches the regurgitant orifice, and the zone of jet expansion within the LA (Figure 6-17).

KEY POINTS

Step 1
- The VC may vary in width in orthogonal planes, so it is best to average the two measurements.
- A confounding factor when using the VC method is that small differences in measurements of diameter translate into large differences in severity of MR. In addition, the resolution of the equipment is approximately 1 mm.
- A width of less than 3 mm corresponds to mild MR, between 3 and 6 mm is moderate, and more than 6 mm corresponds to severe MR.

Step 2
- The accuracy of measurements of VC width can be optimized when the zoom function is used, the frame rate is high, and the VC is in the near field (see Figure 6-17).

Proximal Isovelocity Surface Area (PISA)

Basic Principles

- As a laminar flow stream approaches a finite regurgitant orifice, it accelerates, and in doing so creates a series of hemispheres (Figure 6-18) that are seen by color flow Doppler as alternating bands of blue and red, the surface areas of which share fixed flow velocity—known as isovelocity surface areas (see Figure 6-18).
- The color bands alternate each time the flow velocity exceeds the Doppler Nyquist limit, and each subsequent surface area has a progressively greater isovelocity surface with a progressively smaller surface area.
- The flow rate at every isovelocity shell surface area is the same as that at the regurgitant orifice in accordance with the law of conservation of mass.
- Assuming the isovelocity surface area to be hemispherical, flow rate equals the surface area of the hemisphere ($2\pi r^2$) × the aliasing velocity, where r is the radius of the first aliased hemisphere (Figure 6-19). This flow rate is the

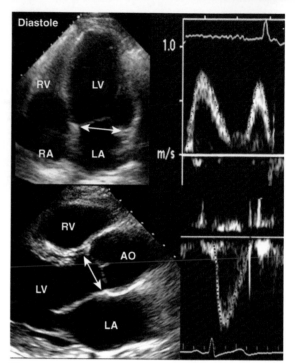

Figure 6-16. *Top panels:* Measurement of the diameter of the MV annulus (*top left panel*) and the VTI of the mitral inflow (*top right panel*). *Bottom panels:* The diameter of the LV outflow tract (*bottom left panel*) and the aortic VTI (*bottom right panel*). The transmitral volume flow and the transaortic volume flow can be quantified. The difference between aortic and mitral flow equals the mitral regurgitant flow.

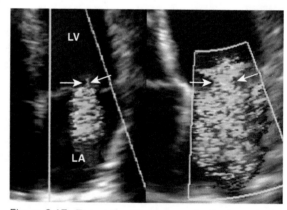

Figure 6-17. The width of the vena contracta shown in the *left panel* is consistent with mild MR while that in the *right panel* is consistent with severe MR.

regurgitant flow rate across the MV, from which the mitral regurgitant orifice area (ROA), regurgitant volume (RV), and regurgitant fraction (RF) can be calculated:

$$ROA = PISA \text{ flow rate}/MR \text{ velocity}$$

$$RV = ROA \times VTI \text{ of the MR jet}$$

$$RF = RV/SV$$

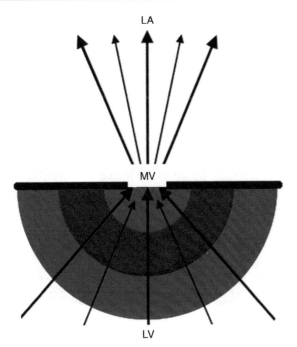

Figure 6-18. Schema showing isovelocity surfaces as flow approaches a regurgitant orifice.

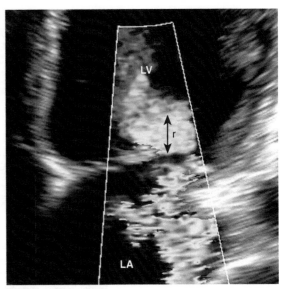

Figure 6-19. Measurement of the radius *r* of the first aliased hemisphere that enables the ROA, RV, and RF to be calculated.

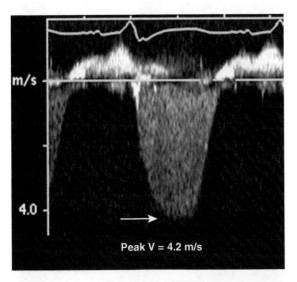

Peak V = 4.2 m/s

Figure 6-20. Continuous wave Doppler velocity signal of the mitral regurgitant jet that must be clear and continuous so that it can be carefully digitized to obtain an accurate mitral regurgitant VTI.

KEY POINTS

- It is important to reduce the aliasing velocity to between 30 and 40 cm/s by shifting the baseline because this enhances the aliasing signal.
- The angle between the insonating Doppler beam and the direction of blood flow must be as close to 0 degrees as possible in the apical 4-chamber and the apical 2-chamber imaging planes.
- The MV plane must be identified unequivocally because the radius to be measured is from the MV plane to the first aliasing isovelocity surface area.

- The accuracy of PISA is compromised when the flow field is incomplete or hemi-ellipsoidal rather than hemispherical.
- PISA measures instantaneous flow rate and has to be integrated over time to obtain volume flow.
- The continuous wave Doppler velocity signal must be of the highest quality so it can be confidently traced throughout systole to obtain the mitral regurgitant VTI (Figure 6-20).
- The ROA can be estimated by dividing the PISA instantaneous volume flow by the peak MV regurgitant jet velocity.

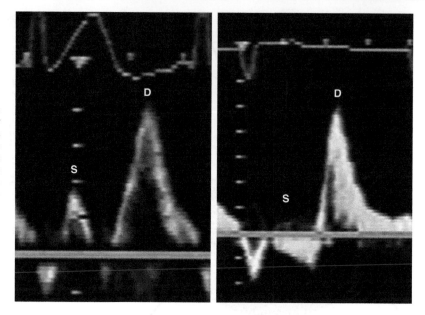

Figure 6-21. Marked attenuation of the systolic blood flow velocity signal (s) in the pulmonary veins (*left panel*) caused by moderate MR as compared with diastolic blood flow velocity (d). There is reversal of systolic blood flow in the pulmonary vein (*right panel*) consistent with severe MR.

Flow Reversal

Basic Principles

- Blunting or reversal of the blood flow velocity in the pulmonary veins during systole is a qualitative means of assessing the severity of MR. The flow velocity signal shows either systolic blunting or reversal of flow (Figure 6-21).

KEY POINTS
- Small MR jets are occasionally directed into the lumen of one pulmonary vein, resulting in the classic systolic reversal of flow, while flow in the remaining pulmonary veins is normal. Thus, the severity of MR necessitates surveillance of two or more pulmonary vein flow velocity signals. - Detection of reversed flow is best achieved with low wall filtering, reduced gain to minimize channel cross-talk, and the scale adjusted for the appropriate range of velocities.

Pericardial Effusion

Basic Principles

- Pericardial effusions occasionally complicate acute HF (Figure 6-22), usually resulting from an ST-segment elevation MI (STEMI), and in so doing may compromise the already unfavorable and unstable hemodynamics.
- Pericardial tamponade rarely intervenes in acute HF, and only occasionally does the

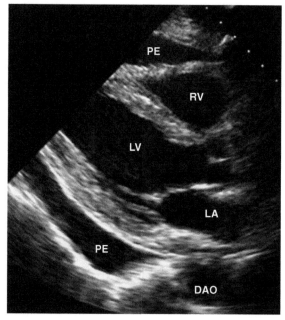

Figure 6-22. There is a modest circumferential pericardial effusion (PE) seen in the left parasternal LV long-axis view anteriorly and posteriorly in a patient with an acute STEMI. Note that the anteroseptal LV wall has not yet thinned out. It is important to determine whether intra-pericardial pressure is elevated and whether there is tamponade.

increased pericardial pressure necessitate percutaneous pericardiocentesis.
- Patients with cardiac rupture and rapid onset of tamponade, whether in the hospital or in the field, do not survive unless there is "contained rupture" due to prior fusion of the parietal and visceral pericardium from pericarditis.

- Contained rupture—also known as LV pseudo-aneurysm—is uncommon, usually arising from the inferobasal LV wall (Figure 6-23).
- Pseudo-aneurysm can be differentiated from true LV aneurysm by echocardiography by the relatively narrow neck that represents the rupture site via which blood gains access to the pericardial space (see Figure 6-23). Blood flow into the pericardium can usually be demonstrated by color flow Doppler velocity mapping.
- By contrast, a true ventricular aneurysm has a wide neck, and there is no breach of the LV wall (Figure 6-24). There is either akinesis or dyskinesis with wall thinning that appears highly echo-reflective because of the formation of a fibrous scar post–MI repair.

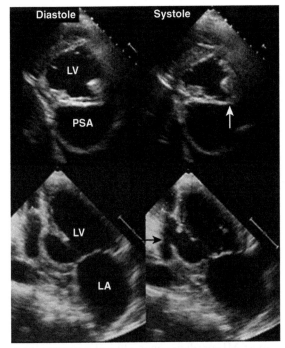

Figure 6-23. *Upper panels:* An old inferior MI with scarring and fibrous replacement of the inferior LV wall, behind which is a fluid collection due to a pseudo-aneurysm. *Lower panels,* A scarred posteroinferior LV wall including the papillary muscle (*lower left panel*) and a fluid collection subjacent to the inferior MI. In the *lower right panel,* a pseudo-aneurysm (contained myocardial rupture) is seen that has a narrow neck and communicates with the pericardial space (*black arrow*).

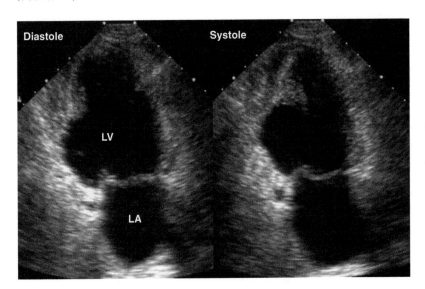

Figure 6-24. In contrast with a pseudo-aneurysm, a true aneurysm seen here in the proximal inferior wall has a wide neck shown in diastole (*left panel*) and in systole (*right panel*) that does not involve myocardial rupture.

RV Infarction

Basic Principles

- HF due to RV infarction may occur from right coronary artery occlusion as an isolated RV event or, more commonly, in association with inferior or inferoposterior LV infarction.
- Recognition of RV infarction is important because the treatment of MI involving the LV presenting with HF is aimed at reducing intravascular volume. Appropriate volume repletion is the optimal treatment strategy in RV infarction. Intravenous diuretics following RV infarction may induce severe hypotension and shock.

KEY POINTS

- RV infarction can be diagnosed unequivocally by echocardiography as new RV RWMAs involving the RV free wall, RV dilatation, and severe global contractile dysfunction (Figure 6-25) usually measured as percent change in cavity area (*A*) from diastole (DA) to systole (SA) because there is no accepted algorithm for computing RV volumes:

$$\%\Delta A = (DA - SA)/DA \times 100\%$$

- RV longitudinal shortening results in reduction in tricuspid annular plane systolic excursion (TAPSE) that is often accompanied by abnormal septal motion.
- There is a wide spectrum of severity of tricuspid regurgitation with reversal of flow in the dilated middle hepatic veins and the similarly dilated inferior vena cava.
- On occasion in pure RV infarcts, there is a discrepancy between good LV function compared with the severe RV dysfunction, but RV MI must be distinguished from acute major pulmonary embolism.

Chronic Heart Failure

Basic Principles

- Chronic HF resulting from CAD can be caused by a discrete clinically recognized acute MI or, less commonly, be the cumulative effect of recurrent episodes of myocardial ischemia associated with recurrent minor myocardial damage that remains clinically unrecognized.
- LV dilatation may be global or regional, resulting in ischemic dilated cardiomyopathy (Figure 6-26) or discrete LV aneurysm formation, respectively (Figure 6-27). LV aneurysms are most common in the antero-apical region from occlusion of the proximal to mid-LAD (see Figure 6-26). Inferior LV aneurysms are less common and result from occlusion of either the right coronary artery or a dominant left circumflex coronary artery (Figure 6-28). Aneurysms must be carefully examined by 2D or 3D echocardiography for retained thrombus as described above.
- LV remodeling results in asymmetric mural hypertrophy induced by regional disparities in stress distribution.
- As the LV enlarges, it assumes an abnormal shape, transitioning from an ellipsoidal to a spherical shape that can be quantified echocardiographically as the LV short- and long-axis ratio (see Figure 6-14). Distortion of LV shape post-MI predicts poor clinical outcome over and above that of LV size.
- The LV dilatation and distortion also disrupts the MV apparatus and annular geometry, causing MR. It is important to ascertain the severity of MR and determine whether MV repair can be achieved safely in HF patients with already compromised LV function.

Figure 6-25. This apical 4-chamber view of a patient who sustained an isolated RV MI shows a dilated right ventricle with almost no change in cavity size from diastole (*left panel*) to systole (*right panel*), denoting severe contractile dysfunction with akinesis of the free wall. The right atrium is moderately enlarged because the RV is dilated and the tricuspid valve leaflets fail to coapt, resulting in important tricuspid regurgitation.

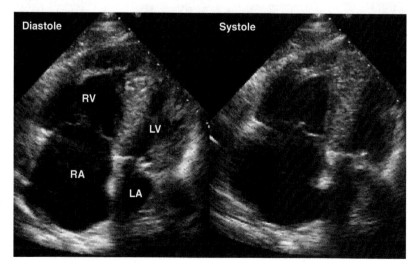

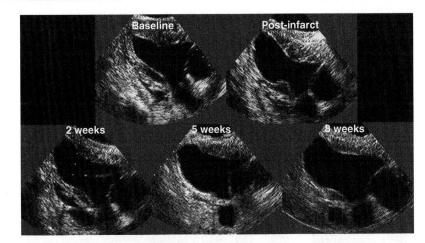

Figure 6-26. Antero-apical MI in an ovine model following ligation of the mid-LAD resulting in progressive LV dilatation and distortion of LV cavity shape that are both associated with a poor prognosis.

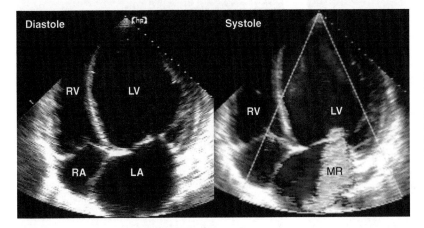

Figure 6-27. Severely dilated LV with little change in size from diastole (*left panel*) to systole (*right panel*) with at least moderate MR and bowing of the interatrial septum to the right because of increased LA pressure.

Assessment of MR in chronic HF is the same as in acute HF as described above.
- Chronic HF that develops post-MI begins the process known as LV remodeling, which may continue for months to several years. LV remodeling has been fully characterized by Doppler echocardiography as a progressive increase in LV volume with a decrease in the LV mass/volume ratio because LV hypertrophy can no longer normalize wall stress. Increased wall stress stretch-activates a portfolio of neurohormones and local tropic factors that further drive the remodeling process to ischemic dilated cardiomyopathy and terminal HF (see Figure 6-26).
- Simultaneous with the structural and functional remodeling, there is the development of prolongation of the QRS duration in 35% to 50% of HF patients that is associated with inter- and intraventricular dyssynchrony. Doppler echocardiography can readily detect LV dyssynchrony, its impact on LV architecture and function, and MR and its reversal with cardiac resynchronization therapy.

KEY POINTS

- Myocardial velocities by TDI in the normal heart vary in magnitude from the LV apex to the base of the heart, and this consistent gradient is maintained. However, the time to peak velocity during LV ejection in the normal heart is similar from all regions of the myocardium, demonstrating the exquisite temporal coordination during contraction. This temporal coordination is typically lost and the magnitudes of the peak velocities are lower and vary by myocardial region, being lowest in areas of infarction, in HF of ischemic etiology. In ischemic HF, some regions attain peak myocardial velocities early while other regions peak late (see Figure 6-6). If the difference between the time to peak for two opposing LV walls is greater than 65 ms, dyssynchrony is present.
- Measuring a time interval between peak septal excursion and peak posterior LV wall excursion

Continued

KEY POINTS—cont'd

by M-mode echocardiography in HF patients of greater than 135 ms is consistent with dyssynchrony.
- It is important to ensure that the sample volumes track the myocardium throughout the cardiac cycle, because tracking from within the cavity or from outside the epicardium results in spuriously low myocardial velocities.
- Speckle tracking enables fiducial tracking of the myocardium so that regional displacement and regional strain can be measured accurately.

- The time to peak displacement (Figure 6-29) and time to peak strain (Figure 6-30) can be compared by region, which in the normal heart is closely coordinated in time. By contrast, in ischemic HF some regions attain peak values early while in some regions the peak velocities are considerably delayed c/w dyssynchrony.
- LV dyssynchrony is associated with an incrementally worse prognosis after adjustment for LV size and function.

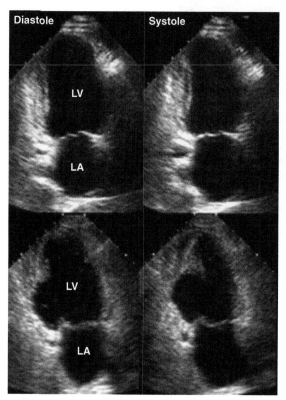

Figure 6-28. Examples of an antero-apical LV aneurysm (*upper panels*) and an inferior basal LV aneurysm (*lower panels*).

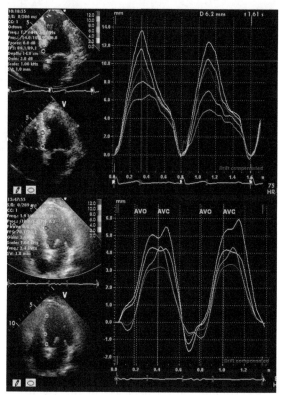

Figure 6-29. *Upper panels:* A normal subject with multiple sample volumes located in the septum (*upper left panel*) showing displacement tracings that peak almost simultaneously (*upper right panel*), which characterizes synchronized contraction and the range of normal values. *Lower panels:* By contrast, in the patient with ischemic heart failure, the magnitude of displacement is markedly decreased (*lower left panel*) and, in addition, the time to peak displacement occurs over a wider range than normal (*lower right panel*), consistent with LV dyssynchrony.

Treatment of Ischemic HF

Basic Principles

Doppler echocardiography provides an array of easily quantifiable metrics that facilitate diagnosis and assessment of the severity of changes during LV structural and functional remodeling in HF patients. These same metrics are equally important for assessing the impact of a number of therapeutic strategies during reverse remodeling.

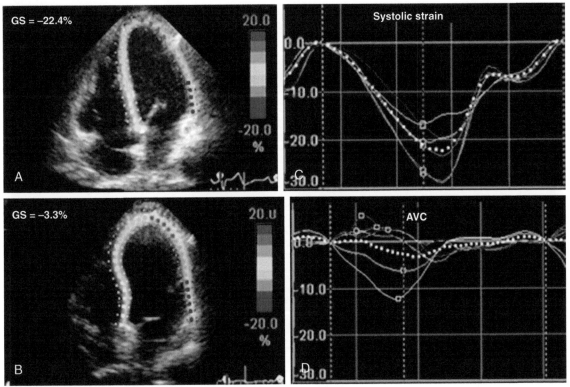

Figure 6-30. Graphic display of systolic strain in a normal subject (*top panels*) and a patient with an antero-apical LV aneurysm (*bottom panels*). Global and regional myocardial strain are both severely reduced in the patient with CAD compared to normal, and the normal exquisite synchrony of the time to peak strain is lost, which typifies patients with heart failure due to ischemic heart disease.

Suggested Readings

1. Otto CM. *The Practice of Clinical Echocardiography*. 3rd ed. Philadelphia: Saunders Elsevier; 2007.
   This is a very comprehensive textbook that provides additional information on the diagnosis and investigation of various causes of right and left HF.
2. Oh JK, Seward JB, Tajik AJ. *The Echo Manual*. Philadelphia: Lippincott Williams & Wilkins, 2005.
   This text provides an excellent source of basic clinical and technologic echocardiology.
3. Grigioni F, Enriquez-Sarano M, Zehr KJ, et al. Ischemic mitral regurgitation: Long-term outcome and prognostic implications with quantitative Doppler assessment. *Circulation*. 2001;103:1759-1764.
   The authors demonstrate that the degree of ischemic MR, defined as effective ROA or RV, is a predictor of mortality independent of the degree of LV systolic function in the postinfarction setting.
4. Lang RM, Bierig M, Devereux RB, et al. Recommendations for chamber quantification: A report from the American Society of Echocardiography's Guidelines and Standards Committee and the Chamber Quantification Writing Group, developed in conjunction with the European Association of Echocardiography, a branch of the European Society of Cardiology. *J Am Soc Echocardiogr*. 2005;18:1440-1463.
   This paper provides the American Society of Echocardiography's recommendations for the standardization of quantitation of LV size, function, and mass and also for RV and LA measurements.

5. Bansal M, Cho G-Y, Chan J, et al. Feasibility and accuracy of different techniques of two-dimensional speckle based strain and validation with harmonic phase magnetic resonance imaging. *J Am Soc Echocardiogr*. 2008;21: 1318-1325.
   This article compares speckle-based strain to velocity vector imaging in 30 patients with known or suspected ischemic heart disease.
6. Kahlert P, Plicht B, Schenk IM, et al. Direct assessment of size and shape of non-circular vena contracta area in functional versus organic mitral regurgitation using three-dimensional echocardiography. *J Am Soc Echocardiogr*. 2008; 21:912-921.
   3D echocardiography was used to directly measure the VC area in 57 patients with MR from different etiologies. The asymmetrical shape of the VC in patients with functional MR resulted in poor estimations of the effective ROA by 2D echocardiography in this group.
7. St. John Sutton M. A comprehensive non-invasive assessment of systolic function heart failure with echocardiography. *Circ Heart Failure*. 2010;3:337-339.
   This editorial suggests using a panel of echocardiographic investigations for risk stratification of patients with acute and chronic systolic HF.
8. Caereji S, La Carrubba S, Canterin FA, et al. The incremental prognostic value of asymptomatic Stage A heart failure. *J Am Soc Echocardiogr*. 2010;23:1025-1034.
   This study demonstrated that pre-clinical functional or structural myocardial abnormalities could be detected by echocardiography in asymptomatic subjects with two or more

cardiovascular risk factors and without electrocardiogram abnormalities (stage A of HF). The presence or absence of LV systolic dysfunction or LV diastolic dysfunction, as demonstrated by echocardiography, has an incremental value to cardiovascular risk factors in predicting more severe HF stage C and the occurrence of cardiovascular events.

9. St. John Sutton M, Pfeffer MA, Plappert T, et al. Quantitative two dimensional echocardiographic measurements are major predictors of adverse cardiovascular events following acute myocardial infarction: The protective effects of captopril. *Circulation.* 1994;89:68-75.
This study describes post-MI LV remodeling using quantitative echocardiography in a double-blind randomized clinical trial of an angiotensin-converting enzyme inhibitor (SAVE Trial) and the impact of a number of echocardiographic parameters on clinical outcome beyond 1 year.

Hypertrophic Cardiomyopathy

Sean Jedrzkiewicz and Anna Woo

7

Background

- Hypertrophic cardiomyopathy (HCM) is defined as the presence of left ventricular hypertrophy occurring in the absence of a cardiac or systemic disorder (e.g., valvular aortic stenosis or systemic hypertension).[1]
- HCM is a genetic disease caused by a mutation of one of the cardiac sarcomeric proteins.
- This condition has an autosomal dominant pattern of inheritance.
- Initially regarded as a rare disorder, the prevalence of HCM in the general population is now estimated to be approximately 1 in 500.
- HCM is a heterogeneous disorder with a spectrum of clinical findings, ranging from completely asymptomatic individuals to severely affected patients.
- Clinical manifestations of HCM include dyspnea, chest pain, presyncope, and/or syncope.
- HCM may occasionally present as sudden cardiac death.
- The symptoms of HCM are largely attributable to diastolic filling abnormalities, dynamic left ventricular outflow tract (LVOT) obstruction, atrial or ventricular arrhythmias, and/or myocardial ischemia.
- Individuals with HCM are most commonly identified by echocardiography.
- Echocardiography is the modality of choice for the diagnosis, screening, and serial monitoring of patients with known or suspected HCM.

Overview of Echocardiographic Approach

- Echocardiography plays a vital role in the evaluation and management of patients with HCM (Box 7-1).
- Multiple echocardiographic techniques are used to assess patients with HCM:
  - M-mode echocardiography
  - Two-dimensional (2D) echocardiography
  - Color Doppler imaging
  - Pulsed and continuous wave Doppler
  - Tissue Doppler imaging
  - Strain imaging

Step-by-Step Approach to the Evaluation of HCM

Step 1: Establish the Diagnosis of HCM

KEY POINTS

- The traditional echocardiographic criteria for the diagnosis of HCM are the presence of the following[1]:
  - Wall thickness ≥ 15 mm (any myocardial segment)
  - Asymmetrical septal hypertrophy (defined as septal/posterior [inferior] wall thickness ratio > 1.3)
- In addition, the diagnosis of HCM requires the exclusion of cardiac or systemic conditions that could explain the degree of increased wall thickness detected (see Step 2 below).

Step 2: Exclude Other Causes of Increased Wall Thickness

- The presence of increased left ventricular wall thickness is not pathognomonic of HCM.[2]
- Left ventricular hypertrophy caused by a genetic defect of the cardiac sarcomeric proteins needs to be distinguished from other important causes (Box 7-2).

KEY POINTS

- The main categories in the differential diagnosis of left ventricular increased wall thickness are the following:
  - Nongenetic causes of left ventricular hypertrophy
  - Disproportionate hypertrophy of ventricular septum

Continued

KEY POINTS—cont'd

- Congenital syndromes associated with HCM
- Storage diseases/metabolic disorders
- Infiltrative cardiomyopathies
- Common causes of left ventricular hypertrophy are systemic hypertension and other conditions causing pressure-overload hypertrophy, such as valvular aortic stenosis, fibrous subaortic stenosis, and coarctation of the aorta.
- These non-monogenetic forms of left ventricular hypertrophy typically have a concentric (rather than asymmetrical) pattern of hypertrophy.
- However, they may be associated with a degree of focal septal hypertrophy (especially in the elderly) and/or the presence of systolic anterior motion (SAM) (see Step 4 below).
- Causes of disproportionate hypertrophy of the ventricular septum may occur with right ventricular hypertrophy and also with D-transposition of the great arteries.

BOX 7-1 Summary of Role of Echocardiography in Evaluation of Patients with HCM

- Diagnosis
  - Evaluation of probands
  - Screening of family members
- Left ventricular hypertrophy
  - Degree of hypertrophy
  - Extent and pattern of hypertrophy
- LVOT obstruction
- Mitral regurgitation
  - Presence of SAM
  - Independent mitral valve disease
- Left ventricular diastolic function
- Left ventricular systolic function
- Left atrial size
- Selection of septal reduction therapy
- Intraprocedural monitoring during septal reduction therapy
- Prognostication

Athlete's Heart[3]

- Wall thickness may be ≥ 13 mm (up to 15 to 16 mm) in 2% of elite athletes, raising the possibility of underlying mild HCM.
- Differentiation between athlete's heart and HCM may be difficult.

KEY POINTS

- The diagnosis of HCM is favored over the diagnosis of athlete's heart in the presence of the following:
  - Family history of HCM
  - Bizarre electrocardiographic patterns
  - Asymmetrical (or other unusual) pattern of left ventricular hypertrophy
  - Small left ventricular cavity size (<45 mm)
  - Left atrial enlargement
  - Abnormal left ventricular filling pattern
- Findings suggestive of athlete's heart (rather than HCM) include the following:
  - Left ventricular end-diastolic dimension >55 mm
  - Regression of hypertrophy with deconditioning
  - Maximum VO₂ greater than 45 mL/kg/min (or >110% predicted) on cardiopulmonary testing

BOX 7-2 Differential Diagnosis of HCM on Echocardiography

Other Causes of Left Ventricular Hypertrophy
- Athlete's heart
- Systemic hypertension
- Aortic valve stenosis
- Fibrous subaortic stenosis
- Supravalvular stenosis

Disproportionate Ventricular Septal Hypertrophy
- Right ventricular hypertrophy
- D-transposition of the great arteries

Syndromic HCM
- Noonan's syndrome
- LEOPARD syndrome
- Friedreich's ataxia

Storage Diseases
- Fabry's disease
- Glycogen storage disease (PRKAG2 cardiomyopathy, Danon's disease, Pompe's disease)
- Mucopolysaccharide storage disorders

Infiltrative Cardiomyopathy
- Amyloidosis
- Sarcoidosis

Storage Diseases[4]

- The intramyocardial accumulation or infiltration of abnormal metabolic products in various storage diseases may mimic HCM on echocardiography (Figure 7-1).
- Fabry's disease is an X-linked recessive disorder of glycosphingolipid metabolism due to a deficiency of the lysosomal enzyme α-galactosidase A.
- Patients with Fabry's disease may have multisystem involvement, especially of the skin, kidneys, nervous system, and heart.
- A cardiac-specific variant of Fabry's has been identified.
- Diagnosis of Fabry's is made with the measurement of α-galactosidase levels.

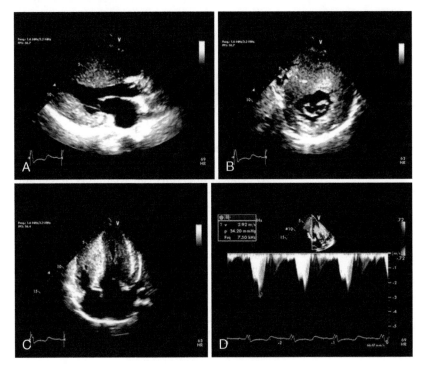

Figure 7-1. Parasternal long-axis (**A**) and apical 4-chamber (**C**) views reveal impressive hypertrophy in an 18-year-old female patient. There is asymmetrical septal hypertrophy with extension to almost all left ventricular segments and right ventricular involvement. **B,** The wall segments measured the following: basal anteroseptum = 27 mm, mid-anteroseptum = 31 mm, basal anterior wall = 24 mm, and basal anterolateral wall = 21 mm. There was no SAM. **C,** Left ventricular cavity obliteration in systole with midventricular obstruction (**D**) noted at rest. The patient had an underlying diagnosis of glycogen storage disease type III.

- Genetic testing for the causative gene in Fabry's, the α-galactosidase (*GLA*) gene, is also available.
- The detection of patients with Fabry's disease is important since enzyme replacement therapy is available for the treatment of this condition.
- Mutations of genes regulating glycogen metabolism may also result in increased wall thickness on echocardiography.
  - Mutations of the regulatory γ2 subunit of AMP-activated protein kinase (*PRKAG2*) gene cause a glycogen storage cardiomyopathy, which may be associated with ventricular preexcitation.
- Mutations of the lysosome-associated membrane protein 2 (*LAMP2*) gene (X-linked) cause Danon's disease.
- Danon's disease is a lysosomal glycogen storage disease characterized clinically by cardiomyopathy, electrophysiologic abnormalities, myopathy, and variable mental impairment.
- Mutations of the acid α-1,4-glucosidase gene cause Pompe's disease, a glycogen storage disease.

KEY POINTS

- The prevalence of Fabry's disease has ranged from 3% in all male patients with left ventricular hypertrophy to as much as 6% in male patients with presumed late-onset HCM (defined as diagnosis at age ≥ 40 years).
- In a cohort of 24 patients with increased wall thickness and ventricular preexcitation, mutations of the *PRKAG2* and *LAMP2* genes were detected in 29% and 17% of patients, respectively.
- Clinical features distinguishing patients with *LAMP2* mutations from patients with HCM caused by sarcomeric gene mutations included the following: male sex, early onset of disease (<17 years of age), ventricular preexcitation on electrocardiography, severe concentric hypertrophy, and elevation of two serum enzymes: creatine kinase (CK) and alanine aminotransferase (ALT).
- These storage diseases typically have a concentric pattern of left ventricular wall thickening.
- However, they occasionally manifest as disproportionate septal thickening and may have associated LVOT or intracavitary obstruction.

Infiltrative Cardiomyopathies
- Conditions such as cardiac amyloidosis or sarcoidosis are associated with increased wall thickness and may occasionally mimic HCM on echocardiography.
- In general, the infiltrative cardiomyopathies usually have the following distinguishing features compared with HCM:
  - Electrocardiographic pattern of diffuse low voltages (in cardiac amyloidosis)
  - A concentric pattern of increased wall thickness
  - SAM or LVOT obstruction is typically absent
  - Restrictive filling pattern
- See Chapter 3 on "Infiltrative/Restrictive Cardiomyopathies" for further details.

Septal Hypertrophy in the Elderly
- It may be difficult to distinguish between elderly patients with HCM and those with hypertensive heart disease.
- Elderly subjects may develop a sigmoid-shaped septum as an age-related phenomenon.
- Terms that have been used to describe this finding are "sigmoid septum," "septal bulge," and "discrete upper septal hypertrophy."
- It is controversial whether this finding should be considered a subtype of HCM or whether it represents a benign anatomic variant.
- Findings on echocardiography that are more compatible with a septal bulge rather than HCM include the following:

- Focal hypertrophy limited to less than 3 cm of the length of the basal anterior septum
- Protrusion of the focal hypertrophy into the LVOT
- A normal left ventricular end-diastolic diameter
- Absence of other characteristic echocardiographic findings of HCM

Step 3: Assess Pattern and Severity of Left Ventricular Hypertrophy
- 2D echocardiography can accurately detect and characterize the degree and extent of hypertrophy in patients with HCM.

KEY POINTS
- Asymmetrical septal hypertrophy (septal/posterior [inferior] wall thickness ratio > 1.3) is the classic echocardiographic pattern detected in patients with HCM.
- The predominant site of hypertrophy is the interventricular septum (usually the anterior portion of the septum), which occurs in greater than 90% of cases.

Anatomic Imaging
Acquisition
- Multiple transthoracic echocardiographic (TTE) views are necessary to assess the extent and severity of left ventricular hypertrophy (Figure 7-2).
  - Parasternal long-axis view

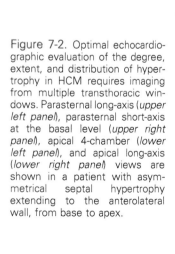
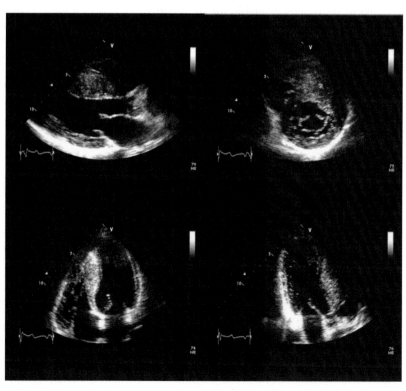

Figure 7-2. Optimal echocardiographic evaluation of the degree, extent, and distribution of hypertrophy in HCM requires imaging from multiple transthoracic windows. Parasternal long-axis (*upper left panel*), parasternal short-axis at the basal level (*upper right panel*), apical 4-chamber (*lower left panel*), and apical long-axis (*lower right panel*) views are shown in a patient with asymmetrical septal hypertrophy extending to the anterolateral wall, from base to apex.

- Parasternal short-axis views at three levels (base, midventricle, apex)
- Apical four-chamber view
- Apical long-axis view
- Measurements of cavity dimensions should be made in the parasternal long-axis view.[5]
- Measurements of the left ventricular wall segments (anteroseptal, inferoseptal, anterior, anterolateral, inferolateral, inferior) should be made in the parasternal short-axis views at the basal and midventricular levels.
- The apical septal, anterior, lateral, and inferior segments should be measured in the parasternal short-axis views at the apical level.
- Hypertrophied segments usually have either similar or slightly increased echogenicity in comparison with myocardial segments with normal wall thickness.
- In addition, diffuse bright echoes may be seen throughout the myocardium and may give a ground-glass appearance.

Analysis
- Septal involvement may be limited to the basal level or the hypertrophy may extend to the left ventricular apex.

KEY POINTS

- Two different septal morphologic subtypes have been described:
  - "Reverse septal curvature"—the maximal thickness of the septum occurs at the midventricular level, predominant midseptal convexity toward the left ventricular cavity, with the cavity itself having an overall crescent shape (Figure 7-3A)
  - "Basal septal morphologic subtype"—basal septal bulge, generally ovoid left ventricular cavity with the septum being concave toward the left ventricular cavity
- Young patients with HCM characteristically demonstrate the reverse septal curvature subtype, whereas older patients typically have the basal septal morphologic subtype.

- Patients with HCM and asymmetrical septal hypertrophy may have hypertrophy confined to the septum, or they commonly have hypertrophy of both the ventricular septum and the free wall (anterolateral wall segments).
- The distribution of hypertrophy can be in any pattern and can involve any myocardial segment (including the right ventricle).
- Other uncommon morphologic variants of HCM include asymmetrical apical HCM (predominant hypertrophy at the apical segments) and a concentric pattern of left ventricular hypertrophy.
- An ultrasound contrast agent should be administered when nonenhanced images are suboptimal for definitive diagnosis, such as in patients with suspected apical HCM.[6]

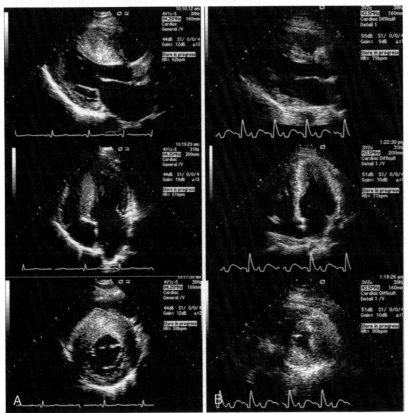

Figure 7-3. Spectrum and variation of HCM in two patients with this condition on 2D echocardiographic parasternal long-axis (*top row*), apical 4-chamber (*middle row*), and parasternal short-axis (*bottom row*) views. **A,** The patient had a typical pattern of asymmetrical septal hypertrophy (with maximal hypertrophy at the midventricular level). **B,** The patient had asymmetrical apical HCM.

Severity of Left Ventricular Hypertrophy

- Since there is considerable variability in the thickness of the different septal and posterior wall segments in patients with HCM, the conventional calculations of left ventricular mass are not applicable in these patients.[5]
- Therefore, a number of echocardiographic indices have been developed to measure the distribution, extent, and/or burden of left ventricular hypertrophy.[7]
  - **Wigle's score:** Incorporates the degree of septal thickness at the basal anteroseptum, the extent of septal involvement, and the presence or absence of anterolateral wall involvement (Table 7-1).
  - **Wall thickness (Spirito-Maron) index:** Obtained by adding the maximal wall thickness (at either the basal or midventricular level) of four left ventricular regions (anterior septum, posterior septum, lateral wall, and posterior wall).
  - **Maximal left ventricular wall thickness:** The most clinically relevant measurement is the determination of the maximal thickness of all the left ventricular myocardial segments. The presence of massive left ventricular hypertrophy, defined as a wall thickness of ≥ 30 mm, has considerable implications for patients' management and prognosis (see "Key Measurements for Predicting Prognosis in Patients with HCM" below).[1]

Other Morphologic Subtypes of HCM
Apical HCM
- This subtype of HCM was originally described in Japan in the 1970s (Figure 7-3B).
- The apical variant occurs in less than 10% of all patients with HCM.

TABLE 7-1 EXTENT OF HYPERTROPHY ACCORDING TO ECHOCARDIOGRAPHIC POINT SCORE

Extent of Hypertrophy	Points
Septal thickness, mm (basal third of septum)	
15–19	1
20–24	2
25–29	3
>30	4
Extension to papillary muscles (basal two thirds of septum)	2
Extension to apex (total septal involvement)	2
Anterolateral wall extension	2
Maximum total	10

- Prominent findings of patients with apical HCM include the presence of giant negative T waves (≥ 10 mm) in the precordial leads on electrocardiography and an "ace of spades" configuration to the left ventricle seen on imaging studies.
- Echocardiography can also identify potential complications of this condition, such as left atrial enlargement, impaired diastolic filling, apical infarction, or apical aneurysm formation.

HCM with Midventricular Obstruction
- The presence of midventricular obstruction is also an uncommon variant of HCM.
- Morphologic features of this condition include the following:
  - "Hourglass"-shaped left ventricular cavity
  - Midventricular obliteration in systole
  - A distinct apical chamber
  - Color turbulence at the midventricle
  - Systolic pressure gradient at the midventricular level

Pitfalls
- Oblique cuts of the left ventricle can overestimate wall thickness and produce the appearance of asymmetrical septal hypertrophy.
- Apical or lateral wall hypertrophy can be poorly visualized due to foreshortening of the apex, poor transthoracic windows, and other technical limitations.
- Echocardiographic contrast agents can better define wall thickness, especially in patients with suspected apical HCM.

Step 4: Determine if There Is LVOT Obstruction
- LVOT obstruction is an important contributor to symptoms in patients with HCM.[1]
- Studies of cohorts of patients with HCM have shown that approximately 25% of patients have LVOT obstruction at rest.
- One recent study has suggested that 70% of patients with HCM have either resting or provocable LVOT obstruction.
- Early M-mode echocardiographic studies demonstrated the abnormalities in morphology of the LVOT and in the mitral apparatus that contribute to the development of dynamic LVOT obstruction.
- LVOT obstruction is due to SAM of the anterior mitral leaflet (Box 7-3).
- The mitral leaflets in patients with HCM may be elongated.
- These mitral leaflets coapt abnormally in the body of the leaflets, rather than at the tip.
- Rapid early left ventricular ejection out of the LVOT also contributes to the development of SAM and LVOT obstruction.

BOX 7-3 Factors Contributing to Dynamic LVOT Obstruction

Narrowing of LVOT
- Septal hypertrophy
- Anterior displacement of mitral apparatus
- Anterior displacement of papillary muscles

Hydrodynamic Forces (Venturi and Drag Forces) Causing SAM
- Rapid early left ventricular ejection
- Elongated mitral leaflets

- Morphologic features of HCM that contribute to SAM and LVOT obstruction include narrowing of the LVOT by the following:
  - Septal hypertrophy
  - Anterior displacement of the mitral apparatus
  - Anterior malposition of the papillary muscles

KEY POINTS

- Although the nature of the hydrodynamic forces on the anterior mitral leaflet remains controversial, it is believed that the distal anterior mitral leaflet is subjected to Venturi and/or drag forces.[2]
- Therefore, SAM occurs and the tip of the anterior mitral leaflet typically develops a sharp anterior and superior angulation, leading to mitral leaflet–septal contact in early to midsystole (Figure 7-4).
- Simultaneous cardiac catheterization and M-mode echocardiographic studies have shown that mitral leaflet–septal contact occurs almost simultaneously with the onset of the LVOT pressure gradient.
- Furthermore, there is a linear relationship between the time of onset of SAM and the severity of LVOT obstruction.
- SAM of the anterior leaflet leads to an interleaflet gap, which results in a posteriorly directed jet of mitral regurgitation (see Step 5 below).

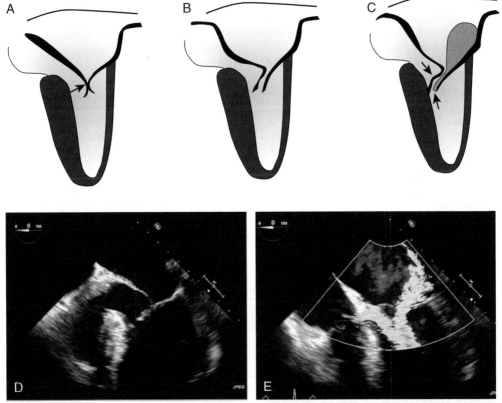

Figure 7-4. **A–C,** Schematic diagram of a transesophageal echocardiogram (TEE) in the frontal long-axis plane demonstrates the anterior and basal motion of the anterior mitral leaflet leading to leaflet-septal contact and failure of leaflet coaptation in midsystole. At the onset of systole (**A**), the coaptation point (*arrow*) is in the body of the mitral leaflets. During early systole (**B**) and midsystole (**C**), there is anterior and basal movement of the residual length of the anterior mitral leaflet (*upper arrow*) with septal contact and failure of leaflet coaptation (*lower arrow*). The interleaflet gap (*lower arrow*) results in a posteriorly directed jet of mitral regurgitation into the left atrial cavity (*shaded area*). **D** and **E,** Corresponding 2D TEE views with color flow imaging in a patient with obstructive HCM show septal hypertrophy, anterior motion of the anterior mitral leaflet, and color turbulence in the outflow tract with the posteriorly directed mitral regurgitation. (*A–C Reprinted with permission from Grigg LE, Wigle ED, Williams WG, et al. Transesophageal Doppler echocardiography is obstructive hypertrophic cardiomyopathy: clarification of pathophysiology and importance in intraoperative decision making. J Am Coll Cardiol. 1992;20:42-52.*)

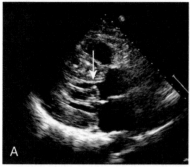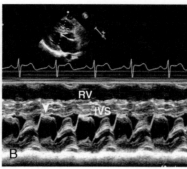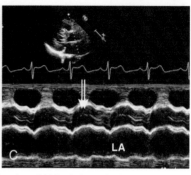

Figure 7-5. **A,** Parasternal long-axis view in a patient with obstructive HCM, showing SAM of the mitral valve (*arrow*). **B,** M-mode echocardiographic recording at the level of the mitral leaflet tips demonstrates increased septal thickness, prolonged contact of the anterior mitral leaflet with the septum during systole, and severe SAM (*arrowhead*). **C,** M-mode recording at the aortic valve showing systolic notching of the aortic valve cusps (*double arrow*). IVS, interventricular septum; LA, left atrium; RV, right ventricle.

Step 4A: Assess for the Presence of LVOT Obstruction at Rest

Anatomic Imaging
- Determine if there is SAM at rest (optimal views are parasternal long-axis view or apical views) (Figure 7-5).
- The severity of SAM can be classified into the following three categories:
  - **Mild:** SAM septal distance greater than 10 mm
  - **Moderate:** SAM septal distance less than 10 mm or brief mitral leaflet–septal contact
  - **Severe:** Prolonged SAM septal contact, lasting more than 30% of echocardiographic systole
- SAM may infrequently also involve the posterior mitral leaflet.
- **Three-dimensional echocardiography** has provided some additional insight regarding the mechanism of SAM.[8]
- Three-dimensional echocardiography has been used to assess the LVOT area following invasive septal reduction therapy.

Physiologic Data
Acquisition
- Pulsed wave and continuous wave Doppler techniques are used to determine the pressure gradient across the LVOT in patients with HCM.
- Pulsed wave Doppler signals can be recorded sequentially from the left ventricular apex toward the outflow tract.
- Peak velocity increases as the sample volume approaches the site of contact between the anterior mitral leaflet and the septum.
- Continuous wave Doppler assessment from an apical window with the beam directed

across the LVOT can be used to determine the peak velocity (V) at the site of obstruction.
- Color flow imaging can be used to determine the level of obstruction, either in the LVOT or in the midventricle.

Analysis

KEY POINTS

- The peak gradient (ΔP) in the outflow tract can be estimated using the modified Bernoulli equation:

$$\Delta P = 4V^2$$

  where V is peak velocity in the LVOT.
- By convention, patients with HCM are considered to have resting LVOT obstruction when the LVOT gradient measures **≥ 30 mm Hg.**
- The characteristic continuous wave Doppler spectral profile of dynamic LVOT obstruction has an asymmetrical leftward concave shape (Figure 7-6).
- This results from a relative rapid initial rise in velocity followed by a more gradual increase in the outflow tract velocity to cause a peak in late systole, leading to a dagger-shaped configuration.
- There is an excellent correlation between the LVOT gradient determined by continuous wave Doppler measurements and by high-fidelity micromanometer recordings during cardiac catheterization.

Pitfalls
- There are important technical considerations in the performance and interpretation of Doppler studies in patients with HCM.

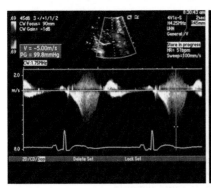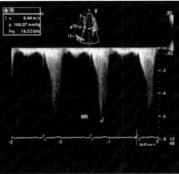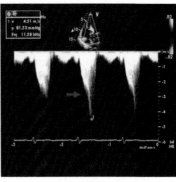

Figure 7-6. Continuous wave Doppler signals from the LVOT at the site of obstruction (*left panel*) in a patient with obstructive HCM. Obstructive outflow tract jet starts after the QRS wave and has characteristic change in acceleration velocity (resulting in a dagger-shaped configuration). Conversely, the jet of mitral regurgitation seen in a different patient (*middle panel*) is typically of higher velocity and starts earlier in systole. One must avoid contamination of the LVOT jet (*red arrow*) with mitral regurgitation (*right panel*).

- It is not always possible to obtain a clear spectral display from the LVOT in these patients.
- Suboptimal continuous wave Doppler signals from the LVOT may be secondary to inadequate transthoracic echocardiographic windows or distortion of left ventricular geometry.
- Importantly, it is crucial to distinguish the high-velocity systolic signal coming from the outflow tract from the signal of the mitral regurgitant jet (see Figure 7-6).
- The spectral profile of mitral regurgitation has an earlier onset, a more abrupt initial increase in velocity, and a higher peak velocity than that of an outflow tract signal.
- Systolic jets with a peak velocity of greater than 5.5 m/s (i.e., LVOT gradient > 120 mm Hg) most likely represent mitral regurgitation.
- Orienting the transducer more medially and anteriorly away from the mitral regurgitant jet can help avoid contamination from the mitral regurgitant jet.
- This pitfall is more common in patients with intrinsic mitral valve disease and a more centrally directed jet of mitral regurgitation (as opposed to the posteriorly directed jet of SAM-related mitral regurgitation).
- Despite consideration of the differences in the timing and contour of these systolic jets, the distinction between the LVOT and mitral regurgitant signals may still occasionally be difficult.

Step 4B: In Patients without Resting LVOT Obstruction, Determine if There Is Provocable LVOT Obstruction

- When there is HCM and a resting LVOT gradient of less than 30 mm Hg, patients should undergo investigations to assess for the presence of provocable LVOT obstruction.
- Determination of the existence of a provocable LVOT gradient is especially important in patients with exertional (or postprandial) symptoms, a history of presyncope or syncope, and/or a dynamic systolic murmur during bedside maneuvers.

KEY POINTS	

- Provocable LVOT obstruction is defined as a resting LVOT gradient of less than 30 mm Hg and a provocable LVOT gradient of ≥ 30 mm Hg.
- Several methods can be used in the echocardiography laboratory to elicit a provocable LVOT gradient in patients with HCM[2]:
  - Valsalva maneuver
  - Inhalation of amyl nitrate
	- Sublingual administration of nitroglycerin
	- Dobutamine infusion
	- Exercise (upright or supine)
	- Some of the advantages and disadvantages of these provocative maneuvers are as follows.
	- **Valsalva maneuver:**
	  - The Valsalva maneuver is the simplest method of eliciting a provocable LVOT gradient.

Continued

KEY POINTS—cont'd

- Assessment of SAM and LVOT gradient (by continuous wave Doppler measurement) is done at rest and then during the strain phase of the Valsalva maneuver.
- Disadvantages of this technique include the fact that some patients cannot perform a Valsalva and the fact that the LVOT Doppler signal may be obscured during the Valsalva maneuver.
- Therefore, Valsalva-induced gradients tend to underestimate the degree of provocable LVOT obstruction when compared with exercise-induced gradients.
- Furthermore, there is not a good correlation between Valsalva- and amyl nitrate–induced LVOT gradients.
- **Dobutamine infusion:**
  - Dobutamine infusion is useful in patients who are unable or unwilling to exercise.
  - The infusion protocol starts with an infusion of 5 µgm/kg/min, increasing to 20 µgm/kg/min.
- **Exercise echocardiography:**
  - Exercise echocardiography is the method of choice since exercise most closely replicates physiologic stress.

- Furthermore, other relevant clinical data, such as the reproducibility of symptoms, exercise duration and capacity, blood pressure response with exercise, and/or oxygen consumption may also be obtained during exercise testing (also see "Additional Testing in Patients with HCM" below for further discussion of exercise testing).
- Upright exercise echocardiography is preferred to supine exercise (using a supine bicycle) since it most resembles upright typical physical activity in most patients.
- In addition, the LVOT gradient obtained by supine exercise may be systematically lower than that obtained with treadmill exercise since the supine position increases venous return and may blunt the magnitude of the exercise-induced LVOT gradient.
- However, the Doppler assessment of exercise-induced LVOT obstruction is generally easier with supine exercise than with upright treadmill testing.
- For discussion of the treatment options for LVOT obstruction, see Step 8.

Step 5: Assess the Mechanism of Mitral Regurgitation

- SAM of the anterior mitral leaflet results in failure of coaptation with the posterior mitral leaflet, creating a funnel-shaped gap through which mitral regurgitation can develop.
- The mitral regurgitant jet is typically posteriorly directed and occurs in mid- to late systole.
- The presence of a nonposterior jet of mitral regurgitation suggests intrinsic disease of the mitral leaflets (or mitral apparatus) independent of SAM.
- Independent mitral valve disease may occur in approximately one fifth of patients with HCM.
- Causes of independent mitral valve disease in this patient population include the following:
  - Mitral valve prolapse
  - Ruptured chordae
  - Mitral annular calcification
  - Anomalous insertion of papillary muscle into anterior mitral leaflet

- Leaflet trauma from repeated anterior mitral leaflet–septal contact
- Infective endocarditis
- In patients referred for surgery, surgical myectomy alone is generally successful in relieving posteriorly directed mitral regurgitation, without the requirement for replacement of the mitral valve with a prosthetic valve.

Step 6: Assess Left Ventricular Diastolic Function

- Diastolic filling of the left ventricle is frequently compromised in HCM and may result in exertional dyspnea, elevated filling pressures, and progressive left atrial enlargement.
- These diastolic filling abnormalities, which are multifactorial in origin, include impairment in left ventricular relaxation and/or worsening left ventricular stiffness.

Step 6A: Measure Diastolic Filling Parameters and Determine E/e′ Ratio

KEY POINTS

- The mitral inflow pattern typically demonstrates a prolonged isovolumic relaxation time (IVRT), reduced early rapid filling (E), a prolonged deceleration time (DT), and increased atrial filling (A) (Figure 7-7).
- Pulmonary venous inflow abnormalities may include systolic blunting, elevation of the

pulmonary venous atrial reversal velocity, and an increased difference in duration between the pulmonary venous and mitral atrial filling velocities (Ar-A).
- However, studies of simultaneous echocardiographic and invasive hemodynamic assessments showed no significant correlation between filling

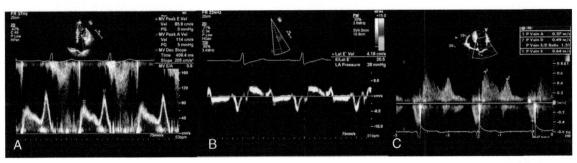

Figure 7-7. Echocardiographic-Doppler evaluation of diastolic function in patients with HCM. **A,** Pulsed wave Doppler recording of E (early diastolic) and A (late diastolic) flow velocities at mitral leaflet tips. **B,** Tissue Doppler imaging from the lateral mitral annulus reveals a reduced early diastolic velocity (e'). **C,** Pulsed wave Doppler recording from the right upper pulmonary vein shows pulmonary venous peak systolic, diastolic, and atrial reversal velocities.

KEY POINTS—cont'd

pressures and various mitral inflow or pulmonary venous flow parameters.
- An integrated approach using a number of diastolic parameters is required in the assessment of diastolic filling in patients with HCM.

- Two echocardiographic techniques, tissue Doppler imaging and color M-mode, are useful for the estimation of left ventricular filling pressures in patients with HCM.

Tissue Doppler Imaging
Acquisition
- Tissue Doppler imaging of mitral annular motion is recorded in the apical 4-chamber view by placing a 5-mm sample volume at the septal and lateral corners of the mitral annulus.
- The early (e') and late (a') diastolic tissue Doppler velocities at the septal and lateral corners of the mitral annulus can be determined.
- All measurements should be made over three cardiac cycles, at end-expiration, using a sweep speed of 50 to 100 mm/s.
Analysis
- The e' velocities at the lateral and septal annulus are lower in patients with HCM (see Figure 7-7).
- A significant increase in e', suggestive of improved left ventricular relaxation, was demonstrated in patients 6 months following septal ethanol ablation.
- The septal e' has been shown to be an independent predictor of death and ventricular arrhythmias in children with HCM.
- E/e', the ratio of the mitral inflow early diastolic velocity to the tissue Doppler early diastolic velocity (using lateral e'), correlates well with left ventricular filling pressures (pre-A pressure).
- The E/e' ratio has correlated with exercise tolerance in patients with HCM.
Pitfalls
- It is important to be careful with sample volume placement and to avoid excessive angulation with annular motion.

- Gain and filter settings should be adjusted to ensure reliable measurements.
- The presence of pronounced mitral annular calcification, mitral stenosis, mitral annular rings, and prosthetic mitral valves contributes to reduced e' velocities.

Color M-mode Flow Propagation Velocity
Acquisition
- The M-mode scan line is placed in the center of the color flow pattern from the mitral valve to the left ventricular apex.
- Then the Nyquist limit is lowered to ensure that the central highest velocity jet is blue.
- The flow propagation velocity (Vp) is measured as the slope of the first aliasing velocity during early filling.
Analysis
- One study has shown that the ratio of E/Vp correlates with left ventricular filling pressures in patients with HCM.
Strain Studies
- Studies using speckle training have demonstrated delayed untwisting in patients with HCM.[7]
- The delay correlated with left ventricular end-diastolic pressure and volume.

Step 6B: Determine Left Atrial Volume
- Mechanisms of left atrial enlargement include chronically abnormal ventricular filling pressures, elevated left atrial pressures, mitral regurgitation (secondary to SAM and independent mitral valve disease), and, possibly, atrial myopathy.

- 2D anteroposterior linear dimensions of the left atrium in the parasternal long-axis view fail to represent accurately true left atrial size.
- The left atrium from the parasternal long-axis view does not appreciate left atrial enlargement in the superior-inferior and medial-lateral dimensions.
- Measurement of the left atrial volume provides an estimation of the true size of the left atrial cavity.

Acquisition
- The left atrial volume indexed to body surface area (LAVI) should be obtained, as outlined by guidelines of the American Society of Echocardiography.[5]
- The biplane methods (area-length and Simpson's method of disks) are very reproducible and are the recommended techniques for obtaining the left atrial volume.
- The equation for obtaining the left atrial (LA) volume using the area-length method is as follows:

$$\text{LA volume} = 8/3\pi[(A_1)\times(A_2)/L]$$

where A_1 is the left atrial area (by planimetry) on apical 4-chamber view, A_2 is the left atrial area (by planimetry) on apical 2-chamber view, and L is the length (shortest) measured from apical 4- or 2-chamber view.

Analysis
- In addition, the left atrial volume provides important prognostic information.[8]
- An increased left atrial volume has been associated with greater hypertrophy, higher filling pressures, and an increased prevalence of cardiovascular events.

Pitfalls
- The left atrial cavity can be foreshortened.
- Since the left atrium is located in the far field of the apical views, the lower lateral resolution may result in apparently thicker left atrial walls.
- Transducer angle or location may need to be modified until the image of the left atrium is optimized.

Step 7: Assess Left Ventricular Systolic Function
- Left ventricular systolic function is usually normal or hyperdynamic in patients with HCM.
- Overt left ventricular systolic dysfunction is usually defined as a left ventricular ejection fraction (LVEF) of less than 50% in this patient population.
- Left ventricular systolic dysfunction occurs in 2% to 5% of patients with HCM.
- The development of an apical aneurysm is an uncommon complication, occurring in 2% of patients.

Step 7A: Determine LVEF

KEY POINTS
- The LVEF can be determined with the biplane modified Simpson's method.[5]
- Patients should be assessed for the presence of an apical aneurysm.
- In patients with suboptimal apical windows, contrast echocardiography may be used if an apical aneurysm is suspected.

Step 7B: Assess Myocardial Mechanics
- Myocardial strain imaging (derived from tissue Doppler imaging) allows for the assessment of regional myocardial function and myocardial deformation.
- Strain rate imaging has been shown to be useful in differentiating nonobstructive HCM from hypertensive heart disease.
- However, tissue Doppler–derived strain imaging has technical limitations due to its angle dependence and need for optimal alignment for Doppler measurements.

KEY POINTS
Speckle Tracking Echocardiography (STE)
- Left ventricular contraction is characterized by complex deformation of the myocardium, including longitudinal myocardial fiber shortening, radial thickening, circumferential shortening, and left ventricular twist or torsion.[8]
- Speckle tracking (or 2D strain) echocardiography directly assesses myocardial motion from B-mode (2D) images and is not subject to angle dependence.
- This is a promising technique that may provide incremental information regarding subclinical systolic impairment in this patient population.
- Studies have shown a reduction in strain in patients with HCM.
- Although speckle tracking evaluates myocardial function, there are significant differences between strain values across the 17 left ventricular segments.
- Therefore, the variation of regional strain across the left ventricle necessitates the use of site-specific normal ranges.
- In terms of rotational motion, STE allows for quantification of the twisting (or wringing) motion of the heart.
- In normal subjects, the base rotates clockwise while the apex rotates counterclockwise, creating the wringing or torsional motion of the left ventricular cavity.
- Left ventricular rotation at the midventricular level occurs in a clockwise direction in HCM, which is opposite to the direction seen in normal subjects.

Step 8: Use Echocardiographic Data in the Management of Obstructive HCM

- The main classes of pharmacologic agents used in the treatment of obstructive HCM are beta blockers, disopyramide, and calcium channel blockers.
- Medical management in HCM is determined by symptomatic response and can be optimized using serial echocardiographic and Doppler studies.
- Important serial echocardiographic measurements include the assessment of SAM of the mitral valve and the degree of LVOT obstruction.
- Despite optimal medical therapy, patients may still have New York Heart Association Class III/IV symptoms and a significant LVOT gradient.
- In these cases, patients should be referred for invasive septal reduction therapy.
- Current options for invasive septal reduction therapy are septal ethanol ablation and surgical myectomy.
- Dual-chamber permanent pacing was previously advocated in drug-refractory symptomatic obstructive patients, but this technique is now infrequently performed because of the lack of long-term effectiveness of this procedure.

- Echocardiography plays an important role in septal reduction therapy:
  - Selection of patients for either septal ethanol ablation or myectomy
  - Intraprocedural echocardiographic guidance of septal ethanol ablation and myectomy
  - Serial monitoring following septal reduction therapy

Septal Ethanol Ablation

- Septal ethanol ablation involves the selective injection of ethanol into a septal perforator branch of the left anterior descending coronary artery.
- The resulting septal branch occlusion causes an acute deterioration of basal septal function at the site of anterior mitral leaflet–septal contact, which abolishes SAM and the LVOT obstruction.
- This occlusion of the septal branch results in localized infarction of the basal septum, which leads to gradual focal septal thinning, widening of the LVOT, and progressive resolution of the LVOT obstruction.
- Intraprocedural transthoracic imaging has become essential for the guidance and monitoring of septal ethanol ablation (Figure 7-8).

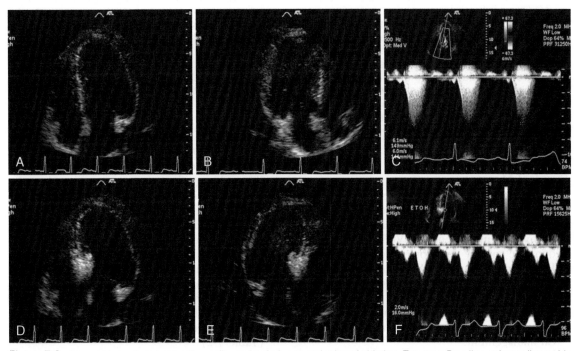

Figure 7-8. Intraprocedural contrast echocardiography during septal ethanol ablation. Top row: Baseline echocardiographic images in the apical 4-chamber (**A**) and apical 3-chamber (**B**) views in a patient with a significant LVOT gradient (**C**) identified using continuous wave Doppler. Bottom row: Following injection of echocardiographic contrast agent into the first septal perforator of the left anterior descending coronary artery in the patient, a contrast depot is identified in the region of the basal septum on the transthoracic apical 4-chamber (**D**) and 3-chamber (**E**) views highlighting the target area for therapeutic infarction. Repeat continuous wave Doppler recording shows a nonsignificant resting gradient across the LVOT (**F**).

- This procedure has traditionally been performed with the intra-arterial administration of an ultrasonic contrast agent into the target septal branch.
- Intra-arterial injection of a contrast agent allows for the specific localization of the vascular bed perfused by the individual septal perforator branch.
- The targeted vascular territory is the region of contact of the anterior mitral leaflet with the basal septum, which leads to LVOT obstruction.
- The site of leaflet-septal contact is identified by the zone of flow acceleration and color turbulence in the LVOT.

KEY POINTS

- Contrast-guided echocardiography has been demonstrated to be safe and effective and results in fewer procedural complications.
- Because of recent concerns regarding the safety of ultrasonic contrast agents, the Food and Drug Administration of the United States has stated that the intracoronary use of ultrasonic contrast agents is contraindicated.[6]
- As an alternative, the use of agitated radiographic contrast agents is possible for the identification of the target septal branch, and it is associated with an acceptable degree of myocardial opacification.
- Echocardiographic and Doppler studies are beneficial in the serial noninvasive follow-up of patients after septal ethanol ablation.
- Multiple studies have documented a significant progressive reduction in the basal septal thickness, a decrease in the magnitude of the resting and provocable LVOT gradients, and an improvement in diastolic filling parameters in the 1 to 2 years following this procedure (Figure 7-9).

Surgical Myectomy

- Septal myectomy is an established surgical technique for severe obstructive HCM.
- Surgical resection of the hypertrophied subaortic myocardium widens the LVOT and decreases dynamic outflow tract obstruction.
- Echocardiography is useful in the identification of patients suitable for surgical myectomy.
- Echocardiography also plays an important role in detecting additional lesions requiring surgical management.
- Preoperative echocardiographic imaging in patients referred for surgical myectomy includes the evaluation of independent mitral valve disease and concomitant aortic valve disease, and the assessment of additional levels of

obstruction (midventricular or right ventricular outflow tract).
- Intraoperative TEE has been used to guide surgical myectomy since the 1980s.
- Intraoperative TEE guides the surgical intervention(s), assesses immediate results, and excludes important complications (e.g., creation of iatrogenic ventricular septal defect).

KEY POINTS

- Intraoperative TEE enables careful assessment of the septal morphology (detailed interrogation of the depth, width, and length of the required myectomy), degree of SAM, and the mechanism and degree of mitral regurgitation (Figure 7-10).
- The length of septal hypertrophy is measured from the base of the right coronary cusp of the aortic valve.
- The targeted length of resection is 1 cm below the point of contact between the anterior mitral leaflet and the septum.
- The LVOT gradient can be measured by transgastric imaging in the long-axis view with the continuous wave Doppler beam aligned parallel to the LVOT.
- Following surgical excision, intraoperative TEE can provide real-time determination of the adequacy of the myectomy: the residual LVOT gradient and the degree of mitral regurgitation are reassessed prior to leaving the operating room (Figure 7-11).
- Monitoring with serial echocardiographic studies after the myectomy shows an immediate and persistent reduction in the magnitude of LVOT obstruction.

Selection of Invasive Septal Reduction Therapy

- There is significant controversy regarding the relative merits versus long-term risks of septal ethanol ablation, which was introduced in the 1990s, as compared with surgical myectomy, which has been performed since the 1960s and is regarded as the gold standard of invasive treatment in this condition.[1]
- In terms of the outcomes of septal ethanol ablation compared with myectomy, there have been a number of nonrandomized studies that have compared these two treatment strategies (Table 7-2).[9]
- There were no significant differences in short-term or long-term mortality between the ethanol ablation and myectomy cohorts.
- The two groups were similar in terms of post-procedure functional class.

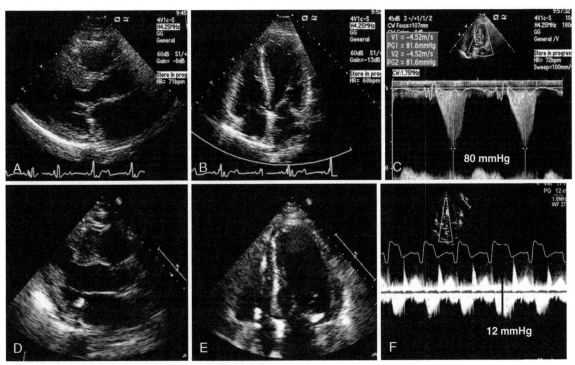

Figure 7-9. TTE studies in a patient prior to (*top row*) and 1 year following (*bottom row*) septal ethanol ablation for symptomatic obstructive HCM. Parasternal long-axis (**A**) and apical 4-chamber (**B**) views obtained prior to the procedure demonstrate septal hypertrophy and a resting LVOT gradient of 80 mm Hg (**C**). Repeat echocardiogram 1 year following septal ethanol ablation in the parasternal long-axis (**D**) and apical 4-chamber (**E**) views shows localized thinning of the anterior septum and a resting outflow tract gradient of only 12 mm Hg (**F**).

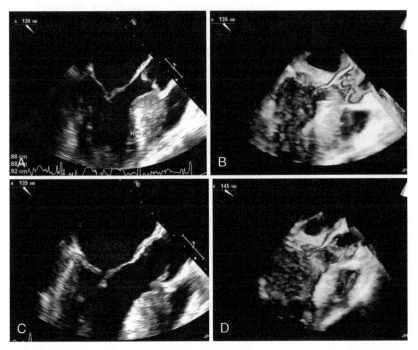

Figure 7-10. Intraoperative TEE in the long-axis view prior to (*top row*) and following (*bottom row*) myectomy using both 2D (**A** and **C**) and three-dimensional techniques (**B** and **D**). The depth, width, and length of the hypertrophied septum (measured from the base of the right coronary cusp of the aortic valve) and the point of anterior leaflet–septal contact are obtained to guide the resection.

- The major differences between patients undergoing ethanol ablation versus those undergoing myectomy were the following: (1) an increased need for permanent pacing following ethanol ablation and (2) a higher residual LVOT gradient following ethanol ablation.
- Both procedures need to be performed at centers with both technical and echocardiographic expertise.[10]

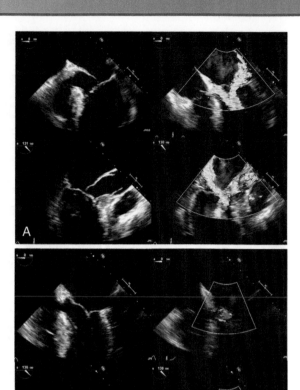

Figure 7-11. Intraoperative TEE before and after myectomy in a patient with obstructive HCM. **A,** Preoperative study. *Upper left,* Transesophageal 2D systolic frame in the 4-chamber view demonstrating anterior leaflet–septal contact with failure of mitral leaflet coaptation. *Upper right,* Same view with Doppler color flow imaging demonstrating turbulent left ventricular outflow and a large jet of posteriorly directed mitral regurgitation arising from the gap between the two mitral leaflets. *Lower left,* 2D systolic frame in the long-axis view highlights the septal hypertrophy at the basal level and the anterior leaflet SAM. *Lower right,* Same view with Doppler color flow imaging showing the LVOT obstruction and the jet of posteriorly directed regurgitation. **B,** Postoperative TEE study following surgical resection of basal septum. Transesophageal 2D systolic frame in the 4-chamber view (*upper left*) and long-axis view (*lower left*) now demonstrate a widened LVOT and abolition of SAM of the anterior mitral leaflet. Same frames with color flow imaging in the 4-chamber view (*upper right*) and long-axis view (*lower right*) show no significant turbulence in the outflow tract and resolution of the mitral regurgitation.

TABLE 7-2 STUDIES COMPARING LVOT GRADIENTS (LVOTG) FOLLOWING SEPTAL ETHANOL ABLATION (SEA) AND MYECTOMY

Study	N	Rest LVOTG—SEA (mm Hg)		Rest LVOTG— Myectomy (mm Hg)		Follow-up Time	P Value
		Pre	Post	Pre	Post		
Qin et al.	51	64 ± 39	24 ± 19	62 ± 43	11 ± 6	3 months	$p < 0.01$
Nagueh et al.	82	76 ± 23	8 ± 15	78 ± 30	4 ± 7	1 year	NS
Firoozi et al.	44	91 ± 18	21 ± 12	83 ± 23	17 ± 12	1 year	NS
Ralph-Edwards et al.	102	74 ± 36	15	64 ± 27	5	1.8 ± 1.1 years (SEA) 2.3 ± 1.5 years (myectomy)	$p < 0.001$
Van der Lee et al.	72	101 ± 34	23 ± 19	100 ± 20	17 ± 14	1 year	NS

NS, not significant.
Adapted from Agarwal S, Tuzcu EM, Desai MY, Smedira N, Lever HM, Lytle BW, Kapadia SR. Updated meta-analysis of septal alcohol ablation versus myectomy for hypertrophic cardiomyopathy. *J Am Coll Cardiol.* 2010;55:823–834.

- Conditions that favor the selection of myectomy over ethanol ablation include the following[10]:
  - Presence of a coexistent cardiac lesion (e.g., epicardial coronary artery disease)
  - Presence of coronary anatomy not amenable to septal ethanol ablation

- Requirement for an acute reduction in the LVOT gradient
- Echocardiography is helpful in identifying additional abnormalities that favor the selection of myectomy over septal ethanol ablation:

- Intrinsic abnormalities of the mitral apparatus (which contributes to the development of LVOT obstruction)
- Independent mitral valve disease (which may require surgical attention)
- Papillary muscle abnormalities
- Extreme septal hypertrophy
- Selection of the appropriate technique requires consideration of patient-specific clinical and echocardiographic characteristics and consideration of local expertise.

Key Measurements for Predicting Prognosis in Patients with HCM

- The most ominous complication of HCM is the occurrence of sudden cardiac death (SCD).[1]

- Early studies of HCM reported high rates of HCM-related death, in the range of 3% to 6% per year.
- However, in the last 2 to 3 decades, multiple long-term studies, especially from community-based cohorts, have shown that the overall prognosis of HCM is more benign.
- The annual mortality rate in this patient population is in the range of 1% per year.
- The most common mechanism of SCD in HCM appears to be the development of ventricular tachyarrhythmias originating from an abnormal myocardial substrate.
- SCD most commonly occurs in young individuals under the age of 30 to 35 years.

KEY POINTS

- Risk stratification of patients with HCM has become increasingly important in the past decade since the prophylactic insertion of an implantable cardioverter-defibrillator (ICD) has been shown to be an effective tool in this patient population.[1]
- Clinical and echocardiographic data can provide important information regarding the long-term prognosis of patients with HCM.
- The major risk factors for sudden death in HCM are the following[1]:
  - Family history of premature HCM-related SCD
  - Unexplained syncope
  - Nonsustained ventricular tachycardia
  - Abnormal blood pressure response to exercise
  - Maximal left ventricular thickness ≥ 30 mm
- The risk factors that are considered to be potentially important (or regarded as minor risk factors) in the occurrence of SCD are the following[1]:
  - Atrial fibrillation
  - Myocardial ischemia
  - High-risk mutation
  - Intense (competitive) physical exertion
  - LVOT obstruction

- One of the main challenges with identifying high-risk individuals in this patient population is that the positive predictive value of the "major risk factors" is actually relatively low, given that the incidence of SCD is low (Table 7-3).[11]
- Therefore, the mere presence of one risk factor does not mean that a patient will die suddenly.
- Furthermore, the major risk factors have a fairly high negative predictive value (see Table 7-3)—thus the absence of these risk factors should be reassuring.
- Echocardiographic indices of prognosis have gained acceptance since they are noninvasive and reproducible.
- The only major risk factor identified by echocardiography is the maximal left ventricular wall thickness.
- Other important echocardiographic findings that are considered to be poor prognostic markers are the following[8]:
  - LVOT gradient ≥ 30 mm Hg
  - Left ventricular dysfunction (LVEF < 50%)
  - Left atrial dilatation

TABLE 7-3 PREDICTIVE VALUE OF RISK FACTORS FOR SCD IN HCM

Risk Factor	SENS (%)	SPEC (%)	PPV (%)	NPV (%)
Abnormal blood pressure response (<40 years old)	75	66	15	97
Nonsustained ventricular tachycardia (<45 years old)	69	80	22	97
Syncope (*unexplained*)	35	82	25	86
Family history (at least 1 premature SCD)	42	79	28	88
Maximal left ventricular wall thickness ≥ 30 mm	26	88	13	95

NPV, negative predictive value; PPV, positive predictive value; SENS, sensitivity; SPEC, specificity.

Left Ventricular Wall Thickness

- Two independent groups have demonstrated a direct association between the magnitude of the maximal left ventricular wall thickness and the risk of SCD in HCM.[1]
- The risk of sudden death increases progressively in relation to left ventricular wall thickness.
- In one multicenter study of 480 patients followed for 6.5 years, the risk of sudden death was 0 per 1000 person-years (95% confidence interval, 0 to 14.4) in patients with maximal left ventricular wall thickness ≤ 15 mm, whereas the risk of sudden death was 18.2 per 1000 person-years (95% confidence interval, 7.3 to 37.6) in patients with maximal left ventricular wall thickness ≥ 30 mm.[12]
- The cumulative 20-year risk of sudden death was almost 40% for patients with a wall thickness of ≥ 30 mm (Figure 7-12).
- In another study of 630 patients followed for nearly 5 years, there was a higher probability of sudden death with increasing wall thickness

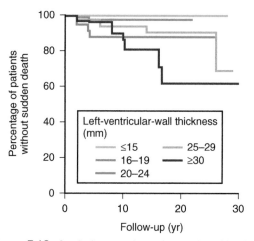

Figure 7-12. Survival curves for patients with HCM illustrating the importance of the maximal left ventricular wall thickness.

(relative risk per 5-mm increment was 1.31; 95% confidence interval, 1.03 to 1.66).
- Left ventricular wall thickness (≥30 mm) is regarded as a strong independent risk factor for sudden death.

LVOT Obstruction

- In one study of over 1000 patients with HCM, the risk of death related to HCM was twofold higher in patients with a resting LVOT gradient of ≥ 30 mm Hg (Figure 7-13).[13]
- The risk of SCD in this study was also higher in patients with obstructive (resting LVOT gradient ≥ 30 mm Hg) versus nonobstructive HCM (relative risk of 2.1).
- However, the difference in the annual rate of sudden death between obstructive and nonobstructive patients was small (1.5% vs. 0.9%).
- In this study, LVOT obstruction was associated with a low positive predictive value for SCD (7%) and a high negative predictive value (95%).

LV Systolic Dysfunction

- Left ventricular systolic dysfunction occurs infrequently in patients with HCM.
- Recent studies suggest that systolic dysfunction occurs in 2% to 5% of this patient cohort.
- Terms used to denote systolic dysfunction in HCM include "dilated phase of hypertrophic cardiomyopathy," "end-stage hypertrophic cardiomyopathy," or "burnt-out hypertrophic cardiomyopathy."[1]
- Systolic dysfunction is associated with wall thinning and cavity dilatation, and has been attributed to interstitial fibrosis, ischemia, infarction, and small vessel disease.[8]
- Long-term prognosis is markedly worsened in the presence of left ventricular systolic dysfunction.
- End-stage HCM is associated with increased mortality (up to 11% per year) and an increased risk of SCD.

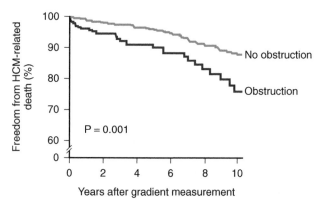

Figure 7-13. Survival curves demonstrating worsened survival in patients with LVOT obstruction (resting LVOT gradient at least 30 mm Hg) compared with nonobstructive patients.

Left Atrial Enlargement

- Left atrial enlargement, as determined by 2D echocardiographic measurements of the left atrial diameter, has been associated with an adverse long-term prognosis (increased risk of atrial fibrillation and increased risk of death).[8]
- However, the anteroposterior linear dimension may misrepresent the true left atrial size since the left atrial cavity may remodel asymmetrically.
- Left atrial volumes (indexed to body surface area) overcome the above limitation.
- The left atrial volume is a good marker of disease severity in patients with HCM.
- A left atrial volume (indexed to body surface area) greater than 34 mL/m^2 has been associated with a greater degree of hypertrophy, a higher E/e' ratio, and an increased number of adverse cardiac outcomes.[8]

Additional Testing in Patients with HCM

Exercise Testing and Exercise Echocardiography

- Exercise testing has an important role in the work-up and management of patients with HCM.[1]
- Pertinent information can be obtained by exercise testing:
  - Reproduciblity of symptoms
  - Exercise duration and functional capacity
  - LVOT gradient with exercise
  - Blood pressure response with exercise

Provocable LVOT Obstruction

- All patients with presumed nonobstructive HCM should be tested for the presence of a provocable (or latent) LVOT gradient.

KEY POINTS

- Patients who should be specifically targeted for exercise echocardiography include patients with the following:
  - Exertional or postprandial symptoms
  - History of presyncope or syncope
  - Dynamic systolic murmur during bedside maneuvers
  - Left atrial dilatation in the absence of overt mitral regurgitation
- Upright exercise testing most accurately simulates physical stress and daily activities in patients with HCM.[2]
- Provocable LVOT obstruction elicited by exercise echocardiography is more reliable and reflective of symptomatology than provocable

---

KEY POINTS—cont'd

LVOT gradients elicited by the Valsalva maneuver or amyl nitrate inhalation.
- Approximately half the patients without LVOT obstruction at rest will develop an LVOT gradient greater than 30 mm Hg with exercise.
- Once provocable LVOT obstruction has been established, serial exercise testing may be used to guide the response to therapy (pharmacologic and nonpharmacologic).

Blood Pressure Response to Exercise

- An abnormal blood pressure response to exercise is seen in up to one third of patients with HCM.[1]
- An abnormal blood pressure response during exercise is defined as either:
  - Absence of a rise in systolic blood pressure greater than 20 mm Hg
  - Decrease in systolic blood pressure greater than 20 mm Hg from peak blood pressure
- Young patients (<40 years old) with HCM with an abnormal blood pressure response to exercise are at higher risk for SCD (see Table 7-3).

Cardiovascular Magnetic Resonance Imaging in HCM

- Advances in cardiovascular magnetic resonance imaging (CMRI) have the following potential applications in patients with HCM[2]:
  - Diagnosis
  - Characterization of left ventricular hypertrophy
  - Left ventricular volume and LVEF
  - Tissue characterization
  - Monitoring following invasive septal reduction therapy
  - Prognostication and risk stratification

Diagnosis of HCM and Characterization of Hypertrophy

- CMRI can provide very accurate measurements of wall thickness at any myocardial segment.
- Determination of the absolute wall thickness and the pattern of hypertrophy is important in the diagnosis of HCM.
- CMRI offers reliable imaging of the epicardial border of the myocardium in regions that often have poor echocardiographic visualization.
- CMRI can identify segmental hypertrophy not always appreciated by echocardiography.

KEY POINTS

- CMRI can appreciate full left ventricular myocardial thickness at wall segments that are traditionally difficult to visualize (e.g., anterolateral wall, apical region).
- In patients in whom there is a strong clinical suspicion of apical HCM and in whom the standard 2D echocardiographic study is nondiagnostic, subsequent testing with either contrast echocardiography or CMRI should be performed (Figure 7-14).
- Other subtypes or variants of HCM that can be detected by CMRI include the following:

- Symmetrical HCM (i.e., concentric pattern of hypertrophy)
- End-stage HCM
- HCM associated with apical aneurysm
- CMRI is useful in differentiating cases of HCM from other cases of unexplained increased wall thickness, such as Fabry's disease or cardiac amyloidosis.
- CMRI can also help demonstrate prominent trabeculations in the condition known as left ventricular noncompaction cardiomyopathy, which may help distinguish it from the apical form of HCM.

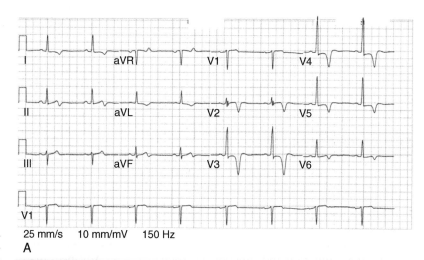

25 mm/s   10 mm/mV   150 Hz

A

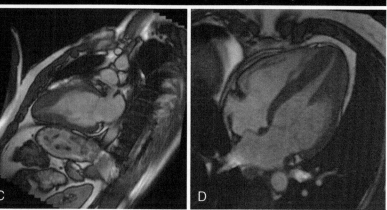

Figure 7-14. **A,** Electrocardiogram in a 50-year-old patient presenting with chest pain. The prominent inverted T waves raised the suspicion of the apical form of HCM. **B,** Suboptimal endocardial definition of the apical segments on TTE. **C** and **D,** CMRI with 2-chamber view (**C**) and 4-chamber view (**D**) of the same patient. The spade-shaped configuration of the left ventricular cavity and the hypertrophy predominantly at the left ventricular apex are compatible with the diagnosis of apical HCM.

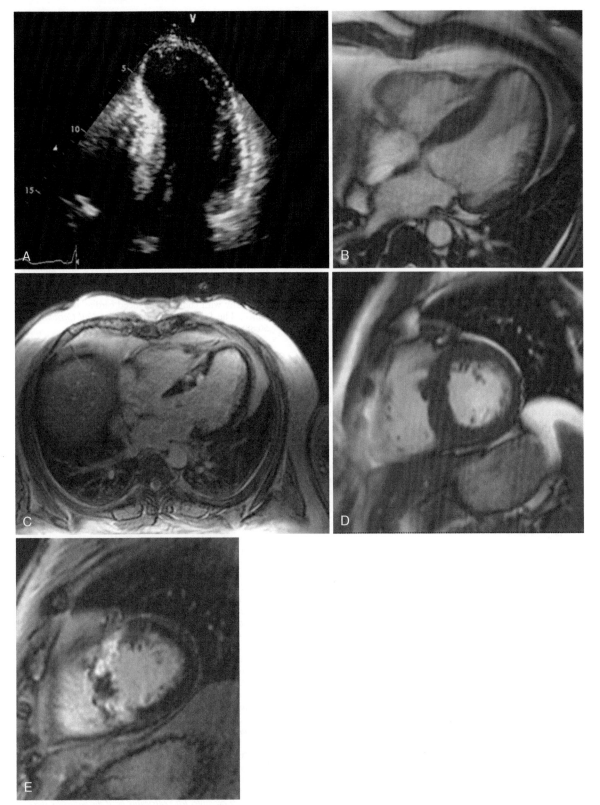

Figure 7-15. **A,** TTE imaging was performed in a 41-year-old man referred for evaluation due to a history of palpitations and a family history of HCM. The patient was diagnosed with HCM. **B** and **C,** Four-chamber view on CMRI showing non–contrast-enhanced (**B**) and gadolinium-enhanced (**C**) images of this patient with HCM. **D** and **E,** Corresponding CMRI short-axis views of the same patient with non–contrast-enhanced (**D**) and gadolinium-enhanced (**E**) images demonstrating significant hyperenhancement following the administration of gadolinium.

Identification of Fibrosis in HCM and Prognostication

- CMRI can be performed with the administration of gadolinium, which permits the detection and quantification of myocardial fibrosis in patients with HCM.[2]
- Following intravenous injection, gadolinium is temporarily deposited in the extracellular space of the myocardium.
- CMRI images with late gadolinium enhancement (LGE) show gadolinium deposition as bright or hyperenhanced.
- Areas within the myocardium with fibrosis or scarring are revealed by hyperenhancement of gadolinium (Figure 7-15).
- LGE occurs predominantly in a patchy, multifocal midwall distribution in hypertrophied regions.[14]
- Multiple large studies have shown a variable but generally high prevalence of LGE in patients with HCM.
- The presence of LGE in patients with HCM has been associated with other risk factors for sudden death and with ventricular arrhythmias.
- The majority of recent studies have demonstrated that the presence of LGE is associated with an increased risk of adverse cardiovascular outcomes, although LGE was not found to be an independent predictor of SCD.[14]

References

1. Maron BJ, McKenna WJ, Danielson GK, et al. Clinical expert consensus document on hypertrophic cardiomyopathy: A report of the American College of Cardiology Foundation Task Force on Clinical Expert Consensus Documents and the European Society of Cardiology Committee for Practice Guidelines. *J Am Coll Cardiol.* 2003; 42:1687-1713.
2. Nagueh SF, Mahmarian JJ. Noninvasive cardiac imaging in patients with hypertrophic cardiomyopathy. *J Am Coll Cardiol.* 2006;48:2410-2422.
3. Maron BJ, Pelliccia A. The heart of trained athletes: Cardiac remodeling and the risks of sports, including sudden death. *Circulation.* 2006;114:1633-1644.
4. Arad M, Maron BJ, Gorham JM, et al. Glycogen storage diseases presenting as hypertrophic cardiomyopathy. *N Engl J Med.* 2005;352:362-372.
5. Lang RM, Bierig M, Devereux RB, et al. Recommendations for chamber quantification: A report from the American Society of Echocardiography's Guidelines and Standards Committee and the Chamber Quantification Writing Group, developed in conjunction with the European Association of Echocardiography, a branch of the European Society of Cardiology. *J Am Soc Echocardiogr.* 2005;18:1440-1463.
6. Mulvagh SL, Rakowski H, Vannan MA, et al. American Society of Echocardiography Consensus Statement on the clinical applications of ultrasonic contrast agents in echocardiography. *J Am Soc Echocardiogr.* 2008;21:1179-1201.
7. Losi MA, Nistri S, Galderisi M, et al. Echocardiography in patients with hypertrophic cardiomyopathy: Usefulness of old and new techniques in the diagnosis and pathophysiological assessment. *Cardiovasc Ultrasound.* 2010;8:7.
8. Afonso LC, Bernal J, Bax JJ, Abraham TP. Echocardiography in hypertrophic cardiomyopathy: The role of conventional and emerging technologies. *J Am Coll Cardiol Imag.* 2008;1:787-800.
9. Agarwal S, Tuzcu EM, Desai MY, Smedira N, Lever HM, Lytle BW, Kapadia SR. Updated meta-analysis of septal alcohol ablation versus myectomy for hypertrophic cardiomyopathy. *J Am Coll Cardiol.* 2010;55: 823-834.
10. Maron BJ, Dearani JA, Ommen SR, et al. The case for surgery in obstructive hypertrophic cardiomyopathy. *J Am Coll Cardiol.* 2004;44:2044-2053.
11. McKenna WJ, Behr ER. Hypertrophic cardiomyopathy: Management, risk stratification, and prevention of sudden death. *Heart.* 2002;87:169-176.
12. Spirito P, Bellone P, Harris KM, et al. Magnitude of left ventricular hypertrophy and risk of sudden death in hypertrophic cardiomyopathy. *N Engl J Med.* 2000;342: 1778-1785.
13. Maron MS, Olivotto I, Betocchi S, et al. Effect of left ventricular outflow tract obstruction on clinical outcome in hypertrophic cardiomyopathy. *N Engl J Med.* 2003;348: 295-303.
14. Salerno M, Kramer CM. Prognosis in hypertrophic cardiomyopathy with contrast-enhanced cardiac magnetic resonance: The future looks bright. *J Am Coll Cardiol.* 2010; 56:888-889.

Suggested Readings

1. Maron BJ, Maron MS, Wigle ED, Braunwald E. The 50-year history, controversy, and clinical implications of left ventricular outflow tract obstruction in hypertrophic cardiomyopathy: From idiopathic hypertrophic subaortic stenosis to hypertrophic cardiomyopathy. *J Am Coll Cardiol.* 2009;54:191-200.
   The history and controversies surrounding the diagnosis and management of HCM are summarized in this review article. The role and contributions of echocardiographic imaging in this condition are also outlined.
2. Drinko JK, Nash PJ, Lever HM, Asher CR. Safety of stress testing in patients with hypertrophic cardiomyopathy. *Am J Cardiol.* 2004;93:1443-1444.
   The safety and risks of exercise echocardiography are examined in this study of 263 patients with HCM.
3. Maron MS, Olivotto I, Zenovich AG, et al. Hypertrophic cardiomyopathy is predominantly a disease of left ventricular outflow tract obstruction. *Circulation.* 2006;114: 2232-2239.
   This large study of stress echocardiography in patients with HCM showed that the majority of presumed nonobstructive HCM patients actually had some degree of provocable LVOT obstruction.
4. Nagueh SF, Appleton CP, Gillebert TC, et al. Recommendations for the evaluation of left ventricular diastolic function by echocardiography. *J Am Soc Echocardiogr.* 2009;22:107-133.
   The evaluation of diastolic function by echocardiography and recommendations for reporting diastolic function are outlined in this comprehensive document issued by the American Society of Echocardiography.
5. Wang J, Buergler JM, Veerasamy K, Ashton YP, Nagueh SF. Delayed untwisting: The mechanistic link between dynamic obstruction and exercise tolerance in patients with hypertrophic obstructive cardiomyopathy. *J Am Coll Cardiol.* 2009;54:1326-1334.
   This study examines left ventricular twist mechanics by speckle tracking echocardiography in patients with HCM. Untwisting is shown to be delayed and longest in patients with obstructive HCM and improves in patients following septal reduction therapy.

6. Yang H, Woo A, Monakier D, et al. Left atrial enlargement in hypertrophic cardiomyopathy: The importance of left ventricular segmental hypertrophy and diastolic dysfunction. *J Am Soc Echocardiogr.* 2005;18:1074-1082.
Left atrial volumes are assessed in this large study of patients with HCM. The degree of left atrial enlargement is found to be associated with the severity of hypertrophy, mitral regurgitation, and diastolic dysfunction.

7. Serri K, Reant P, Lafitte M, et al. Global and regional myocardial function quantification by two-dimensional strain. *J Am Coll Cardiol.* 2006;47:1175-1181.
This paper is the first major study of 2D strain imaging in patients with HCM.

8. Elliott PM, Gimeno JR, Thaman R, et al. Historical trends in reported survival rates in patients with hypertrophic cardiomyopathy. *Heart.* 2006;92:785-791.
Historical trends in the survival rates of patients with HCM are reviewed in this paper. The survival of patients with this condition has markedly improved compared with initial reports 5 decades earlier.

9. Maron BJ. Contemporary insights and strategies for risk stratification and prevention of sudden death in hypertrophic cardiomyopathy. *Circulation.* 2010;121:445-456.
The risk stratification of patients with HCM is outlined in this review. Sudden death and the efficacy and issues surrounding treatment with ICDs are also summarized.

10. Nagueh SF, Bierig M, Budoff MJ, et al. American Society of Echocardiography clinical recommendations for multimodality cardiovascular imaging of patients with hypertrophic cardiomyopathy. Endorsed by the American Society of Nuclear Cardiology, Society for Cardiovascular Magnetic Resonance, and Society of Cardiovascular Computed Tomography. *J Am Soc Echocardiogr.* 2011; 24:473-498.
The imaging of patients with HCM is summarized in this comprehensive document, which summarizes and outlines recommendations for the use of echocardiography and other imaging techniques in this patient population.

Role of Echocardiography in Patients Treated with Cardiotoxic Drugs

8

Bonnie Ky

Basic Principles

- Several anti-neoplastic agents are associated with significant cardiotoxicity.
- Agents most commonly associated with cardiotoxic risk include anthracyclines (doxorubicin), as well as the tyrosine kinase inhibitors trastuzumab, sunitinib, and sorafenib (Table 8-1).
- Cardiotoxicity associated with anti-cancer therapy is typically associated with a global decline in left ventricular ejection fraction (LVEF), although early manifestations may include diastolic dysfunction.
- Radiation therapy is also associated with significant cardiotoxic effects.
- Echocardiography is important to assess both systolic and diastolic cardiac function, extent of valvular disease, and evidence for any pericardial disease.

Anthracycline Cardiotoxicity

- Anthracyclines (e.g., doxorubicin) are widely known to be associated with cardiotoxic effects.
- Doxorubicin cardiotoxicity can occur early or late during therapy. Early changes occur acutely or within the first year of therapy. Late dysfunction occurs months or many years after the initial exposure.
- Overall, doxorubicin cardiotoxicity is indistinguishable from other forms of heart failure with LV dilatation, wall thinning, and decreased contractility (Figure 8-1).
- An increased risk of cardiotoxicity is associated with higher cumulative dosages of doxorubicin (particularly > 550 mg/m^2) and with pre-existing cardiac disease, including hypertension, valvular disease, and ischemic heart disease.

Trastuzumab Cardiotoxicity

- Trastuzumab is a humanized monoclonal antibody targeting the ErbB2 receptor.
- Cardiotoxicity risk is increased in the setting of prior exposure to anthracyclines as well as concomitant cardiovascular disease such as hypertension or coronary disease.
- Cardiotoxicity is often observed during the treatment phase and can be reversible with cessation of therapy or institution of cardioprotective medications.
- Trastuzumab cardiotoxicity is also echocardiographically indistinguishable from other forms of systolic heart failure (Figure 8-2).

Radiation Therapy

- Radiation can induce myocardial fibrosis and vascular changes, pericardial disease, valvular stenoses, and coronary atherosclerosis. The conduction system is also sensitive to fibrosis.
- Restrictive cardiomyopathy with fibrosis and diastolic dysfunction can be seen in radiotherapy-treated patients.
- Pericardial involvement includes acute or chronic effusions, pericarditis, and pericardial constriction. Constriction is a late manifestation often occurring at greater than 18 months (Figure 8-3).
- In terms of valvular disease, the left-sided valves (mitral and aortic) are most frequently involved, with manifestations of regurgitation or stenosis occurring late. The mean time from radiation to symptom onset has been noted as greater than 8 years (Figure 8-4).
- Fibrosis of the conduction system can also occur, manifesting as right bundle branch block and rarely more advanced heart block.
- Premature coronary disease with accelerated atherosclerosis is also observed (Figure 8-5).

TABLE 8-1 COMMON CHEMOTHERAPY AND ANTI-CANCER AGENTS ASSOCIATED WITH SIGNIFICANT CARDIOTOXICITY

Type of Agent	Potential Cardiac Complication
Anthracyclines	
Doxorubicin	Early postinfusion, transient, often reversible decline in LVEF; arrhythmias, myopericarditis; more commonly, a decline in LVEF > 1 year after therapy
Tyrosine Kinase Inhibitors	
Trastuzumab	Potentially reversible, significant decline in LVEF
Bevacizumab	Hypertension, arterial thrombosis
Sunitinib	Decline in LVEF, hypertension
Sorafenib	Myocardial infarction, hypertension
Imatinib	Diastolic dysfunction, pericardial effusion
Alkylating Agents	
Cisplatin	Hypertension, vascular dysfunction
Cyclophosphamide	Pericarditis/myocarditis, decline in LVEF with high doses
Antimetabolites	
5-Fluorouracil	Coronary vasospasm, myocardial ischemia
Antimicrotubules	
Paclitaxel	Arrhythmia, heart failure

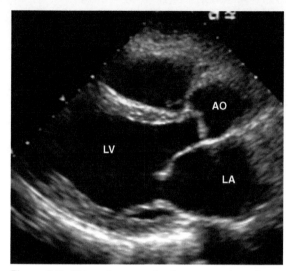

Figure 8-2. This patient sustained trastuzumab cardiotoxicity and had a mild decline in LVEF during trastuzumab therapy.

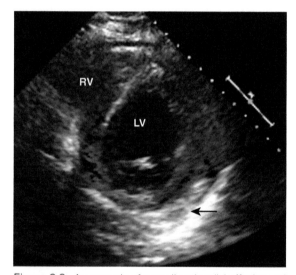

Figure 8-3. An example of a small pericardial effusion and pericardial thickening (*arrow*) related to radiation exposure.

Figure 8-1. **A,** An example of a dilated cardiomyopathy secondary to doxorubicin exposure. **B,** This same patient also suffered from severe functional mitral regurgitation secondary to annular dilatation.

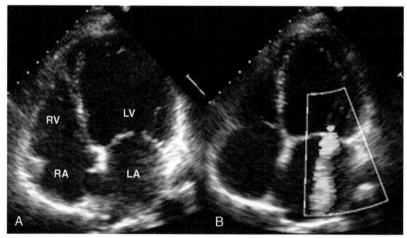

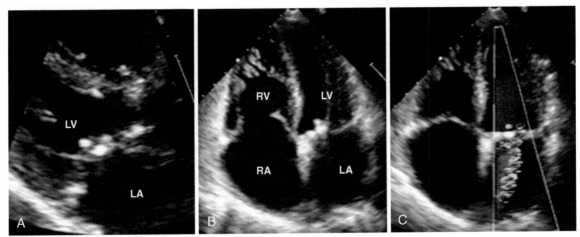

Figure 8-4. **A,** Evidence of severe mitral annular calcification and leaflet thickening secondary to radiation exposure in the distant past. This patient also had severe aortic stenosis from thickened and calcified leaflets. **B,** This apical 4-chamber view from the same patient emphasizes the degree of calcification as well as subvalvular thickening. This patient also developed RV dysfunction secondary to mitral valvular disease. **C,** Color Doppler in this same patient shows moderate mitral regurgitation secondary to leaflet calcification and thickening and failure of adequate coaptation.

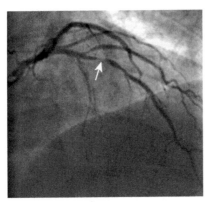

Figure 8-5. Coronary angiogram demonstrating a left anterior descending coronary artery lesion (*arrow*) in a patient who received radiation as a child for lymphoma.

Additional Agents and Cardiotoxic Effects

- Additional tyrosine kinase inhibitors are also known to have off-target effects.
- Sunitinib and sorafenib are associated with an increased incidence of hypertension and LVEF decline. Bevacizumab also results in contractile dysfunction.
- Myocardial ischemia has been seen with 5-fluorouracil (5-FU) alone and in combination with cisplatin.
- Hypertension and vascular dysfunction are common side effects of many of the agents, including bevacizumab, sorafenib, sunitinib, and cisplatin.

- Pericarditis is rarely observed with cyclophosphamide and cytarabine, and effusions can be seen with all-*trans* retinoic acid and imatinib therapy.

Step-by-Step Approach

Step 1: Determine Left Ventricular Size and Systolic Function; Evaluate for Segmental Wall Motion Abnormalities

KEY POINTS
- Anthracyclines, trastuzumab, sorafenib and sunitinib cause a global decrease in LVEF that is indistinguishable echocardiographically from other forms of systolic heart failure.
- Myocardial ischemia and focal wall motion abnormalities may be observed with other agents, including 5-FU.
- Accurate, reproducible estimation of cardiac function is essential, and quantitative assessment should also be performed if image quality is adequate.
- Additional cardiac stress, such as hypertension or ischemic heart disease, may increase cardiotoxic risk.

Step 2: Determine Diastolic Function

KEY POINTS
- Diastolic dysfunction may be an early marker of chemotherapy or anti-cancer therapy–associated cardiotoxicity.
- Restrictive cardiomyopathy can be seen with radiation-induced disease.

Step 3: Determine Degree of Valvular Disease

> **KEY POINTS**
>
> - The valvular disease that occurs in the setting of chemotherapy cardiotoxicity is typically functional.
> - However, radiation therapy is associated with an increased risk of aortic and mitral valvular disease most typically secondary to leaflet abnormalities.

Step 4: Determine Extent of Pericardial Disease

> **KEY POINTS**
>
> - Radiation therapy can be associated with acute or chronic pericarditis, and pericardial effusions.

New, Sensitive Echocardiographic Indices to Detect Cardiotoxicity

- Once a global reduction in cardiac function is observed, there may be irreversible dysfunction and it may be necessary to interrupt anticancer therapy.
- LVEF is also not a robust predictor of incident cardiotoxicity.
- There is a need to develop sensitive, predictive markers of incident cardiac dysfunction.
- Strain imaging quantifies myocardial deformation and is a tool under active investigation to determine subclinical ventricular dysfunction before changes in ejection fraction are evident (Figure 8-6).
- Exercise or dobutamine stress testing has also been proposed as a means of assessing contractile reserve and subclinical dysfunction.

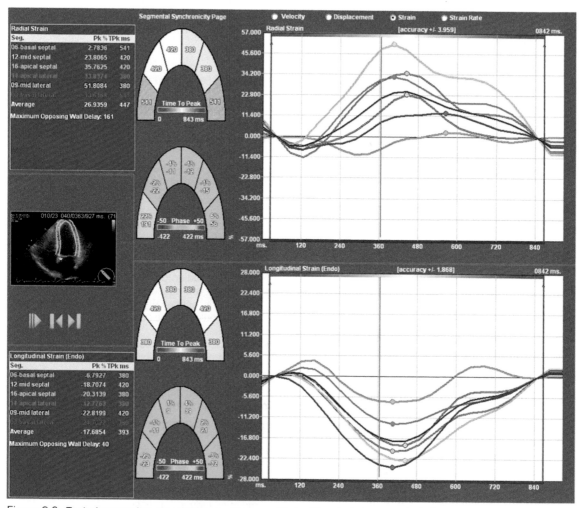

Figure 8-6. Typical output that one might derive from speckle tracking strain image analysis from an apical 4-chamber view.

Suggested Readings

1. Altena R, Perik PJ, van Veldhuisen DJ, de Vries EG, Gietema JA. Cardiovascular toxicity caused by cancer treatment: Strategies for early detection. *Lancet Oncol.* 2009;10:391-399.
   This is an excellent summary regarding the current imaging and biomarker strategies used in the detection of cardiotoxicity.

2. Bird BR, Swain SM. Cardiac toxicity in breast cancer survivors: Review of potential cardiac problems. *Clin Cancer Res.* 2008;14:14-24.
   This is a comprehensive review of the potential cardiotoxicities associated with breast cancer therapies.

3. Chu TF, Rupnick MA, Kerkela R, et al. Cardiotoxicity associated with tyrosine kinase inhibitor sunitinib. *Lancet.* 2007;370:2011-2019.
   This is a very interesting cohort study, which finely details the changes in cardiac function observed with sunitinib.

4. Suter TM, Procter M, van Veldhuisen DJ, et al. Trastuzumab-associated cardiac adverse effects in the Herceptin Adjuvant trial. *J Clin Oncol.* 2007;25:3859-3865.
   This study describes the early cardiac effects observed with trastuzumab in a large adjuvant randomized clinical trial. The late effects were also published and noted below (see Suggested Reading 9).

5. Yeh ET, Bickford CL. Cardiovascular complications of cancer therapy: Incidence, pathogenesis, diagnosis, and management. *J Am Coll Cardiol.* 2009;53:2231-2247.
   This is an excellent summary of the potential cardiotoxicities observed with a diverse panel of cancer therapies.

6. Berry GJ, Jorden M. Pathology of radiation and anthracycline cardiotoxicity. *Pediatr Blood Cancer.* 2005;44: 630-637.
   This is a comprehensive review of the effects of radiation on the cardiac system.

7. Floyd JD, Nguyen DT, Lobins RL, Bashir Q, Doll DC, Perry MC. Cardiotoxicity of cancer therapy. *J Clin Oncol.* 2005;23:7685-7696.
   This is an interesting review of the cardiotoxic effects and proposed mechanisms of cardiotoxic chemotherapies.

8. Barry E, Alvarez JA, Scully RE, Miller TL, Lipshultz SE. Anthracycline-induced cardiotoxicity: Course, pathophysiology, prevention and management. *Expert Opin Pharmacother.* 2007;8:1039-1058.
   This is a well-written review of anthracycline-associated cardiotoxicity.

9. Procter M, Suter TM, de Azambuja E, et al. Longer-term assessment of trastuzumab-related cardiac adverse events in the Herceptin Adjuvant (HERA) trial. *J Clin Oncol.* 2010;28:3422-3428.
   This article details the cardiac substudy from a large adjuvant clinical trial of trastuzumab and describes the natural history of trastuzumab on cardiac function.

10. Chen MH, Kerkela R, Force T. Mechanisms of cardiac dysfunction associated with tyrosine kinase inhibitor cancer therapeutics. *Circulation.* 2008;118:84-95.
    This is a state-of-the-art review of the potential mechanisms and cardiotoxicities observed with the tyrosine kinase inhibitors.

Echocardiographic Assessment of Treatment for Systolic Congestive Heart Failure

Rory B. Weiner and Judy Hung

9

Introduction

The echocardiographic assessment of heart failure (HF) yields important diagnostic and prognostic information. Once diagnosed, numerous medical and device therapies exist to reduce symptoms and mortality in patients with congestive HF secondary to systolic dysfunction. These therapies can also produce favorable changes in left ventricular (LV) structure and function. Additionally, novel therapies are under investigation. The echocardiographic assessment of systolic HF and review of the established and developing treatment options for systolic HF are the focus of this chapter.

Echocardiographic Assessment of Systolic HF

- Echocardiography is an appropriate diagnostic test to investigate symptoms and signs of suspected HF.[1] Echocardiography is also appropriate for guiding therapeutic decisions in HF patients and evaluating changes in clinical status.[1] In addition to diagnosis, results from an echocardiogram (i.e., left ventricular ejection fraction [LVEF]) can provide important prognostic information.[2]
- In addition to LVEF, other echocardiographic parameters provide prognostic information. Specifically, in a study of cardiac mortality in HF patients with LVEF less than 40%, a restrictive transmitral flow pattern (Figure 9-1) by Doppler echocardiography was the best clinical predictor of cardiac death. Relative risk for cardiac death was estimated as 4.1 at 1 year and 8.6 at 2 years in the restrictive group compared with the nonrestrictive group.[3] Several other markers of LV size and function (i.e., end-diastolic and end-systolic volume, myocardial performance index) and diastolic properties of the LV (i.e., pseudo-normal mitral inflow pattern) predict adverse prognosis in systolic HF.

- Three-dimensional (3D) echocardiography is a newer modality for measurement of LV volumes and LVEF. Studies have demonstrated that LV volumes measured by 3D echocardiography compare favorably with cardiac magnetic resonance imaging as a reference standard.[4]
- Novel echocardiographic measures of regional LV function, such as global longitudinal strain by speckle tracking echocardiography, may have superior prognostic value in HF patients over traditional measures of global function such as LVEF.[5] Longitudinal and circumferential strain rates were independent predictors of outcome in myocardial infarction patients with LV dysfunction and/or HF.[6] The effect of HF therapies on these novel echocardiographic measures represents an important area of ongoing investigation.

Medications

Several classes of medications are approved for symptom relief and mortality benefit in systolic HF. These medications are summarized below.

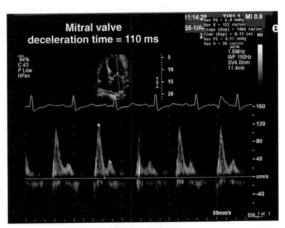

Figure 9-1. Echocardiograhic example of a restrictive transmitral Doppler pattern (deceleration time < 150 ms).

Beta Blockers

- Once thought to be detrimental, several beta-adrenergic blocking agents (beta blockers) are known to provide mortality benefits for systolic HF.
- Bisoprolol, carvedilol, and metoprolol are the beta blockers for which studies have documented mortality benefits in systolic HF.
- Improvement in LVEF with carvedilol in systolic HF results from decreased heart rate, improved chamber contractility, and afterload reduction.[7]

KEY POINTS

- Large mortality trials of beta blockers in systolic HF are highlighted in Table 9-1. Beta blockers are essential first-line therapy in patients with HF and LV systolic dysfunction. Beta blockers are typically started at low doses and titrated to target doses.

- In the MDC trial, beta blockers produced favorable LV remodeling, with a larger increase in LVEF compared to placebo (13.0% vs. 6.0%, $p < 0.0001$). In general, treatment with beta blockers improves systolic function (increase in LVEF of 5% to 10%) and reduces symptoms.

TABLE 9-1 LARGE MORTALITY TRIALS OF BETA BLOCKERS IN SYSTOLIC CONGESTIVE HF

Beta Blocker	Trial (Citation)	Mortality Benefit	NYHA Class	Target Dose
Metoprolol tartrate	MDC (*Lancet.* 1993;342:1441)	No • Improved clinical status and decreased need for heart transplantation	II/III	100–150 mg
Bisoprolol	CIBIS I (*Circulation.* 1994;90:1765)	No • Low mortality in placebo group decreased the statistical power	III/IV	5 mg
Carvedilol	US Carvedilol (*N Engl J Med.* 1996;334:1349)	Yes	II/III	50–100 mg
Bisoprolol	CIBIS II (*Lancet.* 1999;353:9)	Yes • Greatest reduction in sudden death • No benefit in death from pump failure	III/IV	10 mg
Metoprolol succinate	MERIT-HF (*Clin Cardiol.* 1999;22:V30)	Yes • Significant decrease in suddent death and death from pump failure	II–IV	200 mg
Carvedilol	COPERNICUS (*N Engl J Med.* 2001;344:1651)	Yes	"Severe HF"	50 mg
Bucindolol	BEST (*N Engl J Med.* 2001; 344:1659)	No	III/IV	100–200 mg
Carvedilol vs. metoprolol tartrate	COMET (*Lancet.* 2003;362:7)	Carvedilol: Yes	II–IV	Carvedilol: 50 mg Metoprolol: 100 mg
Carvedilol	CAPRICORN (*Lancet.* 2001;357:1385)	Yes	I (post–acute myocardial infarction patients)	50 mg

Angiotensin-Converting Enzyme (ACE) Inhibitors

- Neurohormonal blockade of the renin-angiotensin-aldosterone system with ACE inhibitors has proven mortality benefit in systolic HF.
- Although ACE inhibitors have vasodilator properties, the main mechanism of benefit in HF patients is the prevention of angiotensin II–mediated LV remodeling. ACE inhibitors are first-line therapy for all patients with systolic HF.

Angiotensin II Receptor Blockers (ARBs)

- ACE inhibitors do not completely inhibit renin-angiotensin activation, suggesting that alternative or additional strategies for inhibition (e.g., ARBs) may be useful. Since ARBs are generally more expensive, they are most commonly used as an alternative to ACE inhibitors in patients in whom a cough develops as the result of ACE inhibitor therapy.

KEY POINTS

- Large mortality trials of ACE inhibitors in systolic HF are highlighted in Table 9-2.
- ACE inhibitors reduce ventricular size, increase the LVEF modestly, and reduce symptoms. In the CONSENSUS trial, treatment with enalapril resulted in reduction in LV size. Furthermore, captopril has been shown to attenuate LV dilatation after anterior myocardial infarction.[8]

KEY POINTS

- Large mortality trials of ARBs in systolic HF are highlighted in Table 9-3.
- ARBs can be used in addition to ACE inhibitors in patients with persistent symptoms despite an optimal dose of ACE inhibitor and beta-blocker. However, the risk of adverse effects (e.g., hyperkalemia, increase in serum creatinine, or hypotension) may be increased.
- The Valsartan Heart Failure Trial (Val-HeFT) echocardiographic substudy of 5010 patients with moderate HF demonstrated that valsartan therapy, taken with either an ACE inhibitor or a beta blocker, reversed LV remodeling (decrease in LV end-diastolic dimension and increase in LVEF).[9]

TABLE 9-2 LARGE MORTALITY TRIALS OF ACE INHIBITORS IN SYSTOLIC CONGESTIVE HF

ACE Inhibitor	Trial (Citation)	Mortality Benefit	NYHA Class	Target Dose
Enalapril	CONSENSUS (*N Engl J Med.* 1987;316:1429)	Yes • Mortality reduced by 31% at 1 year	IV	20–40 mg
Enalapril	SOLVD-T (*N Engl J Med.* 1991;325:293)	Yes • Mortality reduced by 16% • Largest reduction among deaths attributed to progressive HF	I–III	20 mg
Enalapril	SOLVD-P (*N Engl J Med.* 1992;327:685)	No • Reduced incidence of HF and hospitalizations	Asymptomatic LV dysfunction	20 mg
Captopril	SAVE (*N Engl J Med.* 1992;327:669)	Yes • 20% relative reduction in mortality	Asymptomatic post–myocardial infarction	150 mg
Ramipril	AIRE (*Lancet.* 1993;342:821)	Yes • 27% relative reduction in mortality	Post–myocardial infarction	10 mg
Trandolapril	TRACE (*N Engl J Med.* 1995;333:1670)	Yes • 22% relative reduction in mortality	Post–myocardial infarction	4 mg

TABLE 9-3 LARGE MORTALITY TRIALS OF ARBS IN SYSTOLIC CONGESTIVE HF

ARB	Trial (Citation)	Mortality Benefit	NYHA Class	Target Dose
Valsartan	VALIANT (*N Engl J Med.* 2003;349:1893)	• Valsartan noninferior to captopril • Combining agents increased risk of adverse effects	Myocardial infarction complicated by LV systolic dysfunction	320 mg
Valsartan	Val-HeFT (*N Engl J Med.* 2001;345:1667)	No • Decreased risk of combined endpoint including HF hospitalizations	II–IV	320 mg
Candesartan	CHARM-Alternative (*Lancet.* 2003;362:772)	Yes • 14% relative reduction in mortality at 1 year in patients intolerant to ACE inhibitors	II–IV	32 mg
Candesartan	CHARM-Added (*Lancet.* 2003;362:767)	Yes • 12% relative reduction in mortality at 1 year in patients also taking ACE inhibitors	II–IV	32 mg

Aldosterone Antagonists

- Aldosterone antagonists can be used as an adjunct for further neurohormonal blockade in patients with systolic HF.

KEY POINTS

- In the RALES trial, there was a 30% decrease in mortality when spironolactone was added to the therapeutic regimen for patients with New York Heart Association (NYHA) class III/IV HF and LVEF ≤ 35%. Spironolactone may exhibit this clinical benefit as a result of improvement in LV volumes and function.[10]
- In the EPHESUS trial, the addition of eplerenone to optimal medical therapy in patients with HF caused by acute myocardial infarction (LVEF ≤ 40%) resulted in a 15% decrease in mortality.[11]
- Recently, the addition of spironolactone in NYHA class I/II HF resulted in beneficial effects on LV remodeling and diastolic function. Specifically, in the spironolactone group, LVEF increased significantly from 35% to 39%, with a decrease in LV end-diastolic and end-systolic volumes and myocardial mass and an improvement in LV diastolic filling pattern.[12]

Hydralazine and Isosorbide Dinitrate

- In African American patients, the response to ACE inhibitors may not be as strong, and hydralazine and isosorbide dinitrate

may have an expanded role in this patient group.
- In the A-HeFT trial, a 40% decrease in mortality was observed in African Americans with NYHA class III/IV HF when isosorbide dinitrate and hydralazine were added to standard treatment.[13]

Diuretics

- Diuretics are used for the relief of dyspnea and fluid retention but do not modify the course of the disease in systolic HF.

Digoxin

- In a trial of systolic HF patients in sinus rhythm, digoxin (added to a diuretic and ACE inhibitor) had no effect on mortality but reduced the risk of hospitalization for HF.

Implantable Cardioverter-Defibrillator (ICD)

- About one half of the deaths in patients with systolic HF are attributed to ventricular arrhythmias. An ICD reduces the risk of sudden cardiac death in patients with LV systolic dysfunction. The benefit of ICD therapy may not be apparent until 1 year or more after implantation of the device.

KEY POINTS

- For primary prevention, the current indications for ICD implantation are:
  - LVEF ≤ 35% despite optimal medical therapy
  - NYHA functional class II or III
  - Expected survival of at least 1 year with a reasonable quality of life and functional status[12]
- For secondary prevention, an ICD is indicated for any patient who survives an unprovoked episode of ventricular fibrillation or sustained ventricular tachycardia.[14]
- The benefit of ICDs is documented for ischemic and nonischemic cardiomyopathies. Following myocardial infarction, early (<40 days) implantation of an ICD does not improve survival.[14]

Cardiac Resynchronization Therapy (CRT)

- Intraventricular conduction delay (IVCD), identified by a 12-lead electrocardiogram QRS interval ≥ 120 ms, occurs in up to one third of patients with systolic HF. IVCD is associated with dyssynchronous LV contraction, leading to impaired emptying and possibly mitral regurgitation (MR).
- CRT may improve cardiac performance by increasing stroke volume and producing reverse remodeling, a process characterized by a reduction in LV volumes leading to improved systolic and diastolic function.[15] CRT has also demonstrated a reduction in functional MR.[16]
- In randomized trials of severe systolic HF, CRT resulted in a reduction in symptoms and improved functional capacity, a reduction in the number of hospitalizations for worsening HF, and increased survival.[17]
- Current guidelines recommend CRT in patients with NYHA functional class III/IV HF, LVEF ≤ 35%, sinus rhythm, and a QRS duration ≥ 120 ms.[14]

KEY POINTS

- In the MADIT-CRT trial,[18] CRT in addition to an ICD in patients with NYHA functional class I/II, LVEF ≤ 30%, and QRS duration ≥ 130 ms resulted in improved LV function and reduced risk of worsening HF, compared to those who received an ICD alone. These effects were most pronounced in patients with a QRS complex ≥ 150 ms.
- In the RethinQ trial,[19] CRT was not shown to increase the primary outcome measure of peak oxygen consumption in patients with NYHA class III symptoms and a narrow (< 120 ms) QRS interval and echocardiographic evidence of dyssynchrony (opposing wall delay > 65 ms; see below).
- Several echocardiographic parameters have been investigated as measures of mechanical dyssynchrony. These involve M-mode measurements as well as tissue Doppler imaging (TDI) for measurement of longitudinal tissue velocity or deformation (strain) of the myocardium. Several of the well-studied parameters of intraventricular dyssynchrony are described here:
  - **M-mode echocardiography:** Septal-posterior wall motion delay (SPWMD), the time difference between peak inward motion of the ventricular septum and the posterior wall, can be obtained from parasternal short axis M-mode images (Figure 9-2A). An initial study showed SPWMD ≥ 130 ms predicted reduction in LV-end systolic volume index greater than 15% with a sensitivity of 100% and specificity of 63% in 20 patients after 1 month of CRT, and predicted improvement in LVEF greater than 5% and better prognosis at 6 months after CRT.[20] However, this parameter was feasible in only one half of patients, and in follow-up reports SPWMD did not predict outcome after CRT.[21]
  - **TDI:** The standard deviation of time to peak systolic velocity among 12 basal segments and mid-LV segments (Ts-SD) has been proposed as a dyssynchrony index.[22] Ts-SD greater than 32.6 ms predicted reverse remodeling 3 months after CRT with a sensitivity and specificity of 100% in the initial 30 patients.[22] A Ts-SD greater than 31.4 ms had a sensitivity of 96% and specificity of 78% in a subsequent 54 patients.[23] Ts-SD was shown to correlate better with reverse remodeling after CRT compared to other dyssynchrony parameters.
  - **TDI:** A basal septal-lateral delay greater than 60 ms in time to peak systolic velocity predicted a short-term improvement in LVEF,[24] and a similar dyssynchrony index (maximum difference in opposing basal segment delay greater than 65 ms; Figure 9-2B) predicted reverse remodeling at 6 months after CRT.[25]
- Interventricular dyssynchrony can also be evaluated to assess coordinated ventricular contraction. It is measured by the preejection period difference between pulsed wave Doppler flow in the aorta and pulmonary artery. This measure correlates with QRS duration and typically exceeds 40 ms in patients with a QRS greater than 150 ms. The CARE-HF research group found that a cutoff value of 49.2 ms separated event-free curves after CRT.[26]
- Although numerous echocardiographic parameters of mechanical dyssynchrony have been

Continued

proposed, no large prospective trial to date has proven the clinical utility of these indices for selecting patients for CRT.

- In the prospective, multicenter PROSPECT trial, 12 echocardiographic parameters of mechanical dyssynchrony were tested to predict CRT response.[27] Indicators of positive CRT response were improved clinical composite score and 15% reduction in LV end-systolic volume at 6 months. The ability of the 12 echocardiographic parameters to predict clinical composite score response varied widely, with sensitivity ranging from 6% to 74% and specificity ranging from 35% to 91%; for predicting LV end-systolic volume response, sensitivity ranged from 9% to 77% and specificity from 31% to 93%.
- At present, no single echocardiographic parameter beyond current guidelines (e.g., LVEF) can be recommended to improve patient selection for CRT. However, ongoing efforts to reduce variability in technical and interpretative factors may improve the predictive powers of these or other newer echocardiographic parameters.
- CRT has been shown to reduce functional MR by producing favorable changes in mitral valve geometry and closing forces on the mitral valve. Specifically, tethering is reduced through reversal of LV remodeling and increasing the systolic duration of peak transmitral closing forces, consistent with improved coordination of LV force generation.[28]
- Potential future directions include the use of real-time 3D echocardiography and 3D speckle tracking echocardiography to assess mechanical dyssynchrony and the site of latest mechanical activation.

Figure 9-2. **A,** M-mode echocardiography with color-coded tissue velocity. *Left panel:* Timing of ventricular septal (VS) wall motion is difficult to define because of its severe hypokinesis and the lack of distinct peaks. *Right panel:* Color coding of tissue velocity helps to identify the exact wall motion timing as the transition point of blue to red color for the septal wall (*arrows*) and red to blue color for the posterior wall (PW; *arrowheads*). **B,** Color-coded tissue Doppler study from three standard apical views of a patient who responded to resynchronization therapy. Time-velocity curves from representative basal or mid-LV levels are shown. Maximum opposing wall delay was seen in the apical long-axis view (140 ms between septum and PW), consistent with significant dyssynchrony (≥ 65 ms). (*A,* Reprinted with permission from Anderson LJ, Miyazaki C, Sutherland GR, Oh JK. Patient selection and echocardiographic assessment of dyssynchrony in cardiac resynchronization therapy. Circulation. 2008;117:2009-2023. *B,* Reprinted with permission from Gorcsan J 3rd, Abraham T, Agler DA, et al. Echocardiography for cardiac resynchronization therapy: recommendations for performance and reporting—a report from the American Society of Echocardiography Dyssynchrony Writing Group endorsed by the Heart Rhythm Society. J Am Soc Echocardiogr. 2008;3:191-213.)

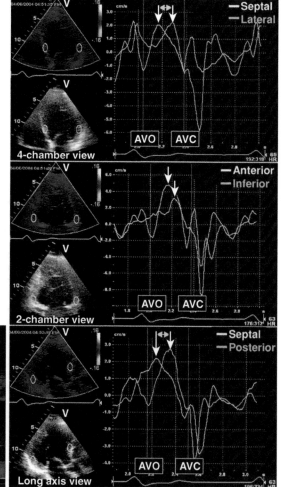

A

B

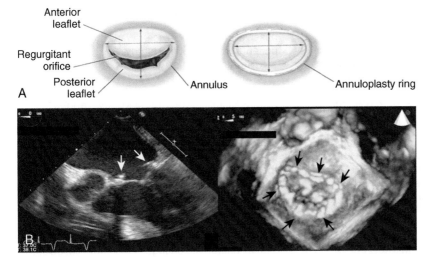

Figure 9-3. **A,** Schematic representation of the position of a mitral annuloplasty ring. **B,** *Left panel:* two-dimensional transesophageal image following mitral ring annuloplasty (*arrows*). *Right panel:* 3D transesophageal echocardiographic image showing mitral valve with ring annuloplasty (*arrows*) as viewed from left atrium. *(Reprinted with permission from www.nature.com/.../v13/n10/images/nm1645-F4.jpg.)*

Novel Devices

MR Reduction and Direct Ventricular Remodeling

- Chronic ischemic MR results from ischemic ventricular distortion with papillarly muscle (PM) displacement and restricted mitral leaflet closure resulting from tethering. The mitral leaflets are structurally normal. *Functional MR* is a more general term to describe MR resulting from ischemic disease or cardiomyopathy. Ischemic MR occurs in up to 30% of patients with postinfarct CHF, and increasing MR severity is associated with a progressively worse 5-year survival rate.[29]

- Restrictive annuloplasty (Figure 9-3), combined with coronary artery bypass grafting (CABG), is currently the most commonly performed surgical procedure to treat ischemic MR, although its impact on late survival and functional class is unproven. Alternative methods for ischemic MR reduction, via percutaneous or surgical approaches, are currently under investigation.[30]

KEY POINTS

- Direct remodeling of the PMs is a potential therapeutic target to reduce ischemic MR. Surgical approaches (both experimentally and in human patients) that reposition the PMs to reduce tethering of the mitral leaflets have been developed in small case series (Figure 9-4A).
- The Coapsys device (Myocor Inc.) was designed to treat mitral annular dilatation and PM displacement using two epicardial pads that are approximated through an internal cord (Figure 9-4B and 9-4C). It has the advantage that it can be placed on a beating heart without cardiopulmonary bypass. One-year follow-up of the first 11 patients with a Coapsys device and off-pump CABG showed effective ischemic MR and NYHA class improvement. Preoperative MR grade 2.9 ± 0.5 was reduced to grade 1.1 ± 0.8 at 1-year follow-up ($p < 0.05$). The RESTOR-MV trial (Randomized Evaluation of a Surgical Treatment for Off-pump Repair of the Mitral Valve) demonstrated a greater decrease in LV end-diastolic dimension and improved survival at 2 years of follow-up with the Coapsys device.[31]

- PM remodeling techniques remain investigational or alternative surgical approaches at the present time.
- Alfieri edge-to-edge mitral valve repair has been applied percutaneously with a clip device (Mitra-Clip; Evalve Inc.). Results from the EVEREST II trial show that the novel MitraClip device may lead to fewer early adverse events than traditional valve repair or replacement, with "noninferior" efficacy out to 1 year.[32]
- EVEREST II enrolled a highly selected group of 279 patients with significant MR (3+ to 4+); 27% of patients had ischemic MR and 73% had degenerative MR. Patients were randomized 2 : 1 to the MitraClip procedure or to surgical repair or replacement at the surgeon's discretion.
- The primary safety endpoint (a combination of adverse events including death, major stroke, reoperation, urgent/emergent surgery, myocardial infarction, renal failure, blood transfusions, and others) in the per-protocol analysis significantly favored the percutaneous

Continued

KEY POINTS—cont'd

procedure at 30 days, with less than 10% of patients experiencing a major adverse event, as compared with 57% of the patients treated surgically ($p < 0.0001$). Need for blood transfusions was the main driver of the safety endpoint, with a difference of 8.8% versus 53.2%.

- For the primary efficacy endpoint in the per-protocol analysis, the overall clinical success rate was numerically higher in the surgery group, at 87.8% compared with 72.4%, but this difference, statistically, met the pre-specified noninferiority hypothesis. However, MR reduction was greater in the surgical group.

- Percutaneous coronary sinus-based mitral valve repair remains under study. In the AMADEUS trial of patients with dilated cardiomyopathy, acute MR reduction (grade 3.0 ± 0.6 to 2.0 ± 0.8, $p < 0.0001$) and permanent implantation were achieved in 30 of 43 patients in whom an attempt was made.[33]

- Cardiac support devices that reduce ventricular wall stress and promote beneficial reverse remodeling have been proposed as an adjunct to mitral valve surgery. The Acorn CorCap (Acorn Cardiovascular, St. Paul, MN; Figure 9-5), an LV passive restraint device, was studied in 193 patients in the ACORN study.[34]

- MR grade was not reduced further by the use of the CorCap device; however, addition of the CorCap device led to greater decreases in LV end-diastolic volume and LV end-systolic volume, and a more elliptical LV shape. These changes were maintained at 3 years of follow-up.

- Direct ventricular remodeling was evaluated in the STITCH trial to address the question of whether surgical ventricular reconstruction (SVR) added to CABG would decrease the rate of death or hospitalization for cardiac causes, as compared with CABG alone.[35]

- Adding SVR reduced ventricular volumes, but this anatomic change was not associated with a greater improvement in symptoms or exercise tolerance or with a reduction in the rate of death or hospitalization for cardiac causes.

- The "Batista operation" (partial left ventriculectomy) showed initial promise as a method to achieve direct ventricular reverse remodeling; however, follow-up studies showed early and late failures of this technique and therefore it is not a recommended treatment.

Figure 9-4. **A,** PM approximation by passing a single U-shaped suture reinforced by two patches of autologous pericardium through the bodies of the posterior and anterior PMs. (**A,** *Reprinted with permission from Rama A, Praschker L, Barreda E, Gandjbakhch I. Papillary muscle approximation for functional ischemic mitral regurgitation. Ann Thorac Surg. 2007;84:2130-2131.* **B,** *Reprinted with permission from Fukamachi K, Inoue M, Popović ZB, et al. Off-pump mitral valve repair using the Coapsys device: a pilot study in a pacing-induced mitral regurgitation model. Ann Thorac Surg. 2004; 77:688-692.* **C,** *Reprinted with permission from Grossi EA, Woo YJ, Schwartz CF, et al. Comparison of Coapsys annuloplasty and internal reduction mitral annuloplasty in the randomized treatment of functional ischemic mitral regurgitation: impact on the left ventricle. J Thorac Cardiovasc Surg. 2006;131: 1095-1098.)*

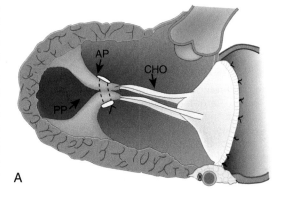

A

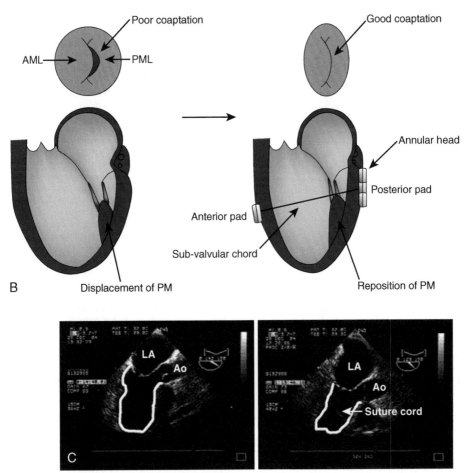

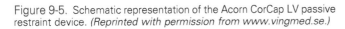

Figure 9-4, cont'd **B,** The Coapsys device (Myocor Inc., Maple Grove, MN) was designed to treat mitral annular dilatation and PM displacement. The device consists of epicardial posterior and anterior pads connected by a flexible subvalvular chord. The two pads are located on the epicardial surface of the heart with the load-bearing subvalvular chord passing through the LV. When the device is tightened under echocardiographic guidance, the annular head increases coaptation and the papillary head repositions the PMs. **C,** Preoperative (*left panel*) and postoperative (*right panel*) echocardiographic views after application of the Coapsys device.

Figure 9-5. Schematic representation of the Acorn CorCap LV passive restraint device. *(Reprinted with permission from www.vingmed.se.)*

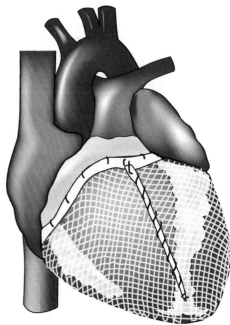

References

1. Douglas PS, Garcia MJ, Haines DE, et al. ACCF/ASE/AHA/ASNC/HFSA/HRS/SCAI/SCCM/SCCT/SCMR 2011 appropriate use criteria for echocardiography. *J Am Coll Cardiol*. 2011;57:1126-1166.
   This document identifies common clinical scenarios in cardiovascular disease and indicates the appropriateness of using echocardiography for diagnosis, treatment, or management. The use of echocardiography is rated as either appropriate, uncertain, or inappropriate.

2. Rihal CS, Nishimura RA, Hatle LK, Bailey KR, Tajik AJ. Systolic and diastolic dysfunction in patients with clinical diagnosis of dilated cardiomyopathy: Relation to symptoms and prognosis. *Circulation*. 1994;90:2772-2779.
   This study reports that, in patients with a clinical diagnosis of cardiomyopathy, LVEF was independently predictive of subsequent mortality. Markers of diastolic function correlated with congestive symptoms.

3. Xie GY, Berk MR, Smith MD, Gurley JC, DeMaria AN. Prognostic value of Doppler transmitral flow patterns in patients with congestive heart failure. *J Am Coll Cardiol*. 1994;24:132-139.
   This study documented that a restrictive transmitral flow pattern by Doppler echocardiography was a predictor of cardiac mortality in patients with congestive HF. Results from this study provided the foundation for making transmitral flow velocity a routine measurement in clinical echocardiography.

4. Sugeng L, Mor-Avi V, Weinert L, et al. Quantitative assessment of left ventricular size and function: Side-by-side comparison of real-time three-dimensional echocardiography and computed tomography with magnetic resonance reference. *Circulation*. 2006;114:654-661.
   3D echocardiography is emerging as a technique to improve quantification of LV geometry and function, and this study is one of the initial clinical studies to show strong correlations between the reference standard of cardiac magnetic resonance imaging with 3D echocardiography (with regard to measurement of LV volumes and LVEF).

5. Nahum J, Bensaid A, Dussault C, et al. Impact of longitudinal myocardial deformation on the prognosis of chronic heart failure patients. *Circ Cardiovasc Imaging*. 2010;3:249-256.
   This study of symptomatic HF patients demonstrated that global longitudinal strain measured by speckle tracking echocardiography was superior to LVEF in predicting major adverse cardiac events. Results from this study indicate that novel echocardiographic measurements may have prognostic significance in HF patients.

6. Hung CL, Verma A, Uno H, et al. Longitudinal and circumferential strain rate, left ventricular remodeling, and prognosis after myocardial infarction. *J Am Coll Cardiol*. 2010;56:1812-1822.
   Participants of the VALIANT (Valsartan in Acute Myocardial Infarction Trial) were studied, and both longitudinal and circumferential strain rates were independent predictors of clinical outcomes after myocardial infarction. Circumferential strain rate was also predictive of ventricular remodeling, indicating that preserved circumferential function may limit ventricular enlargement after myocardial infarction.

7. Maurer MS, Sackner-Bernstein JD, El-Khoury Rumbarger L, Yushak M, King DL, Burkhoff D. Mechanisms underlying improvements in ejection fraction with carvedilol in heart failure. *Circ Heart Fail*. 2009;2:189-196.
   This study used 3D echocardiography to investigate the mechanisms resulting in improved LVEF with chronic beta blocker therapy. In addition to a reduction in heart rate, positive inotropic effects and afterload reduction were shown to contribute to reverse remodeling with carvedilol treatment.

8. Pfeffer MA, Lamas GA, Vaughan DE, et al. Effect of captopril on progressive ventricular dilatation after anterior myocardial infarction. *N Engl J Med*. 1988;319:80-86.
   This double-blind, placebo-controlled study documented that ventricular enlargement after anterior myocardial infarction is progressive, although captopril can prevent ventricular dilatation. Captopril was also shown to reduce filling pressures and improve exercise tolerance.

9. Wong M, Staszewsky L, Latini R, et al. Valsartan benefits left ventricular structure and function in heart failure: Val-HeFT echocardiographic study. *J Am Coll Cardiol*. 2002;40:970-975.
   In this echocardiographic substudy of the large Val-HeFT trial, the addition of an angiotensin receptor blocker to prescribed HF therapy resulted in more favorable cardiac remodeling. The exception was patients already receiving an ACE inhibitor and beta blocker, in whom there was no difference in LV size and function between the angiotensin receptor blocker and placebo groups.

10. Cicoira M, Zanolla L, Rossi A, et al. Long-term, dose-dependent effects of spironolactone on left ventricular function and exercise tolerance in patients with chronic heart failure. *J Am Coll Cardiol*. 2002;40:304-310.
    In an effort to understand the mechanism behind the clinical benefit of spironolactone in HF patients, this study demonstrated that the medication improved LV volumes and function. Exercise tolerance (assessed by cardiopulmonary exercise testing) was also improved.

11. Pitt B, Remme W, Zannad F, et al. Eplerenone, a selective aldosterone blocker, in patients with left ventricular dysfunction after myocardial infarction. *N Engl J Med*. 2003;348:1309-1321.

12. Vizzardi E, D'Aloia A, Giubbini R, et al. Effect of spironolactone on left ventricular ejection fraction and volumes in patients with class I or II heart failure. *Am J Cardiol*. 2010;106:1292-1296.
    The benefits of spironolactone in HF were initially demonstrated in patients with NYHA class III/IV symptoms. This study evaluated NYHA class I or II symptoms and demonstrated improvements in LV volumes as well as measures of systolic and diastolic function.

13. Taylor AL, Ziesche S, Yancy C, et al. Combination of isosorbide dinitrate and hydralazine in blacks with heart failure. *N Engl J Med*. 2004;351:2049-2057.

14. Hunt SA, Abraham WT, Chin MH, et al. 2009 focused update incorporated into the ACC/AHA 2005 Guidelines for the Diagnosis and Management of Heart Failure in Adults: A report of the American College of Cardiology Foundation/American Heart Association Task Force on Practice Guidelines; developed in collaboration with the International Society for Heart and Lung Transplantation. *Circulation*. 2009;119:e391-e479.
    This practice guideline serves as an evidence-based document summarizing the recommendations for care of HF patients. Behavioral, medical, and device-based therapies are addressed.

15. St. John Sutton MG, Keane MG. Reverse remodeling in heart failure with cardiac resynchronization therapy. *Heart*. 2007;93:167-171.
    This review summarizes the role of CRT in the treatment of systolic HF, with a focus on the beneficial effects of CRT on producing favorable changes in LV size and function.

16. St. John Sutton MG, Plappert T, Hilpisch KE, et al. Sustained reverse left ventricular structural remodeling with cardiac resynchronization at one year is a function of etiology: Quantitative Doppler echocardiographic evidence from the Multicenter InSync Randomized Clinical Evaluation (MIRACLE). *Circulation*. 2006;113:266-272.
    In this substudy of the MIRACLE trial, CRT was shown to reduce LV volumes and increase ejection fraction. A reduction in MR was also observed. Findings were more pronounced in patients with nonischemic cardiomyopathy as compared to ischemic cardiomyopathy.

17. Cleland JG, Daubert JC, Erdmann E, et al. The effect of cardiac resynchronization on morbidity and mortality in heart failure. *N Engl J Med.* 2005;352:1539-1549.
In this groundbreaking randomized trial, CRT improved symptoms and quality of life in NYHA class III/IV HF patients, as well as producing a reduction in mortality.

18. Moss AJ, Hall WJ, Cannom DS, et al. Cardiac-resynchronization therapy for the prevention of heart-failure events. *N Engl J Med.* 2009;361:1329-1338.
In this trial of relatively asymptomatic patients (NYHA class I/II), CRT decreased the risk of HF events. This trial supports the recommendation to expand CRT to less symptomatic HF patients with reduced systolic function and a wide QRS complex on electrocardiogram.

19. Beshai JF, Grimm RA, Nagueh SF, et al. Cardiac-resynchronization therapy in heart failure with narrow QRS complexes. *N Engl J Med.* 2007;357:2461-2471.
Since a subset of HF patients have evidence of mechanical dyssynchrony despite a narrow QRS complex, this trial sought to examine the effect of CRT in such patients. However, CRT did not improve peak oxygen consumption in HF patients with a narrow QRS.

20. Pitzalis MV, Iacoviello M, Romito R, et al. Ventricular asynchrony predicts a better outcome in patients with chronic heart failure receiving cardiac resynchronization therapy. *J Am Coll Cardiol.* 2005;45:65-69.
In an effort to predict response to CRT, this study investigated the M-mode echocardiographic parameter defining the time difference between peak inward motion of the ventricular septum and the posterior wall (SPWMD). This parameter predicted response to CRT in this study of 60 patients.

21. Marcus GM, Rose E, Viloria EM, et al. Septal to posterior wall motion delay fails to predict reverse remodeling or clinical improvement in patients undergoing cardiac resynchronization therapy. *J Am Coll Cardiol.* 2005;46: 2208-2214.
In this retrospective analysis of the CONTAK-CD trial, the SPWMD did not predict response to CRT. This study failed to reproduce the findings from previous smaller studies with shorter follow-up.

22. Yu CM, Fung WH, Lin H, et al. Predictors of left ventricular reverse remodeling after cardiac resynchronization therapy for heart failure secondary to idiopathic dilated or ischemic cardiomyopathy. *Am J Cardiol.* 2003;91: 684-688.
This study evaluated a dyssynchrony index (standard deviation to peak systolic velocity among 12 basal and mid-LV segments) and showed that a preimplantation index value of 32.6 ms was able to segregate responders from nonresponders to CRT. Additionally, the dyssynchrony index was an independent predictor of reverse remodeling.

23. Yu CM, Fung JW, Zhang Q, et al. Tissue Doppler imaging is superior to strain rate imaging and postsystolic shortening on the prediction of reverse remodeling in both ischemic and nonischemic heart failure after cardiac resynchronization therapy. *Circulation.* 2004;110:66-73.
This study of nonischemic and ischemic HF patients showed that the TDI parameter of standard deviation to peak systolic velocity among 12 basal and mid-LV segments was a predictor of reverse remodeling at 3 months of follow-up. Strain-rate imaging parameters did not predict reverse remodeling.

24. Bax JJ, Marwick TH, Molhoek SG, et al. Left ventricular dyssynchrony predicts benefit of cardiac resynchronization therapy in patients with end-stage heart failure before pacemaker implantation. *Am J Cardiol.* 2003;92:1238-1240.
In this study of end-stage HF patients, a delay in the time to peak systolic velocity between the basal septum and lateral wall of greater than 60 ms predicted improvement in LVEF.

25. Bax JJ, Bleeker GB, Marwick TH, et al. Left ventricular dyssynchrony predicts response and prognosis after cardiac resynchronization therapy. *J Am Coll Cardiol.* 2004;44: 1834-1840.
This study followed the effect of CRT out to 6 months of follow-up, and demonstrated that a dyssynchrony index (maximal difference in opposing basal segment delay > 65 ms) predicted response to CRT and portended a more favorable prognosis.

26. Richardson M, Freemantle N, Calvert MJ, et al. Predictors and treatment response with cardiac resynchronization therapy in patients with heart failure characterized by dyssynchrony: A pre-defined analysis from the CARE-HF trial. *Eur Heart J.* 2007;28:1827-1834.
In this analysis of the CARE-HF trial, the presence of interventricular dyssynchrony identified patients more likely to respond to CRT. This trial measured the preejection period difference in the aorta and pulmonary artery, a measurement of interventricular dyssynchrony (as opposed to intraventricular dyssynchrony).

27. Chung ES, Leon AR, Tavazzi L, et al. Results of the Predictors of Response to CRT (PROSPECT) trial. *Circulation.* 2008;117:2608-2616.
Given numerous single-center studies reporting the benefit of using echocardiographically derived parameters of dyssynchrony to predict response to CRT, this multicenter study was conducted. This study showed that there was large variability in the analysis of dyssynchrony parameters, and the ability of the parameters to predict CRT response varied widely. Therefore, none of the echocardiographic parameters studied here are currently recommended for use in selecting patients for CRT.

28. Solis J, McCarty D, Levine RA, et al. Mechanism of decrease in mitral regurgitation after cardiac resynchronization therapy: Optimization of the force-balance relationship. *Circ Cardiovasc Imaging.* 2009;6:444-450.
This study sought to evaluate the mechanisms by which CRT can reduce the degree of MR. Results demonstrated that CRT reduces leaflet tethering and increases the systolic duration of peak transmitral closing pressures.

29. Grigioni F, Enriquez-Sarano M, Zehr KJ, et al. Ischemic mitral regurgitation: Long-term outcome and prognostic implications with quantitative Doppler assessment. *Circulation.* 2001;103:1759-1764.
This study of over 300 patients after myocardial infarction helped document the common prevalence of ischemic MR and its association with negative clinical outcomes.

30. Bouma W, van der Horst IC, Wijdh-den Hamer IJ, et al. Chronic ischaemic mitral regurgitation: Current treatment results and new mechanism-based surgical approaches. *Eur J Cardiothorac Surg.* 2010;37:170-185.
This article highlights surgical approaches to reduce the degree of ischemic MR. Visual representations of the anatomy and surgical repair techniques are provided.

31. Grossi EA, Patel N, Woo YJ, et al. Outcomes of the RESTOR-MV Trial (Randomized Evaluation of a Surgical Treatment for Off-Pump Repair of the Mitral Valve). *J Am Coll Cardiol.* 2010;56:1984-1993.
This study evaluated the use of the Coapsys device and demonstrated that ventricular reshaping (in addition to revascularization) decreased adverse outcomes and improved survival in patients with functional MR.

32. Feldman T, Foster E, Glower DD, et al. Percutaneous repair or surgery for mitral regurgitation. *N Engl J Med.* 2011;364:1395-1406.

33. Siminiak T, Hoppe UC, Schofer J, et al. Effectiveness and safety of percutaneous coronary sinus-based mitral valve repair in patients with dilated cardiomyopathy (from the AMADEUS trial). *Am J Cardiol.* 2009;104:565-570.
Coronary sinus-based mitral valve repair represents a novel percutaneous technique designed to reduce the degree of MR. This study demonstrated feasibility of this technique.

34. Acker MA, Bolling S, Shemin R, et al. Mitral valve surgery in heart failure: Insights from the ACORN Clinical Trial. *J Thorac Cardiovasc Surg.* 2006;132:568-577.
This study evaluated the CorCap cardiac support device, which is designed to reduce ventricular wall stress and promote beneficial reverse remodeling. Results showed that the CorCap produced a more elliptical shape of the LV along with decreased volumes.

35. Jones RH, Velazquez EJ, Michler RE, et al. Coronary bypass surgery with or without surgical ventricular reconstruction. *N Engl J Med.* 2009;360:1705-1717.
This landmark study of 1000 patients showed that adding SVR to CABG did not improve clinical outcomes, although it did reduce LV volumes.

Echocardiography in the Patient with Right Heart Failure

10

Anjali Tiku Owens and Martin St. John Sutton

Basic Principles of Right Ventricular Imaging

Step-by-Step Approach
Step 1: Analysis of Right Ventricular Size

KEY POINTS

- Obtain two-dimensional (2D) images utilizing parasternal, right ventricular (RV) inflow, apical 4-chamber, and subcostal views.
- The RV has a crescent shape, with no accurate geometric representation.
  - Measure RV basal, midcavity, and longitudinal dimensions from the apical 4-chamber view (Figure 10-1).
  - The upper reference limits for the RV are: basal dimension, 4.2 cm; midcavity, 3.5 cm; longitudinal dimension, 8.6 cm.
- Assess the size of the RV in relation to the left ventricle (LV) from the apical 4-chamber view.

- Normal size—RV smaller than LV and does not participate in forming the apex of the heart
- Mildly enlarged—RV size still smaller than LV size
- Moderately enlarged—RV size equal to LV size
- Severely enlarged—RV size bigger than LV size
- Measure right ventricular free wall thickness (Figure 10-2).
  - Normal thickness—≤ 0.5 cm in the subcostal view

Step 2: Analysis of RV Volume and Systolic Function

KEY POINTS

- For volume measurements using area-length and Simpson's rule, assumptions of geometric shape are necessary and may not be accurate.
- Estimate RV systolic function qualitatively: normal, mildly reduced, moderately reduced, or severely reduced
- Estimate RV systolic function quantitatively using a combination of the following methods.
  - Right ventricular fractional area change (RVFAC) can be calculated using the following formula:

RVFAC (%) = (end-diastolic area – end-systolic area)/end-diastolic area × 100%

Using the apical 4-chamber view with focus on the RV, trace the RV volume from the tricuspid annulus down the free wall to the apex and back along the septum; tricuspid leaflets, trabeculations, and chords are regarded as cavity.

RVFAC = 35% is the lower limit of normal in reference studies.
- On RV tissue Doppler, normal pulsed wave Doppler peak velocity at the tricuspid annulus is greater than 10 cm/s.
- Tricuspid annular plane systolic excursion (TAPSE) can be calculated from the apical 4-chamber view using M-mode and 2D techniques (see "Measurement of Prognostic Echocardiographic Parameters" below).
- Radionuclide ventriculography has been utilized historically for comparison with newer methods. However, due to the unique shape of the RV, three-dimensional (3D) echocardiography and cardiac magnetic resonance imaging (MRI) are best suited for accurate assessments of volume and systolic function (RV ejection fraction [RVEF]). These methods can be time consuming and are not widely available.

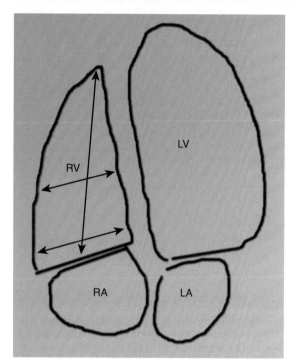

Figure 10-1. Schematic from the apical view of a normal heart showing measurement of RV basal, midcavity, and longitudinal dimensions (*arrows*). *(Courtesy of Ted Plappert.)*

Step 3: Evaluation of RV Wall Motion

KEY POINTS

- Septal and free wall motion should be assessed in multiple 2D views, including parasternal short-axis, apical 4-chamber, and subcostal views.
- RV volume and/or pressure overload can cause septal wall motion abnormality.
  - Pressure overload of the RV causes flattening of the interventricular septum as a result of an abnormal pressure gradient between the RV and the LV, in essence pushing the septum toward the LV during both in systole and in diastole (Figure 10-3). Normally, when viewed in the parasternal short axis, the LV has the appearance of a symmetrical O or "doughnut." With RV pressure or volume overload, the septum is D-shaped.
  - Volume overload of the RV results in flattening of the interventricular septum during diastole only.
  - The degree of septal flattening correlates approximately with the severity of pulmonary hypertension.
- Free wall motion should be assessed for regional wall motion abnormalities suggestive of RV infarction versus global wall motion abnormality.
  - Septal and free wall thickening and endocardial excursion should be examined in multiple 2D views.

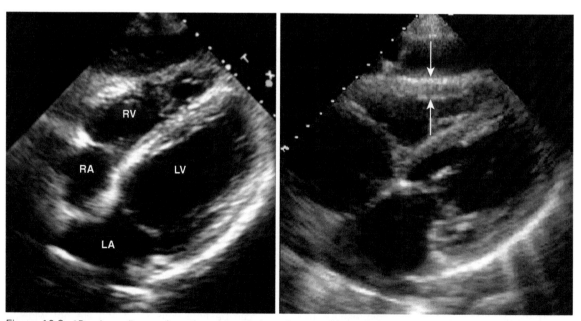

Figure 10-2. 2D echocardiogram from the subcostal view of a normal heart (*left panel*) and the heart in a patient with RV hypertrophy (*right panel*) showing measurement of RV free wall thickness (*arrows*).

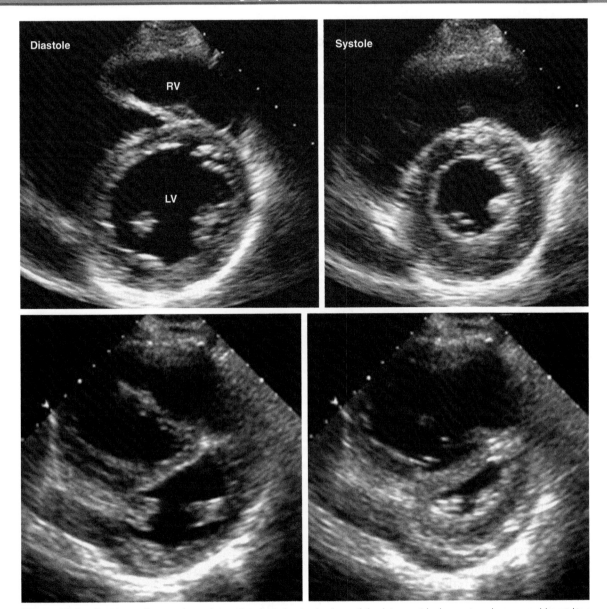

Figure 10-3. 2D echocardiogram from the parasternal short-axis view of the interventricular septum in a normal heart (*top panels*) and the heart from a patient with RV volume and pressure overload (*bottom panels*) during diastole (*left panels*) and systole (*right panels*). Note the D-shaped LV in the *bottom panels,* illustrating shift of the septum toward the LV.

Step 4: Evaluation of Tricuspid Valve Regurgitation

KEY POINTS

- Tricuspid regurgitation often accompanies significant right heart dysfunction and should be assessed along with function of the RV (see Chapters 2 and 6).
- Interrogation of the tricuspid regurgitation jet using Doppler is used to calculate the estimated pulmonary artery systolic pressure (PASP) (see "Measurement of Prognostic Echocardiographic Parameters" below).

Identify the Cause of Right Heart Failure

RV Infarction

- RV infarction is relatively rare. The vast majority of RV infarctions occur in the setting of acute inferior myocardial infarction.
- Obtaining right-sided electrocardiographic (ECG) leads in acute inferior myocardial infarction often helps in making the diagnosis.
- The characteristic hemodynamic sensitivity to alterations in preload is a hallmark of RV infarction and impacts upon treatment strategies.

Step-by-Step Approach
Step 1: Assess LV Wall Motion and Systolic Function, and Look for Mechanical Complications of Myocardial Infarction

KEY POINTS

- Often, the inferior wall motion abnormality is mild, with preserved overall LV function.
- Occasionally, a ventricular septal defect (VSD) resulting in left-to-right shunting, or papillary muscle rupture with severe mitral regurgitation, will complicate an inferior myocardial infarction. In these situations, RV dysfunction can be exacerbated by volume overload.

Step 2: Assess the Right Heart

KEY POINTS

- Dilatation of the RV with global or regional wall motion abnormality is common.
- Acute RV dysfunction can be a result of true myocardial infarction, or more commonly, ischemia that improves in time with supportive care.
- Acute RV dysfunction and dilatation also occur with acute pulmonary embolism.
- Annular dilatation with secondary tricuspid regurgitation is frequently encountered.
- Occasionally, right-to-left shunting through a patent foramen ovale (PFO) will result in oxygen desaturation and clinical deterioration.

Pulmonary Arterial Hypertension

- There are many etiologies of secondary pulmonary hypertension (Box 10-1). When pulmonary hypertension is suspected, a detailed search for an underlying cause should be performed. This section refers specifically to the evaluation of pulmonary arterial hypertension.
- Chronic pressure overload of the RV resulting from high pulmonary vascular resistance (PVR) results in pulmonary hypertension.
- There are echocardiographic signs of pulmonary hypertension that can be helpful in making the diagnosis and assessing disease progression and response to treatment.
- Echocardiography can be used to estimate PASP, pulmonary artery diastolic pressure (PADP), and PVR noninvasively (see "Measurement of Prognostic Echocardiographic Parameters" below).

BOX 10-1   Etiologies of Pulmonary Hypertension

- Diseases that cause elevated pulmonary venous pressure
- Acute and chronic pulmonary embolism
- Intrinsic lung disease
- Disorders that cause intracardiac shunting
- Primary pulmonary hypertension

Step-by-Step Approach
Step 1: Assess RV Size and Function

KEY POINTS

- The RV initially enlarges and hypertrophies as a compensatory response to pressure overload.
- RV function is often preserved or hyperdynamic during this phase of disease and can be assessed using TAPSE and qualitative estimation.
- With progressive increase in RV afterload, the RV initially hypertrophies and then dilates and the normal tricuspid valve geometry is disrupted, resulting in tricuspid regurgitation and systolic dysfunction leading to RV failure (Figure 10-4).

Step 2: Look for Associated Right Heart Findings of Pulmonary Hypertension

KEY POINTS

- Tricuspid regurgitation due to annular dilatation is common.
- Right atrial (RA) enlargement is often present.
- M-mode of the pulmonic valve reveals a diminished or absent *a* wave.
- M-mode of the pulmonic valve reveals midsystolic closure—the "flying W" sign (Figure 10-5).
- Doppler velocity curve of the RV outflow tract (RVOT)/PA has mid-systolic "notching" (Figure 10-6).
- The main PA may be enlarged (>2.5 cm) and should be measured from the left parasternal acoustic window if 2D image quality permits.
- There are septal wall motion abnormalities suggestive of RV pressure overload (described earlier in "Basic Principles of Right Ventricular Imaging").
- Left heart filling abnormalities including reduced mitral valve E/A ratio can be seen.
- In cases of severe pulmonary hypertension and RA enlargement, stretching of the foramen ovale may result in a right-to-left shunt.
- In advanced cases of PA hypertension, a pericardial effusion can be seen. Because of elevated RV pressure and hypertrophy, frank tamponade rarely occurs.
- Compression of the LV with impaired filling is a poor prognostic sign (Figure 10-7).

Step 3: Calculate PASP, PADP, and PVR
- See "Measurement of Prognostic Echocardiographic Parameters" below.

Acute Pulmonary Embolism
- Acute pulmonary embolism can cause right heart failure due to sudden increase in PVR.

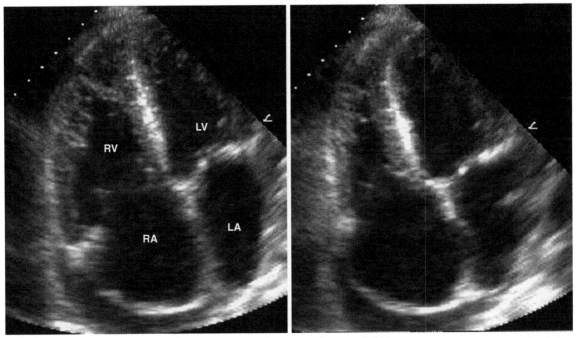

Figure 10-4. 2D echocardiogram from the apical 4-chamber view showing severe RV dilatation that is apex-forming and marked dysfunction typical of end-stage RV failure (*left panel* in diastole, *right panel* in systole).

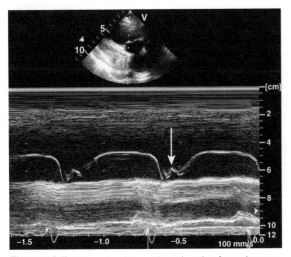

Figure 10-5. M-mode of the pulmonic valve from the parasternal short-axis view. Note the midsystolic closure of the valve (*arrow*) that can be seen with significant pulmonary hypertension. *Courtesy of Amresh Raina, MD.*

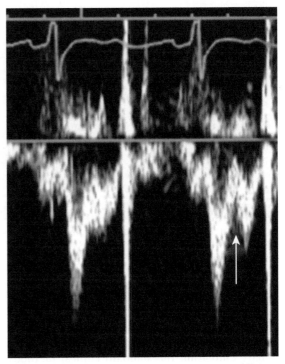

Figure 10-6. Pulsed wave Doppler of the RVOT in a patient with pulmonary hypertension resulting in pulmonary vascular disease. Note the midsystolic "notch" that can be observed with significant pulmonary vascular disease (*arrow*).

- The degree of pulmonary hypertension that occurs acutely is often less severe than that which can occur over time with chronic causes of pulmonary hypertension.
- In acute pulmonary embolism, there is no time for compensatory changes. Moderate to

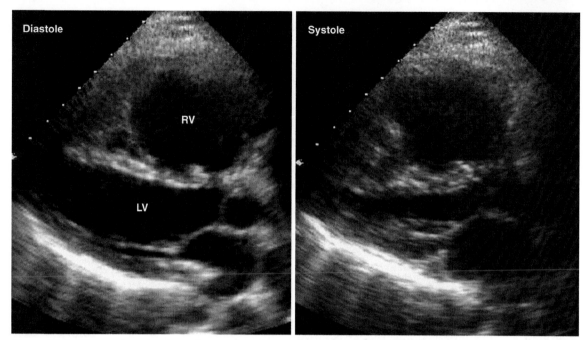

Figure 10-7. 2D transthoracic echocardiogram from the parasternal long-axis view showing a compressed, underfilled LV in a patient with severe RV dilatation and dysfunction.

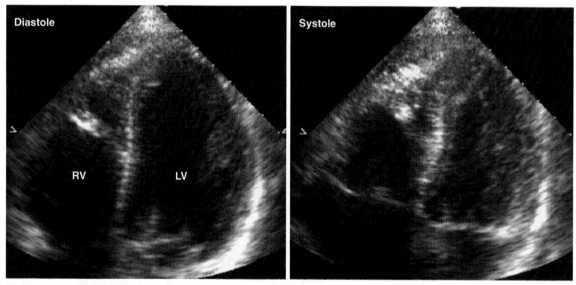

Figure 10-8. 2D transthoracic echocardiogram from the apical 4-chamber view of the RV in the setting of acute pulmonary embolism. Note that the RV forms the apex of the heart (*left panel*). In this example of McConnell's sign, there is preserved systolic function of only the apical segment of the RV (*right panel*).

severe elevations in PASP can be seen in association with clinically relevant right heart failure.

- Although echocardiography can be helpful in the diagnosis and treatment of acute pulmonary embolism, the standard clinical methods of diagnosis are computed tomography of the chest with intravenous contrast or radionuclide lung ventilation-perfusion scan. Only rarely is pulmonary angiography needed for diagnosis.

Step-by-Step Approach
Step 1: Assess RV Size, Shape, and Function

KEY POINTS
• The RV is often dilated with acute systolic dysfunction. • Septal motion reveals signs of pressure and/or volume overload. • A classic finding is McConnell's sign: a dilated, apex-forming RV with preserved systolic function of only the apical segment (Figure 10-8).

Step 2: Look for Associated Findings That Can Accompany Acute Pulmonary Embolism

- The RA may be normal in size due to the acute nature of the insult.
- There may be associated tricuspid regurgitation.
- Rarely, a pulmonary embolus can be visualized in the pulmonary artery from the 2D parasternal short-axis view. Color Doppler may reveal turbulent flow in the PA.
- An attempt should be made to look for thrombus in the RA and inferior vena cava (IVC).
- The LV usually functions normally or is underfilled with hyperdynamic function.

Step 3: Calculate PA Systolic Pressure

- See "Measurement of Prognostic Echocardiographic Parameters" below.

Intracardiac Shunt

- Abnormal intracardiac communications can cause right heart dysfunction and should be looked for carefully in the evaluation of right heart enlargement and pulmonary hypertension.
- If transthoracic images do not adequately exclude intracardiac shunting, transesophageal echocardiography (TEE) should be performed.
- The volume and direction of blood flow are determined by the size of the communication, the pressure gradient between the two chambers, and the resistance to flow in the distal vascular beds.

- Atrial septal defects (ASDs) and partial anomalous pulmonary venous return can cause left-to-right shunting and chronic volume overload of the RA and RV.
- VSDs can cause left-to-right shunting. RV size may remain normal, because blood flows from the LV to the RV and almost immediately into the PA during systole.
- Rarely, a coronary artery fistula to the RV can lead to RV dilatation. Turbulent flow in the RV can be visualized with color Doppler and, if 2D imaging is optimal, a dilated coronary artery is seen.
- Over time, especially if the pulmonary-to-systemic shunt ratio exceeds 2:1, pulmonary pressures and PVR increase. Irreversible pulmonary hypertension and right heart failure can occur.

Step-by-Step Approach
Step 1: Assess RA and RV Size

- With significant left-to-right shunting through an ASD or anomalous pulmonary venous return, the RA and RV should be enlarged. Right heart size is best evaluated from the apical and subcostal views.
- Normal RV size can be seen with VSD.

Step 2: Assess RV Function (described above)
Step 3: Look for Intracardiac Shunting

- ASDs include ostium primum, ostium secundum, sinus venosus, and coronary sinus defects.
- Evaluate the interatrial septum with 2D and color Doppler in the parasternal short-axis, apical 4-chamber, and subcostal 4-chamber views to look for an ASD. Flow across the atrial septum, if present, will be of low velocity because of the small pressure gradient between the left atrium (LA) and RA.
- Identification of pulmonary vein flow into the LA can be evaluated from the apical 4-chamber view. However, in adults, it is usually not possible to visualize all four pulmonary veins. TEE should be performed to visualize pulmonary vein flow if suspicion for partial anomalous pulmonary venous return is high.
- It is often difficult to visualize a sinus venosus ASD using TTE. The suprasternal, apical, and subcostal views should be used, with the subcostal

view most likely to visualize a defect. In addition, sinus venosus ASDs are usually associated with partial anomalous pulmonary venous return. TEE should be performed for adequate visualization.
- Most commonly, the right upper or middle pulmonary veins drain directly into the right atrium or into the superior vena cava.
- Evaluate the interventricular septum with 2D and color Doppler in the parasternal long-axis, parasternal short-axis, apical 4-chamber, and subcostal views to look for a VSD. Because of the large pressure gradient between the LV and RV, interventricular flow is typically high velocity. A notable exception is a large non-restrictive VSD, where pressure has equalized between the LV and RV (Eisenmenger syndrome).
- An estimate of the pressure gradient between the two chambers can be calculated using the peak velocity of the blood flow across the VSD,

Continued

where $\Delta P = 4v^2$. Doppler analysis should be undertaken in multiple views to optimize intercept angle.

- Shunt flow can be quantified noninvasively using the Qp/Qs ratio (see Chapter 6):

$$Qp/Qs = \frac{\text{(cross-sectional area of the PA)} \times \text{(VTI of the PA)}}{\text{(cross-sectional area of the LVOT)} \times \text{(VTI of the LVOT)}}$$

where Qp is blood flow in the pulmonary circulation, Qs is blood flow in the system circulation, VTI is the velocity-time integral, PA is the pulmonary artery, and LVOT is the left ventricular outflow tract.

- Perform agitated saline contrast injection to look for evidence of right-to-left flow across an ASD or PFO.
  - The apical 4-chamber or subcostal view generally works best, keeping in mind that recording should continue for several seconds to ascertain timing of flow.
  - Often, multiple injections of agitated saline are needed, during normal respiration, cough, and/or Valsalva maneuver.
  - If late passage of contrast (after 5 beats) is observed, this suggests the presence of pulmonary arteriovenous malformations rather than an ASD or PFO.

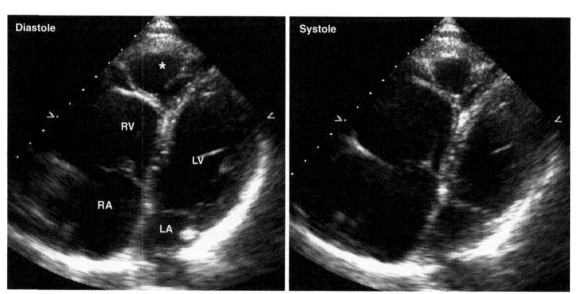

Figure 10-9. 2D transthoracic echocardiogram from the apical view of the RV in ARVC. Note that the RV is severely enlarged and deformed with focal aneurysm (*asterisk*). Fibro-fatty infiltration of the free wall can be seen with MRI. Patients often present with abnormal ECG and ventricular arrhythmias.

Step 4: Calculate PASP, PADP, and PVR

- See "Measurement of Prognostic Echocardiographic Parameters" below.

Right-Sided Valvular Disease

- Primary tricuspid and pulmonary valve disease can cause secondary right heart abnormalities. These entities should be included in the differential diagnosis of right heart failure.

Cardiomyopathy Affecting the RV

- When evaluating potential primary causes of right heart dysfunction, nonischemic dilated cardiomyopathy, arrhythmogenic RV

cardiomyopathy (ARVC), infiltrative disease, and restrictive cardiomyopathy should be in the differential diagnosis.

- Classic findings of ARVC on echocardiography include an enlarged and dysfunctional RV with focal wall motion abnormalities and free wall aneurysms (Figure 10-9). Adipose and fibrous tissue infiltration of the RV free wall is seen on pathology. In a minority of ARVC cases, the LV is also affected. If echocardiography is not conclusive, cardiac MRI can be helpful in establishing the diagnosis noninvasively.
- Infiltrative disease, including hemochromatosis and amyloid, can affect both ventricles.

Measurement of Prognostic Echocardiographic Parameters

PA Systolic Pressure
- PASP can be calculated noninvasively using echocardiography.
- Two components are needed to calculate PASP.
  - The first is the pressure gradient between the RV and RA, which is ascertained by measuring the peak velocity of the tricuspid regurgitation jet (V_{TR}).
  - The second is an estimate of RA pressure (RAP), described below.

Step-by-Step Approach
Step 1: Record Maximum V_{TR}

KEY POINTS
- Using 2D and color-guided continuous wave Doppler in multiple views, find the maximum V_{TR} (Figure 10-10). - Care should be taken to obtain a parallel intercept angle between the regurgitation jet and the ultrasound beam.

Step 2: Estimate RAP Noninvasively

KEY POINTS
- RA pressure can be estimated from the degree of collapse of the IVC during inspiration. - Using 2D from the subcostal window, measure the diameter of the IVC (Figure 10-11). - Using 2D and M-mode, estimate the degree of IVC collapse during inspiration (Figure 10-12). - Estimate the RAP from IVC collapse (Table 10-1). The simplest method of estimating RAP is to look at the degree of inspiratory IVC collapse alone. More sophisticated estimates include IVC size, RA size, and degree of tricuspid regurgitation.

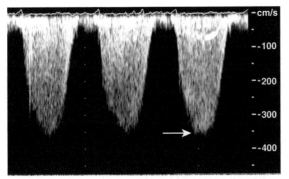

Figure 10-10. Continuous wave Doppler of the tricuspid regurgitation jet. Maximum V_{TR} should be measured (*arrow*) in multiple views to calculate PASP.

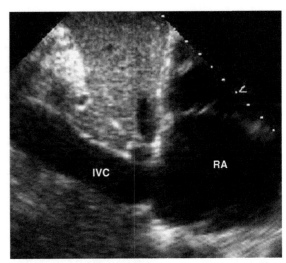

Figure 10-11. 2D echocardiogram from the subcostal view showing the IVC emptying into the RA. The size of the IVC can be measured from this view.

Step 3: Calculate PASP Using V_{TR} and RAP

KEY POINTS

- In the absence of pulmonary valve stenosis, $PASP = RAP + 4(V_{TR})^2$
- Assess severity of pulmonary hypertension.
  - Mild pulmonary hypertension: PASP 30 to 40 mm Hg
  - Moderate pulmonary hypertension: PASP 40 to 60 mm Hg
  - Severe pulmonary hypertension: PASP greater than 60 mm Hg
- Correlation with invasive measurement of PASP using PA catheterization is highly dependent on the presence and quality of the tricuspid regurgitation jet.
- Absence of tricuspid regurgitation does not exclude the presence of significant pulmonary hypertension.
- Agitated saline contrast injection can be used to enhance a faint V_{TR} signal.
- Invasive measurement of PASP should be pursued if pulmonary hypertension is suspected or if there is a discrepancy between clinical findings and noninvasive measurement of PASP.

PA Diastolic Pressure
- PADP can be estimated noninvasively using the spectral Doppler profile of the pulmonary valve regurgitation jet.

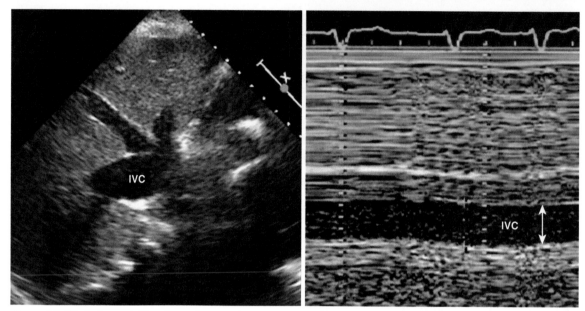

Figure 10-12. *Left panel:* 2D echocardiogram of the IVC from the subcostal view. Collapse of the IVC can be visualized if imaged during inspiration versus expiration. *Right panel:* M-mode through the IVC. M-mode is used to measure the extent of inspiratory IVC collapse (*double-headed arrow*).

TABLE 10-1 ESTIMATES OF RAP FROM IVC COLLAPSE	
Degree of Inspiratory IVC Collapse	**Estimated RAP**
Full collapse	5 mm Hg
Greater than 50% collapse	10 mm Hg
Less than 50% collapse	15 mm Hg
No collapse	20 mm Hg

Step-by-Step Approach
Step 1: Measure the End-Diastolic Velocity of the Pulmonary Valve Regurgitation Jet

KEY POINTS

- Using the parasternal short-axis view, obtain 2D and color Doppler–guided continuous wave Doppler of the pulmonary valve regurgitation jet.
- Measure the end-diastolic velocity of the regurgitation jet.
- Calculate the PADP using the simplified Bernoulli equation:

$$PADP = 4(\text{end-diastolic velocity of pulmonic regurgitation jet})^2 + \text{estimated RAP}$$

Pulmonary Vascular Resistance

- Elevated PASP does not equal elevated PVR in all cases.
- Elevated PA pressure can be due to high flow without elevated PVR, which is an important

distinguishing point when determining therapy for pulmonary hypertension.
- There are noninvasive methods to estimate PVR; however, they are not sufficiently reliable to take the place of invasive measurement by pulmonary artery catheterization, especially in patients with suspected pulmonary vascular disease.

Step-by-Step Approach
Step 1: Measure Peak V_{TR} (described above)
Step 2: Measure the RVOT VTI

KEY POINTS

- The RVOT VTI can be measured best from the parasternal short-axis view.
- Care should be taken to align the Doppler near the center of the RVOT.

Step 3: Calculate Noninvasive PVR

- $PVR = V_{TR}/RVOT\ VTI \times 10 + 0.16$
- A normal noninvasive PVR is less than 1.5 Wood units.

Spectral Doppler of RVOT

- Characteristics of the spectral Doppler of the RVOT can be used to estimate severity of pulmonary hypertension.
- Mid-systolic notching pattern seen in the RVOT spectral Doppler profile is suggestive of significant pulmonary vascular disease (see Figure 10-6).

- Acceleration time, or time to peak systolic velocity, of the RVOT spectral Doppler can also be measured to estimate severity of pulmonary hypertension.

Step-by-Step Approach
Step 1: Record Spectral Doppler from the RVOT from the Parasternal Short-Axis View
Step 2: Measure Time from Onset of Ejection to Peak Systolic Velocity

KEY POINTS

- Usually acceleration time is slower in the RVOT than the LVOT.
- Acceleration time in the RVOT is greater than 140 ms in normal adults and shortens with increasing pulmonary hypertension.
- Acceleration time of less than 70 to 90 ms is suggestive of severe pulmonary hypertension.

Tricuspid Annular Plane Systolic Excursion
- TAPSE measures the distance that the tricuspid annulus moves longitudinally during systole and as such is a measure of RV function.
- It has been validated against other measures of RV function such as radionuclide angiography, RVFAC, and RVEF.
- Normal TAPSE is greater than 1.6 cm.

Step-by-Step Approach
Step 1: Image the RV from the Apical 4-Chamber View with RV Focus
Step 2: Using M-mode through the Lateral Tricuspid Annulus, Measure the Distance of Longitudinal Movement of the Tricuspid Annulus during Systole (Figure 10-13)

Suggested Readings
1. Abbas AE, Fortuin FD, Schiller NB, Appleton CP, Moreno CA, Lester SJ. A simple method for noninvasive estimation of pulmonary vascular resistance. *J Am Coll Cardiol.* 2003;41:1021-1027.
   Simultaneous Doppler echocardiographic examination and right-heart catheterization were performed in 44 patients. The ratio of peak tricuspid regurgitant velocity to the right ventricular outflow tract time-velocity integral was then correlated with invasive measurements of pulmonary vascular resistance.
2. Arkles JS, Opotowsky AR, Ojeda J, et al. Shape of the RV Doppler envelope predicts hemodynamics and right heart function in pulmonary hypertension. *Am J Respir Crit Care Med.* 2011;183:268-276.
   In this referral population, the authors correlated visual inspection of the shape of the RVOT Doppler envelope with invasive hemodynamics. Mid-systolic notching was associated with the most severe pulmonary vascular disease.
3. Armstrong WF, Ryan T, Feigenbaum H. *Feigenbaum's Echocardiography.* 7th ed. Philadelphia: Wolters Kluwer Health/Lippincott Williams & Wilkins; 2010.
   This is a comprehensive textbook of echocardiography.

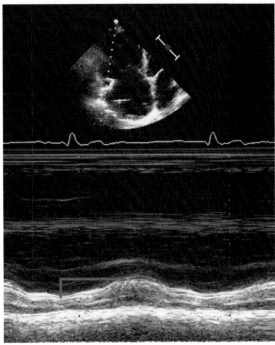

Figure 10-13. *Top panel:* 2D echocardiogram of the RV from the apical view. *Bottom panel:* M-mode through the lateral tricuspid annulus is used to measure the longitudinal TAPSE during systole (vertical segment of L-shaped marker).

4. Ghio S, Klersy C, Magrini G, et al. Prognostic relevance of the echocardiographic assessment of right ventricular function in patients with idiopathic pulmonary arterial hypertension. *Int J Cardiol.* 2010;140:272-278.
   The authors looked at 59 patients referred for idiopathic pulmonary arterial hypertension. They found that assessment of RV systolic and diastolic function based on TAPSE, left ventricular diastolic eccentricity index and degree of tricuspid regurgitation allowed accurate prognostic stratification of patients with idiopathic pulmonary arterial hypertension.
5. Hausmann D, Daniel WG, Mugge A, Ziemer G, Pearlman AS. Value of transesophageal color Doppler echocardiography for detection of different types of atrial septal defect in adults. *J Am Soc Echocardiogr.* 1992;5:481-488.
   This study in 121 patients showed that compared with transthoracic echocardiography, the transesophageal approach was superior for the detection of small secundum atrial septal defects, sinus venosus defects, and partial anomalous pulmonary venous return.
6. Kitabatake A, Inoue M, Asao M, et al. Noninvasive evaluation of pulmonary hypertension by a pulsed Doppler technique. *Circulation.* 1983;68:302-309.
   The authors used pulsed Doppler to examine the flow velocity pattern in the right ventricular outflow tract in 33 adults. In the patients with normal pulmonary artery pressure, ejection flow reached a peak level at midsystole, producing a domelike contour of the flow velocity pattern during systole. In contrast, the flow velocity pattern in patients with pulmonary hypertension was demonstrated to accelerate rapidly and to reach a peak level sooner.
7. Lahm T, McCaslin CA, Wozniak TC, et al. Medical and surgical treatment of acute right ventricular failure. *J Am Coll Cardiol.* 2010;56:1435-1446.
   This review summarizes the general measures, ventilation strategies, vasoactive substances, and surgical as well as mechanical approaches that are currently used or actively investigated in the treatment of the acutely failing RV.

8. Oh JK, Seward JB, Tajik AJ. *The Echo Manual*. 3rd ed. Philadelphia: Lippincott Williams & Wilkins; 2006.
   This is a comprehensive textbook of echocardiography.

9. Otto CM. *Textbook of Clinical Echocardiography*. 4th ed. Philadelphia: Saunders Elsevier; 2009.
   This is a comprehensive textbook of echocardiography.

10. Rudski LG, Lai WW, Afilalo J, et al. Guidelines for the echocardiographic assessment of the right heart in adults: A report from the American Society of Echocardiography endorsed by the European Association of Echocardiography, a registered branch of the European Society of Cardiology, and the Canadian Society of Echocardiography. *J Am Soc Echocardiogr*. 2010;23:685-713.
    This guideline document from the American Society of Echocardiography details the recommended assessment of the right heart.

11. Rydman R, Soderberg M, Larsen F, Caidahl K, Alam M. Echocardiographic evaluation of right ventricular function in patients with acute pulmonary embolism: A study using tricuspid annular motion. *Echocardiography*. 2010;27: 286-293.

This case control study illustrated that both systolic and diastolic RV function are impaired in acute pulmonary embolism, with diastolic function recovering faster than systolic function.

12. Watts JA, Marchick MR, Kline JA. Right ventricular heart failure from pulmonary embolism: Key distinctions from chronic pulmonary hypertension. *J Card Fail*. 2010;16: 250-259.
    This review focuses on mechanisms of right ventricular dysfunction, contrasting mechanisms of RV adaptation and injury in pulmonary embolism versus chronic pulmonary hypertension.

13. Yock PG, Popp RL. Noninvasive estimation of right ventricular systolic pressure by Doppler ultrasound in patients with tricuspid regurgitation. *Circulation*. 1984;70: 657-662.
    In this paper, the authors evaluated the accuracy of a noninvasive method for estimating right ventricular systolic pressures in patients with tricuspid regurgitation. The noninvasive measurement correlated well with values from catheterization.

Heart Failure Caused by Congenital Heart Disease

11

Meryl S. Cohen

Basic Principles

KEY POINTS

- Heart failure occurs frequently in children with congenital heart disease (CHD) and is often an indication for intervention.
- In contrast to adult heart failure, which is often caused by decreased coronary perfusion, children with CHD typically develop heart failure as a result of the underlying cardiac defect or in association with congenital heart surgery.
- Commonly used measures of ventricular performance (Table 11-1) are limited because they are preload and/or afterload dependent. However, in serial assessment of function, these methods are useful clinically.
- Newer echocardiographic modalities to assess ventricular performance (such as strain and strain-rate imaging) are challenging in the CHD population because of the abnormal anatomy.

The Causes of Heart Failure in CHD

Left-to-Right Shunts

- Left-to-right shunt lesions comprise the most common congenital cardiac anomalies in children, excluding bicuspid aortic valve (Box 11-1), and are the most common cause of high-output heart failure.
- Newborn infants with significant left-to-right shunts are typically asymptomatic at birth as a result of high pulmonary vascular resistance. If a left-to-right shunt is large (i.e., a large ventricular septal defect), symptoms usually develop by 4 to 8 weeks of age when the pulmonary vascular resistance normalizes.
- Over this time period, pulmonary blood flow increases, resulting in symptoms that include tachypnea, tachycardia, failure to gain weight,

TABLE 11-1 ECHOCARDIOGRAPHIC INDICES OF VENTRICULAR PERFORMANCE

Shortening fraction (SF)	$SF\ (\%) = \dfrac{\text{left ventricular end-diastolic dimension} - \text{left ventricular end-systolic dimension}}{\text{left ventricular end-diastolic dimension}}$
Ejection fraction (EF)	$EF\ (\%) = \dfrac{\text{left ventricular end-diastolic volume} - \text{left ventricular end-systolic volume}}{\text{left ventricular end-diastolic volume}}$
Heart rate corrected mean velocity of circumferential fiber shortening (Vcf$_c$)	$Vcf_c = \dfrac{\text{left ventricular end-diastolic dimension} - \text{left ventricular end-systolic dimension}}{\text{left ventricular end-diastolic dimension} \times \text{left ventricular ejection time}_c}$ where ejection time$_c = \dfrac{\text{left ventricular ejection time}}{\text{square root of R-R interval}}$
End-systolic wall stress (ESWS)	$ESWS = \dfrac{\text{end-systolic pressure} \times \text{radius}}{\text{wall thickness}}$
Myocardial performance index (MPI)	$MPI = \dfrac{\text{time from closure to opening of atrioventricular valve} - \text{ventricular ejection time}}{\text{ventricular ejection time}}$

BOX 11-1   Left-to-Right Shunt Lesions in Children

- Atrial septal defects
- Partial anomalous pulmonary venous return
- Ventricular septal defects
- Common atrioventricular canal defect
- Patent ductus arteriosus
- Aortopulmonary window
- Truncus arteriosus

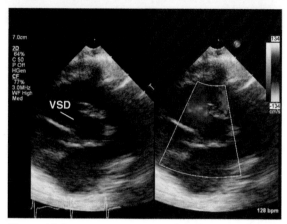

Figure 11-1. Parasternal short-axis view in color compare mode demonstrates a large, unrestrictive perimembranous ventricular septal defect (VSD). Color Doppler demonstrates laminar flow across the defect suggestive of systemic right ventricular pressure.

and diaphoresis with feedings. Feeding is a form of exercise for the newborn, thus nursing or bottle-feeding in a child with a large left-to-right shunt will often result in a catecholamine surge.
- As a rule, surgical repair of left-to-right shunts alleviates the heart failure and growth resumes.

KEY POINTS

- Echocardiography of left-to-right shunts will identify the lesion in multiple views (Figure 11-1).
- If the shunt is large, the pressure in the right and left ventricles will be equal and Doppler color interrogation will demonstrate laminar flow (see Figure 11-1).
- Other indicators of a chronic, large shunt will include chamber dilatation, generally best seen in the subxiphoid and apical 4-chamber views (see Video 11-1 on the Expert Consult website). In ventricular septal defect, common atrioventricular canal defect, truncus arteriosus, and patent ductus arteriosus, the left atrium and left ventricle dilate because of left ventricular volume overload.
- Right ventricular pressure will be systemic or near-systemic with a large left-to-right shunt and can be measured from the tricuspid regurgitation jet or from the velocity across the ventricular septal defect.
- Ventricular systolic performance is typically hyperdynamic (as measured by shortening fraction or ejection fraction) to compensate for the high cardiac output. If left unrepaired for a long time, ventricular dysfunction may occur.
- In contrast, atrial septal defect and partial anomalous pulmonary venous return result in right atrial and right ventricular dilatation. Of note, these two lesions do not typically cause early heart failure.

Left Heart Obstructive Lesions

- Left ventricular systolic dysfunction is seen with higher frequency in certain congenital heart lesions, such as left heart obstructive lesions (Box 11-2).

BOX 11-2   Left Heart Obstructive Lesions

- Valvar aortic stenosis
- Subaortic stenosis
- Supravalvar aortic stenosis
- Coarctation of the aorta
- Hypoplastic left heart syndrome

- The pressure load associated with these obstructive lesions results in ventricular hypertrophy, elevated end-diastolic pressure and eventual systolic and diastolic dysfunction.
- Critical left heart obstruction is a newborn diagnosis, defined as obstruction that is so severe that the infant is dependent on flow from the ductus arteriosus to augment cardiac output. Neonates with critical left heart obstruction require urgent surgical or catheter-directed intervention.
- Left ventricular failure is a component of the diagnosis because of significant pressure overload from the diminutive aortic valve orifice (Figure 11-2; also see Video 11-2 on the Expert Consult website). In addition, some infants with critical aortic stenosis have marked mitral regurgitation, which adds a volume load to the already pressure-loaded left ventricle (see Video 11-2 on the Expert Consult website).
- Critical aortic stenosis is often associated with endocardial fibroelastosis. Endocardial fibroelastosis is a poorly understood phenomenon whereby the left ventricular endocardium becomes fibrotic, likely as a result of longstanding subendocardial ischemia (Figure 11-3; also see Video 11-3 on the Expert Consult website). Children with endocardial

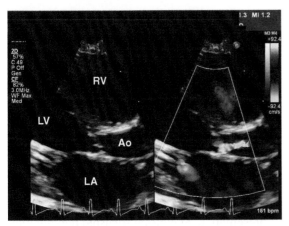

Figure 11-2. Parasternal long-axis view in color compare mode of an infant with critical aortic valve stenosis demonstrates a hypoplastic aortic valve annulus with a thickened and doming aortic valve. The left atrium is dilated. Color Doppler shows a narrow jet of flow across the stenotic valve. Mitral regurgitation is also seen.

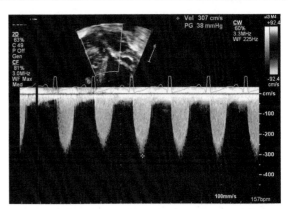

Figure 11-4. Continuous wave Doppler interrogation across the aortic valve in a patient with critical aortic stenosis. Though the peak gradient across the valve is only 38 mm Hg, the obstruction is severe. The poorly functioning left ventricle cannot generate a high pressure across the valve.

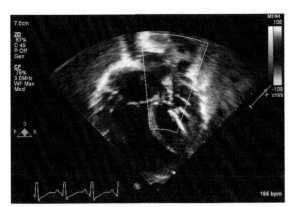

Figure 11-3. Apical 4-chamber view in the same patient as Figure 11-2 with critical aortic stenosis demonstrates a dilated but hypoplastic left ventricle (non–apex forming), with echo-bright papillary muscles consistent with endocardial fibroelastosis. Color Doppler demonstrates mitral regurgitation.

KEY POINTS

- Endocardial fibroelastosis can often be visualized in multiple views, but the sonographer must be cautioned not to mistake increased gain for this disorder.
- In critical aortic stenosis, it must be recognized that the peak instantaneous velocity across the stenotic aortic valve may not be particularly high if there is severe left ventricular dysfunction, because the ventricle cannot generate high pressure (Figure 11-4).
- The mitral regurgitation jet may be measured to estimate peak left ventricular pressure.
- Additional echocardiographic evidence of low cardiac output is a shortened ejection time using pulsed wave Doppler.
- In critical left heart disease, the ductus arteriosus flow pattern will be right to left in systole to augment cardiac output from the right ventricle.
- Adolescents and young adults who had critical aortic stenosis in association with endocardial fibroelastosis as infants may continue to show evidence of significant cardiac disease, which may be manifested as restrictive cardiomyopathy (Figure 11-5; also see Video 11-4 on the Expert Consult website).

fibroelastosis have poor ventricular systolic shortening and high end-diastolic and left atrial pressure, even after the aortic stenosis is relieved.
- After intervention, these infants may remain quite ill because of residual outflow obstruction, poor left ventricular function or the development of new-onset aortic regurgitation as a complication of the intervention.
- Intervention for aortic stenosis in later infancy or childhood tends to have better outcome because the left ventricle has responded over time to the pressure load by developing hypertrophy.

The Systemic Right Ventricle

- Certain forms of CHD, both palliated and unpalliated, result in the right ventricle supporting the systemic circulation.
- Early in life, most children with a systemic right ventricle compensate well; however, ventricular failure is common in adolescence and adulthood.
- Prior to surgical intervention, the most common cardiac lesion with a systemic right ventricle is

congenitally corrected transposition of the great arteries (cc-TGA). cc-TGA is defined as discordant atrioventricular as well as ventriculo-arterial connections such that the right atrium connects to the left ventricle, from which the pulmonary artery arises, and the left atrium connects to the right ventricle, from which the aorta arises (most commonly the aorta is positioned anterior and to the left of the pulmonary artery) (Figure 11-6A; also see Video 11-5 on the Expert Consult website). The circulation remains in series (thus the term "congenitally corrected"), and rarely patients with the simple form of this defect (no additional cardiac anomalies) go unrecognized until adolescence

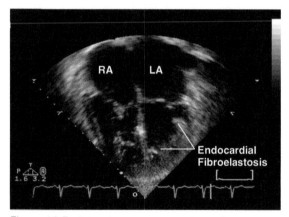

Figure 11-5. Apical 4-chamber view of a young adult who had critical aortic stenosis and had balloon dilatation of the aortic valve in infancy. Both atria are enlarged as a result of marked restrictive cardiomyopathy with elevated atrial pressures. Echo-bright regions on the papillary muscles suggest endocardial fibroelastosis, which may be the etiology of the restrictive cardiomyopathy.

or adulthood because they are initially asymptomatic.

- cc-TGA is frequently associated with Ebstein-like malformation of the tricuspid valve and associated tricuspid regurgitation (see Figure 11-6; see also Video 11-5 on the Expert Consult website). In the more complex form of cc-TGA, additional cardiac defects are common, such as ventricular septal defect, pulmonary outflow obstruction, or systemic outflow obstruction. These findings lead to early clinical presentation.
- The natural history of cc-TGA is variable, with right ventricular failure being the most common presentation. Significant tricuspid regurgitation may accelerate the development of ventricular dysfunction. By the third decade of life, most patients with cc-TGA will have systemic right ventricular failure with decreased exercise capacity on exercise stress testing and advanced New York Heart Association (NYHA) functional classification status.
- Those with additional cardiac defects (e.g., ventricular septal defect, outflow obstruction) develop heart failure and exercise intolerance earlier than those with the simple form.
- Similar findings occur in patients with the more common form of transposition of the great arteries (TGA), whereby there is atrio-ventricular concordance and ventriculo-arterial discordance.
- In the late 1950s through the early 1980s, the primary surgical procedure for TGA was an atrial switch procedure (Senning or Mustard); the atrial switch baffles blood flow at the atrial level with a systemic venous pathway to the mitral valve and a pulmonary venous pathway

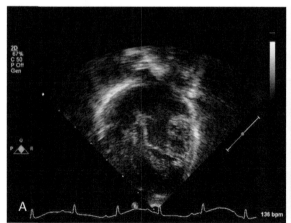

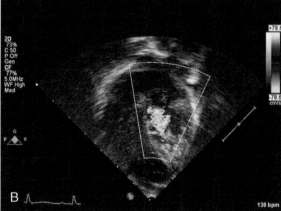

Figure 11-6. **A,** Apical 4-chamber view in a child with cc-TGA in association with Ebstein's malformation of the tricuspid valve. Atrioventricular discordance is seen. The left-sided tricuspid valve exhibits features of Ebstein's anomaly with displacement of the septal leaflet. **B,** Color Doppler in the same patient demonstrating significant tricuspid regurgitation. Note the origin of the tricuspid regurgitation jet is displaced because of the Ebstein's anomaly.

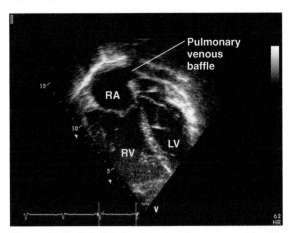

Figure 11-7. Apical 4-chamber view in a young adult with TGA who has undergone an atrial switch operation. The systemic right ventricle is dilated and hypertrophied. The pulmonary venous baffle is seen entering the right atrium. A pacing wire is seen in the left atrium entering the left ventricle.

to the tricuspid valve. This procedure changes the parallel circulation to one in series (Figure 11-7; also see Video 11-6 on the Expert Consult website).

- The long-term consequence of the atrial switch operation is that the right ventricle must support the systemic circulation. With long-term follow-up of these patients, it has recently become clear that right ventricular failure is common in this population, similar to those individuals with cc-TGA.
- The etiology of right heart failure in both cc-TGA and TGA after the atrial switch operation is poorly understood. The morphology of the right ventricle may in part account for the right ventricular failure that develops. Muscle fiber orientation is different in the two ventricles. In those patients with significant tricuspid regurgitation, the volume load burdens the right ventricle and likely leads to decreased systolic and diastolic performance.
- Some studies suggest that low-grade coronary insufficiency occurs in the systemic right ventricle. This has been supported by studies of myocardial perfusion that have shown myocardial fibrosis and regional wall motion abnormalities in these patients.
- Arrhythmias are commonly associated with these cardiac lesions. Patients with cc-TGA have a 2% annual risk for the development of complete heart block, which may cause cardiac dyssynchrony and heart failure.
- Atrial arrhythmias such as sick sinus syndrome, atrial flutter, and atrial fibrillation are common after the atrial switch procedure. Pacemakers are frequently implanted in this patient

population, and this abnormal conduction pathway may be associated with decreased right ventricular function.
- Treatment of heart failure in patients with systemic right ventricles is challenging as there are no specific medical therapies that target the right ventricle.
- As a result of poor long-term outcome in unrepaired cc-TGA, some advocate for the "double switch" operation; this procedure includes an atrial and arterial switch such that the left ventricle becomes the systemic ventricle. The left ventricle often has to be "prepared" for such a procedure by performing a pulmonary artery banding to achieve systemic pressure in the left ventricle.
- The operative mortality for late "double switch" operation is approximately 5% to 6%. Complications may occur from both procedures, including atrial arrhythmias, atrial baffle obstruction and/or baffle leak, left ventricular failure, coronary perfusion abnormalities, and outflow tract obstruction. In some cases, cardiac transplantation becomes the best option if severe heart failure develops.

KEY POINTS

- Echocardiography of the systemic right ventricle is challenging. In contrast to the left ventricle, there are no standard methods for assessing right ventricular performance in this setting.
- Subjective assessment remains the most common method used in echocardiography laboratories. This method is quick and easy to perform, particularly with user experience, but is confounded with regard to interobserver variability and reproducibility.
- Percent fractional area change is a quantitative measure of right ventricular performance. This method is similar to ejection fraction except it uses a planimetric technique to measure right ventricular end-diastolic and end-systolic area. Fractional area change less than 40% is considered abnormal.
- Myocardial performance index (MPI), a measure of global systolic and diastolic function, can be used to assess systemic right ventricular performance. The isovolumic relaxation and contraction time intervals are divided by the ejection time, with a higher MPI indicating worse overall ventricular performance (see Table 11-1). Using MPI to assess right ventricular function has resulted in conflicting data. In addition, MPI may not correlate with right ventricular dysfunction, particularly when there are regional wall motion abnormalities.
- Tricuspid annular plane systolic excursion (TAPSE) has been found to correlate with

Continued

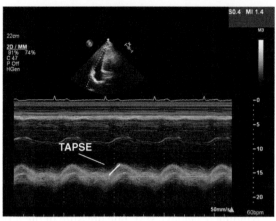

Figure 11-8. TAPSE is seen using M-mode through the right ventricle.

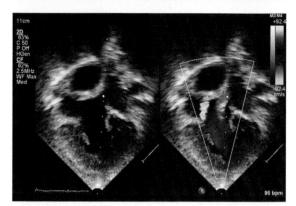

Figure 11-9. Apical 4-chamber view in color compare mode in a patient with hypoplastic left heart syndrome after an extracardiac Fontan operation. There is essentially no left ventricular chamber. The Fontan baffle is readily seen. Color Doppler identifies a fenestration in the Fontan baffle.

The Single Ventricle

- A variety of congenital heart defects comprise the functional single ventricle, including most commonly hypoplastic left heart syndrome, hypoplastic right heart, tricuspid atresia, and double inlet ventricle.
- After initial surgery (depending on the underlying anatomy), patients undergo staged palliation that culminates in the total cavopulmonary anastomosis procedure known as the Fontan operation (Figure 11-9; also see Video 11-7 on the Expert Consult website). In this palliative procedure, the systemic venous blood bypasses the heart and is connected directly to the pulmonary arteries, such that blood flows passively across the pulmonary vascular bed. The single ventricle is thus dedicated to providing the systemic circulation.
- Diastolic dysfunction is common after the Fontan procedure for single-ventricle lesions. Prior to the era of staging with the bidirectional cavopulmonary shunt, children who underwent the Fontan operation often had significant morbidity, including recalcitrant pleural effusions, ascites, electrolyte abnormalities, and low

cardiac output. Echocardiographic assessment in these patients often reveals a ventricle with diminished end-diastolic volume, relaxation abnormalities, and increased ventricular mass in association with good systolic performance.
- The "volume unloading" that occurs with the Fontan procedure results in increased ventricular mass that regresses slowly over time. By staging the Fontan procedure with the interim bidirectional cavopulmonary shunt, the single ventricle adapts over time to the changes in volume with an adequate output to the body via the inferior vena cava.
- In general, children who have had the Fontan operation have lower cardiac output and poorer exercise performance than those with a biventricular circulation. Early- and late-onset heart failure is a common problem after the Fontan operation and can be a result of systolic and/or diastolic dysfunction.
- The ventricle may sustain injury from one of the surgical procedures or from other residual or recurrent cardiac problems (e.g., coarctation of the aorta, significant atrioventricular or semilunar valve regurgitation).
- High filling pressure in the systemic ventricle leads to high Fontan baffle pressure (and thus high systemic venous pressure). Symptoms may include plethora, exercise intolerance, edema, recalcitrant pleural effusions, and hepatic dysfunction.
- Patients who have undergone the Fontan procedure are also at risk for arrhythmias that may affect cardiac performance. Junctional rhythm is common after surgery, and cardiac index may decrease without atrial contraction. Atrial flutter and fibrillation may also occur and impact adversely on ventricular function.

- Few therapies exist for heart failure in association with a functional single ventricle. Routine medical therapies such as afterload reduction and inotropes may be effective. Carvedilol has been effective in the treatment of heart failure in some patients with single ventricle. Even cardiac resynchronization has been attempted in the subset of patients with dyssynchrony. Cardiac transplantation is the only known effective long-term therapy.

KEY POINTS

- Echocardiographic imaging of the single ventricle has challenges similar to those with the systemic right ventricle. Moreover, the ventriculo-ventricular interactions observed in hearts with two ventricles are often not present.
- Subjective evaluation of dysfunction remains the most common method of assessment, although the techniques described for systemic right ventricle are being utilized in the single-ventricle population as well. MPI in patients with single right ventricles has been reported as significantly higher compared to that in normal subjects.
- In patients with fenestrated Fontan baffles, the trans-fenestration gradient can be estimated by Doppler assessment of the mean velocity across the fenestration (Figure 11-10). A higher trans-fenestration mean gradient may indicate high Fontan baffle pressures.

Coronary Insufficiency

- Although unusual in the pediatric population, coronary insufficiency and subsequent heart failure do occur in a subset of congenital heart defects that affect the coronary arteries.
- Anomalous left coronary artery from the pulmonary artery (ALCAPA) is the most common of these lesions. In this defect, the left coronary artery arises from the pulmonary artery instead of the aorta. After pulmonary vascular resistance falls in the neonatal period, a "steal" phenomenon occurs such that blood flows from the left ventricular myocardium into the pulmonary artery. Myocardial ischemia and infarction occur as a result of this coronary insufficiency. The echocardiographic presentation is consistent with endocardial fibroelastosis with echo-bright endocardium and mitral valve dysfunction (Figure 11-11).
- Infants with ALCAPA typically present at 6 to 10 weeks of age with profound heart failure. The most common albeit pathognomonic

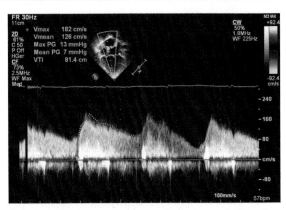

Figure 11-10. Continuous wave Doppler across the fenestration demonstrates a mean trans-fenestration gradient of 7 mm Hg.

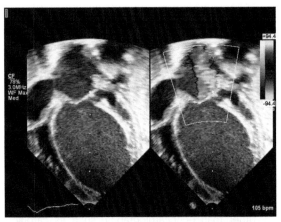

Figure 11-11. Apical 4-chamber view in color compare mode in an infant with ALCAPA. A markedly dilated left ventricle with evidence of papillary muscle ischemia is seen (echo-bright papillary muscle). Color Doppler demonstrates significant mitral regurgitation.

symptom is irritability and sometimes loss of consciousness with exertion (feeding).
- The arterial switch operation performed in patients with TGA may compromise coronary perfusion because the coronary arteries must be transferred to the neo-aorta.
- Some coronary variations in TGA, including single coronary anatomy and, in particular, coronaries that take an intramural course, are associated with left ventricular dysfunction after the arterial switch operation.
- Coronary insufficiency may occur early at the time of surgical repair or late in adolescent years. The presentation may be similar to myocardial infarction in adults, in whom sudden death can be the presenting symptom.
- Routine assessment for coronary insufficiency in children who have had coronary

reimplantation is controversial. If coronary insufficiency is identified, surgical coronary reintervention is usually indicated to preserve ventricular performance. Sudden death is rare but can occur in this population of patients.

KEY POINTS

- Echocardiography of an infant with ALCAPA and heart failure typically demonstrates a markedly dilated and poorly functioning ventricle with echo-bright endocardium and papillary muscles. Significant mitral regurgitation is common from the papillary muscle dysfunction (see Figure 11-11).
- Echocardiographic assessment of the origin of the left coronary artery can be challenging; in ALCAPA, the left coronary artery may appear to arise normally from the aorta (Figure 11-12).
- In many cases, the anomalous connection to the pulmonary artery can be visualized with retrograde flow into the main pulmonary artery. If all other findings point to ALCAPA but the coronary origin is not well seen, cardiac catheterization may be required to make the diagnosis.
- Surgical intervention may include coronary transfer or a baffling procedure (Takeuchi operation).
- Coronary ischemia after the arterial switch operation is typically manifest as regional wall motion abnormalities or global left ventricular dysfunction.
- Assessment of coronary perfusion after the arterial switch operation typically requires modalities other than echocardiography, such as cardiac catheterization, CMRI, and stress echocardiography to assess myocardial perfusion.

Left Ventricular Dysfunction after Biventricular Repair

- Biventricular repair is performed for a variety of congenital heart defects, including ventricular septal defect, tetralogy of Fallot (TOF), common atrioventricular canal defect, double-outlet ventricle, and truncus arteriosus. Left ventricular dysfunction and heart failure may occur early or late after repair.
- Patients with tetralogy of Fallot or truncus arteriosus may develop late-onset left ventricular failure. This is poorly understood but likely related to ventriculo-ventricular interactions and conduction abnormalities.
- The right ventricle is typically exposed to a significant volume load (pulmonary regurgitation) after repair, resulting in significant dilatation and eventually systolic dysfunction (Figure 11-13; also see Videos 11-8A and 11-8B on the Expert Consult website). Left ventricular dysfunction may occur after long-standing right ventricular dilatation and dysfunction.
- Valvuloplasties and valve replacements may also be associated with left ventricular dysfunction and heart failure after surgery.

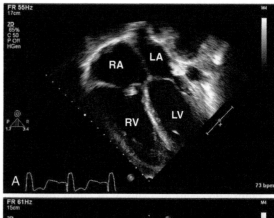

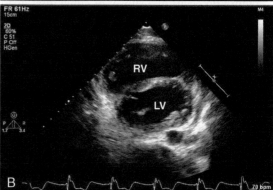

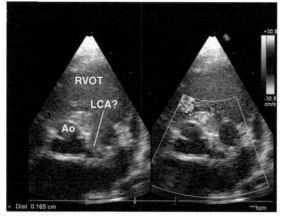

Figure 11-12. Parasternal long-axis view in color compare mode in an infant with ALCAPA. Note that the left coronary artery (LCA) can appear to arise normally from the aorta in this disease. On careful inspection, color Doppler in this patient suggests retrograde flow, which should raise suspicion of the diagnosis. RVOT, right ventricular outflow tract.

Figure 11-13. **A,** Apical 4-chamber view in a young adult with TOF after repair who has pulmonary outflow obstruction and severe pulmonary insufficiency. The right atrium and right ventricle are dilated. **B,** Parasternal short-axis of the ventricles in the same patient shows significant right ventricular dilatation.

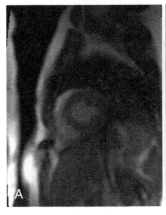
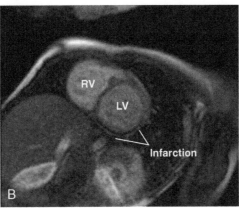

Figure 11-14. CMRI using steady-state free precession gadolinium adenosine stress perfusion. **A,** Image of the ventricles in a child after the arterial switch operation with normal coronary perfusion. **B,** Image of the ventricles in a child with occlusion of the circumflex artery. There is a perfusion defect suggesting infarction (dark stripe within the myocardium in the inferior and posterior distribution). *(Courtesy of Mark Fogel, MD.)*

- Significant mitral regurgitation increases preload to the left ventricle; at the same time, afterload is decreased as the blood empties into the left atrium. Eventually irreversible myocardial damage develops.
- It is often a challenge to determine the ideal timing for mitral valvuloplasty or replacement because left ventricular dysfunction may not become evident until after surgery. Repair of mitral regurgitation results in an acute increase in afterload to the left ventricle. As a result, mitral valvuloplasty and/or replacement continue to have a relatively high morbidity and mortality when compared to other congenital heart defect surgeries.

KEY POINTS

- Strain and strain-rate imaging can be used to detect subtle changes in left ventricular performance in patients with TOF. Moreover, left ventricular dyssynchrony and abnormal strain may occur after TOF repair in association with prolonged QRS complex duration on electrocardiogram.
- Echocardiographic indices of dysfunction prior to atrioventricular valve intervention have been challenging in both the pediatric and adult population. The decreased afterload associated with significant mitral regurgitation may mask ventricular dysfunction. Serial echocardiography to assess left ventricular end-diastolic and end-systolic volume changes is helpful in clinical decision making.
- In a patient with normal myocardium, the systolic performance should be hyperdynamic. If ejection fraction decreases over serial assessments (even if still in the normal range), intervention may be necessary to prevent the development of significant left ventricular dysfunction and heart failure after surgery.

When Are Other Diagnostic Tests Needed?

- There are significant limitations to the use of echocardiography in the detection of heart failure in the setting of CHD, particularly in the assessment of right ventricular function and in the detection of subtle abnormalities in left ventricular performance.
- CMRI provides accurate quantitative information on ventricular performance in children with CHD; this includes measures of ejection fraction, regurgitant fraction, ventricular volumes, and, when appropriate, cardiac index. In addition, CMRI can also be used to assess myocardial viability (Figure 11-14). New techniques have recently been developed to assess ventricular performance and viability during exercise; some CMRI scanners have exercise bicycle equipment for this purpose.
- Cardiac computed tomographic imaging provides some information similar to that from CMRI and requires shorter periods in the scanner. However, there is radiation risk to the patient, particularly if performed multiple times.
- Cardiac catheterization remains the only diagnostic test that accurately measures end-diastolic pressure.

Suggested Readings
1. McDaniel NL, Gutgesell HP. Ventricular septal defects. In: Allen HD, Driscoll DJ, Shaddy RE, Feltes TF, eds. *Moss and Adams' Heart Disease in Infants, Children and Adolescents including the Fetus and Young Adult.* Philadelphia: Wolters Kluwer/Lippincott Williams & Wilkins; 2008: 667-682.
2. McElhinney DB, Lock JE, Keane JF, et al. Left heart growth, function, and reintervention after balloon aortic valvuloplasty for neonatal aortic stenosis. *Circulation.* 2005;111:451-458.
3. Lofland GK, McCrindle BW, Williams WG, et al. Critical aortic stenosis in the neonate: A multi-institutional study

of management, outcomes, and risk factors. Congenital Heart Surgeons Society. *J Thorac Cardiovasc Surg.* 2001;121: 10-27.

4. Hornung TS, Calder L. Congenitally corrected transposition of the great arteries. *Heart.* 2010;96:1154-1161.

5. Graham TP Jr, Bernard YD, Mellen BG, et al. Long-term outcome in congenitally corrected transposition of the great arteries: A multi-institutional study. *J Am Coll Cardiol.* 2000;36:255-261.

6. Tei C, Dujardin KS, Hodge DO, et al. Doppler echocardiographic index for assessment of global right ventricular function. *J Am Soc Echocardiogr.* 1996;9:838-847.

7. Eidem BW, O'Leary PW, Tei C, et al. Usefulness of the myocardial performance index for assessing right ventricular function in congenital heart disease. *Am J Cardiol.* 2000;86:654-658.

8. Gewillig M. The Fontan circulation. *Heart.* 2005;91: 839-846.

9. Mahle WT, Coon PD, Wernovsky G, et al. Quantitative echocardiographic assessment of the performance of the functionally single right ventricle after the Fontan operation. *Cardiol Young.* 2001;11:399-406.

10. Rathod RH, Prakash A, Powell AJ, Geva T. Myocardial fibrosis identified by cardiac magnetic resonance late gadolinium enhancement is associated with adverse ventricular mechanics and ventricular tachycardia late after Fontan operation. *J Am Coll Cardiol.* 2010;55: 1721-1728.

11. Cohen MS, Herlong R, Silverman ND. Echocardiographic imaging of anomalous origin of the coronary arteries. *Cardiol Young.* 2010;20(suppl 3):26-34.

12. Pasquali SK, Hasselblad V, Li JS, et al. Coronary artery pattern and outcome of arterial switch operation for transposition of the great arteries: A meta-analysis. *Circulation.* 2002;106:2575-2580.

13. Cheung EWY, Liang X, Lam WWM, et al. Impact of right ventricular dilation on left ventricular myocardial deformation in patients after surgical repair of tetralogy of Fallot. *Am J Cardiol.* 2009;104:1264-1270.

14. Tzemos N, Harris L, Carasso S, et al. Adverse left ventricular mechanics in adults with repaired tetralogy of Fallot. *Am J Cardiol.* 2009;103:420-425.

15. Gillespie MJ, Marino BS, Cohen MS, et al. Systemic atrioventricular valve surgery in 116 pediatric patients: Risk factors for adverse outcomes. *Cardiol Young.* 2006;16(suppl 3):35-42.

16. Murakami T, Nakazawa M, Nakanishi T, et al. Prediction of postoperative left ventricular pump function in congenital mitral regurgitation. *Pediatr Cardiol.* 1999;20: 418-421.

Echocardiographic Evaluation of Ventricular Support Devices

12

James N. Kirkpatrick

Background

- Ventricular assist devices (VADs) were initially used to stabilize patients with acute cardiogenic shock (particularly post–cardiac surgery).
- Subsequently, they have been used as a "bridge to transplant," "bridge to recovery," or "bridge to decision" (stabilizing patients during work-up to decide transplantation candidacy) and as "destination therapy" (lifelong use).
- Early-generation left ventricular assist devices (LVADs) mimic the pulsatile action of the heart and have inlet and outlet valves (Figure 12-1A; Table 12-1).
- Pulsatile pumps can be set to fixed heart rate or automatic modes.
- Automatic mode on pulsatile pumps varies heart rate to maintain constant volume; therefore, pumping is asynchronous with the electrocardiogram (ECG).
- More recent LVADs are continuous flow, involving axial (rotating propeller) pumps, and have no valves (making them more durable) (see Figure 12-1B; see Table 12-1).
- In continuous-flow LVADs, rotor speed (in rotations per minute, rpm) and pressure difference between inflow chamber and outflow chamber (usually left ventricle and aorta, respectively) determine flow.
- In continuous-flow LVADs, increasing rotor speed leads to ventricular unloading.
- Even in continuous-flow LVADs, pulsatility is present as a result of residual ventricular function and the fact that LVAD flow is higher when the aorta-LV pressure differential is low (systole) and lower when the differential is higher (diastole).
- Third-generation VADs are magnetically or hydrodynamically levitated, continuous-flow centrifugal (rotating plate) pumps with no bearings or valves, theoretically making them even more durable than second-generation VADs (see Table 12-1).

- The dysfunctional RV can respond well to LVAD implantation because of reduced afterload from lower pulmonary pressures.
- Alternatively, the RV function may worsen because of high preload from increased venous return secondary to increased left-sided output.
- Some patients receiving LVADs will require RV mechanical support, either temporarily (separate right ventricular assist device [RVAD]) or permanently (biventricular assist device [BiVAD]).
- Other patients with RV dysfunction can be supported medically with pulmonary vasodilators and inotropes.
- RVADs generally involve an inflow cannula placed in the right atrium and an outflow cannula placed in the proximal pulmonary artery.
- The total artificial heart is an alternative to VADs as a bridge to transplantation and consists of right and left pumping chambers attached to the native atria.
- The intra-aortic balloon pump (IABP) reduces systolic afterload on the left ventricle and can improve diastolic coronary flow via counterpulsation in the descending aorta.
- Percutaneous ventricular assist devices (PVADs) involve cannulae inserted via peripheral arteries and veins.
- PVADs can provide 2 to 6 L/min of cardiac output support and can be placed quickly in acute cardiogenic shock from (usually left but also right) ventricular decompensation and/or acute severe mitral regurgitation.
- PVADs are used primarily as a bridge to recovery and "bridge to bridge" (acute stabilization with subsequent implantation of a standard LVAD).
- PVADs are also used in high-risk percutaneous coronary interventions in patients with severely reduced LV ejection fraction (LVEF), and in percutaneous aortic valve procedures.
- PVADs provide better hemodynamic support than IABPs, but studies have not demonstrated improvements in mortality.

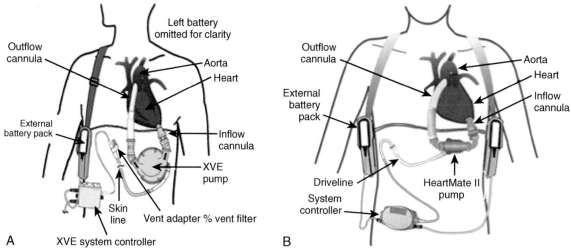

Figure 12-1. Schematic drawings of a pulsatile LVAD (Thoratec XVE; **A**) and a continuous-flow LVAD (HeartMate II, Thoratec Corp.; **B**). Components of each LVAD are labeled. The pump is implanted in the upper abdomen. Inflow cannula connects the left ventricular apex to the pumping chamber, which is connected, in turn, to the ascending aorta via an outflow cannula. A drive line runs from the pump, through the skin, to the externalized system controller. The system controller is connected to battery packs. The pulsatile LVADs employ a compressible chamber that fills with blood via an inlet valve. A pusher plate mechanism then squeezes the chamber to expel blood through an outlet valve. The valves have limited durability and contribute to the reduced longevity of first-generation LVADs. The continuous-flow LVADs use either a rotor device (second generation) or a rotating disk (third generation) to accelerate and expel blood. Continuous-flow VADs do not have valves and have proven to be more durable. *(From Thoratec Corp.)*

TABLE 12-1 EXAMPLES OF VAD GENERATIONS

Examples	Type
First Generation	
HeartMate XVE (Thoratec Corp.)	Pulsatile
Novacor pumps (WorldHeart Corp.)	Pulsatile
Second Generation	
HeartMate II (Thoratec Corp.)	Axial Flow
Jarvik 2000 (Jarvik Heart Corp.)	Axial Flow
Micromed DeBakey (Micromed Cardiovascular Inc.)	Axial Flow
Third Generation	
HeartWare HVAD (HeartWare Inc.)	Centrifugal
Duraheart (Terumo Heart Inc.)	Centrifugal
Levacor (WorldHeart Corp.)	Centrifugal
Total Artificial Heart	
Abiocor (Abiomed Corp.)	
Cardiowest (Syncardia Inc.)	

- The Impella Recover (Abiomed, Danvers, MA) can support the right or left ventricle and consists of a catheter in an inflow port and an outflow port that is advanced retrograde through the aorta or pulmonary artery into the ventricle (Figure 12-2A).

- The inflow port placed below the aortic or pulmonic valve draws blood from the ventricle and ejects it from the outflow port positioned above the valve.
- The TandemHeart (Cardiac Assist, Pittsburgh, PA) involves an inflow cannula placed through the femoral vein in the RA, across an interatrial septotomy, and into the left atrium. The outflow cannula is placed through the femoral artery into the abdominal aorta (see Figure 12-2B).
- The TandemHeart can also be used to support the RV.
- Extracorporeal membrane oxygenation (ECMO) provides temporary cardiopulmonary support for patients with reversible cardiogenic shock and/or severe pulmonary failure.
- ECMO systems include an inflow cannula placed into the right atrium via the femoral vein or right internal jugular vein, and an outflow cannula in the femoral artery or ascending aorta.

Overview of Echocardiographic Approach (Table 12-2)

LVADs
Preimplantation Echocardiographic Assessment
- Echocardiography establishes severely reduced LVEF, one of the criteria for LVAD implantation.

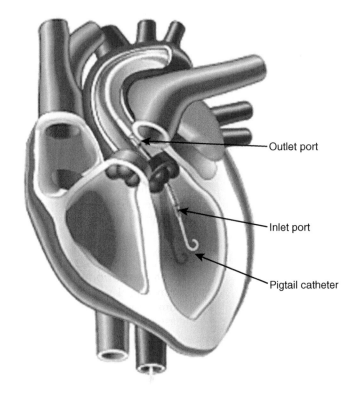

Outlet port

Inlet port

Pigtail catheter

A

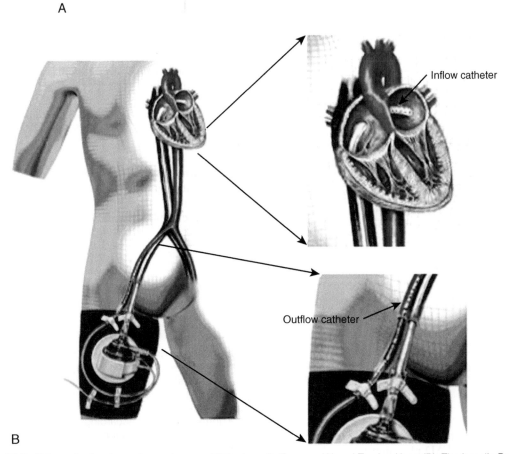

Inflow catheter

Outflow catheter

B

Figure 12-2. Schematic drawings of percutaneous VADs: Impella Recover (**A**) and TandemHeart (**B**). The Impella Recover is advanced retrograde through femoral artery access, across the aortic valve and into the left ventricular cavity. The inlet port (at the tip) is positioned 3 to 4 cm below the aortic valve via a pigtail catheter. The outlet port is positioned 1.5 to 2 cm above the sinus of Valsalva in the proximal ascending aorta. The TandemHeart inflow catheter is advanced through femoral vein access, antegrade into the right atrium and across an interatrial septal puncture, into the left atrium. The separate, outflow catheter is placed in the femoral artery or abdominal or descending aorta. (**A,** *from Abiomed Corp.* **B,** *from CardiacAssist Corp.*)

TABLE 12-2 APPROACH TO ECHOCARDIOGRAPHY IN LVADS

Preoperative
- Establish criteria for VAD candidacy (LVEF < 25%–30%)
- Assess need for RVAD
- Detect intracavitary thrombi
- Detect aortic atheroma, aneurysms, dissection
- Detect shunts
- Evaluate for valvulopathy, esp. mitral stenosis, aortic insufficiency

Intraoperative
- Direct cannulae placement away from potential obstructions
- De-airing

Diagnosis of LVAD dysfunction
Diagnose Obstruction
- Septum shifted toward RV
- LVEDD increased compared to baseline
- Spontaneous echocardiographic contrast
- High velocities in cannulae

Diagnose Underfilling
- Septum shifted toward LV
- LVEDD reduced compared to baseline
- Pericardial effusion with chamber collapse
- Septum shifting into LV

Diagnose Regurgitation
- Aortic regurgitation
- Mitral regurgitation
- LVAD regurgitation
- Tricuspid regurgitation

Detect Vegetations and Thrombi on Valves and Cannulae
LVAD Optimization
- Changes in LVEDD
- Alignment of interventricular septum
- Changes in degree and frequency of aortic valve opening
- Reductions in aortic, mitral, or tricuspid regurgitation
- LVAD weaning
- Changes in LVEDD, LVEF, aortic valve opening with reductions in level of VAD support

Percutaneous VADs
- Aortic abnormalities
- Aortic stenosis and regurgitation
- Ventricular septal defect
- Positioning of Impella Recovery device across aortic valve
- Guidence of trans-septal puncture for TandemHeart
- Positioning of IABP
- Positioning of ECMO cannulae
- Assessment of catheter migration and obstruction

- Echocardiography excludes diagnoses that complicate LVAD placement.
- Echocardiography assesses preimplantation RV function and can predict the need for RVAD.

Implantation/Intraoperative Echocardiographic Assessment
- Echocardiography guides placement of cannulae and de-airing.

Diagnosis of the Causes of LVAD Dysfunction
- Etiologies include obstruction, underfilling, and valvulopathy.
- Comprehensive two-dimensional (2D), M-mode, and color and spectral Doppler echocardiographic examination is crucial for diagnosing the cause of LVAD dysfunction.

Echocardiography-Guided LVAD Optimization
- Optimizing LVAD pumping rates, pumping volumes, or rotor speeds uses echocardiographic measurements to balance proper preload and adequate decompression with excessive unloading leading to "suck-down" events (obstruction of the inflow cannula by trabeculation, chamber walls, papillary muscles, or chordal structures in the setting of an underfilled chamber).

Echocardiography-Guided LVAD Weaning ("Turndown")
- Decrease in LVAD support will lead to increases in afterload and preload.
- A ventricle that maintains its size and improves its function may have recovered to the point that the LVAD can be explanted.

Percutaneous VADs, IABP, and ECMO
- Echocardiography is useful in preimplantation assessment, placement, and follow-up of two of the currently available PVADs, IABPs, and ECMO.

KEY POINTS
- Comprehensive echocardiography is necessary preimplantation to establish criteria for LVAD implantation, uncover findings that complicate LVAD placement, and assess the need for concomitant RVAD.
- Intraoperative echocardiography guides cannula placement and de-airing.
- Postimplantation use of echocardiography includes diagnosis of the cause of LVAD dysfunction, and guidance of LVAD optimization and weaning.

Preimplantation Echocardiographic Assessment

Anatomic Imaging

Acquisition

- Standard echocardiographic imaging techniques are used to evaluate cardiac anatomy, with particular attention to ventricles, the left atrium, the great vessels, and the interatrial and interventricular septae.
- In patients with limited echocardiographic windows, the use of microbubble contrast for LV opacification may be necessary to provide an accurate LVEF assessment.
- Microbubble contrast may be necessary to detect LV thrombi prior to LVAD implantation.
- Transesophageal echocardiography (TEE) is necessary to exclude LA and LA appendage thrombus, especially before planned LA cannulation.
- Agitated saline contrast study is necessary to examine the interatrial septum for evidence of atrial septal defect (ASD) or patent foramen ovale (PFO) prior to implantation. TEE may be required for optimal visualization of the septum.

Analysis

- Standard measurement and interpretation is done, with careful measurements of ventricular size (LV end-diastolic diameter [LVEDD]) and function, and detection of thrombi, aortopathy, and shunts.
- Echocardiography establishes LVEF criteria for LVAD (<25% to 30%).
- Real-time three-dimensional (3D) echocardiography may provide more accurate and reproducible measurements of LV volumes and LVEF.
- Severely enlarged RVs (defined in single-center experiences as > 85-mm end-diastolic diameter, > 200-mL end-diastolic volume, > 177-mL end-systolic volume, or short-axis to long-axis ratio ≥0.6), severe qualitative systolic RV dysfunction, tricuspid annular planar systolic motion (<7.5 mm in one study), or moderate to severe tricuspid regurgitation (TR), may require RVAD support (Table 12-3).

Pitfalls (Box 12-1)

- Placement of a VAD inflow cannula into the apex of a small ventricle risks cannula obstruction from walls, septae, papillary muscles, chordal apparati, ridges, or trabeculae.
- Intracardiac thrombi detected by echocardiography dictate where surgeons can place inflow cannulae (e.g., LA if there is an LV apical thrombus).

TABLE 12-3 PREDICTORS OF THE NEED FOR RVAD

Echocardiographic Finding	Measurement
RV enlargement	• RVEDD > 85 mm • RVEDV > 200 mL • RVESV > 177 mL • RV short-to-long axis ratio ≥ 0.6
Severe RV systolic dysfunction	• Qualitative interpretation • TAPSE < 7.5 mm
Moderate to severe tricuspid regurgitation	
Other predictors (not assessed by echocardiography) • Nonischemic etiology of cardiomyopathy • Female gender • Elevated central venous pressure • Low mean pulmonary artery pressure • Low cardiac output • Low RV stroke work index • Preoperative need for IABP • Elevated pulmonary vascular resistance • Destination therapy VAD	

RVEDD, right ventricular end-diastolic diameter; RVEDV, right ventricular end-diastolic volume; RVESV, right ventricular end-systolic volume; TAPSE, tricuspid annular plane systolic excursion.

BOX 12-1 Pitfalls in VAD Imaging

- Reduced sensitivity to detect PFO preimplantation in setting of high LA pressure.
- Reduced ability to detect significant AI preimplantation due to low systemic pressures and high LV filling pressures, which reduce aortoventricular diastolic gradient.
- Flow paradox is unreliable marker of increased intra-pericardial pressure in VAD.
- Assessment of septal shift as a marker of LV filling is complicated by many other factors that influence septal motion.
- Increased aortic valve opening and pulsatile velocities through the VAD cannulae can be a marker for LV overload, cannulae obstruction, or LV recovery.
- Measurement of changes in LVEDD in diagnosing VAD dysfunction or guiding optimization and weaning require precisely reproduced imaging planes.
- Adequately aligned Doppler interrogation of LVAD cannulae may require off-axis imaging or TEE.

- Protruding and mobile plaques, aneurysms, or dissection in the ascending aorta complicate outflow cannula placement.
- ASDs, PFOs, and ventricular septal defects (VSDs) can cause right-to-left shunting and systemic hypoxia and/or paradoxical embolus after LVAD placement.
- The sensitivity of agitated saline contrast ("bubble") studies to detect PFOs is often reduced because the bubbles cannot pass from right to left due to high left-sided pressures.

Physiologic Data
Acquisition
- Standard echocardiographic imaging techniques are used preimplantation to detect and grade valvulopathy and measure intracardiac pressures.

Analysis
- Significant degree of valvulopathy can change implantation strategy and demonstrate the need for valve repair or replacement at the time of LVAD implantation.

Pitfalls (see Box 12-1)
- Mitral stenosis compromises LVAD inflow through a left ventricular apical cannula and may dictate that the LA be cannulated instead.
- LVAD implantation will worsen baseline aortic insufficiency (AI). Aortic valve replacement or oversewing (which risks thrombus formation) may be necessary.
- In decompensated heart failure (HF), low systemic pressures and high LV pressures may lead to underestimation of AI due to a low aortic-ventricular diastolic gradient.
- Mechanical aortic valves have an increased tendency to form thrombus, despite anticoagulation, when VADs are placed because they may not open or may open minimally. Strong consideration should be given to replacing mechanical aortic valves with bioprosthetic valves at the time of LVAD implantation.

Alternative Approaches
- TEE or contrast-enhanced computed tomography (CT) or magnetic resonance imaging (MRI) may be necessary to exclude aortopathy prior to outflow cannula placement.
- Dobutamine echocardiography may be necessary to differentiate low-gradient aortic stenosis (AS) from pseudo-stenosis in the presence of severely depressed LVEF.
- Invasive hemodynamic measurements may be necessary to confirm or evaluate the severity of valvular lesions.

BOX 12-2 Uses of TEE IN VADs

- Exclude LA appendage thrombus
- Exclude PFO/ASD
- Detect aortic atheroma, aneurysms, dissection
- Detect vegetations and thrombi on valves and cannulae
- Obtain parallel Doppler angle through cannulae
- Assess chamber collapse of atria in setting of pericardial effusion (esp. with total artificial heart)

KEY POINTS

- A careful echocardiographic examination must be performed to exclude LV thrombi, possibly involving the use of microbubble contrast agents.
- Echocardiographic measures can predict the need for mechanical RV support after LVAD placement.
- Aortopathy must be characterized as it can complicate placement of the LVAD outflow cannula.
- ASDs, PFOs, and VSDs can cause right-to-left shunting and systemic hypoxia and/or paradoxical embolus after LVAD placement, but PFOs can be difficult to detect when left atrial pressures are elevated.
- Detection of significant mitral stenosis may necessitate LA cannulation or valve replacement.
- Detection of significant AI may necessitate aortic valve replacement or oversewing but can be difficult to detect in the setting of a reduced aortic-LV diastolic pressure gradient in decompensated HF.

Implantation/Intraoperative Echocardiographic Assessment

Anatomic Imaging (Box 12-2)
- Intraoperative TEE guides placement of inflow cannulae away from walls/trabeculae. 3D TEE may be helpful in delineating the relationship of the cannula to the LV wall, papillary muscle, or trabeculations (Figure 12-3).
- Outflow cannulae can be positioned to avoid aneurysms and protruding plaques and to provide some "washing" of the aortic root to prevent thrombus formation.
- Intraoperative TEE directs de-airing of the heart after VAD insertion. TEE can detect bubbles following cannulae anastomosis and prior to unclamping of the aorta, and before and after termination of cardiopulmonary bypass.
- Anastomotic sites, ascending aorta, RV, and anterior LV (anterior chambers) are important areas to examine for air bubbles.

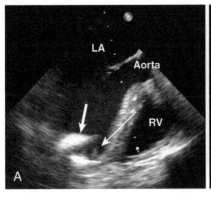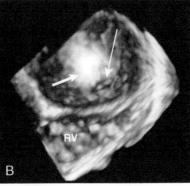

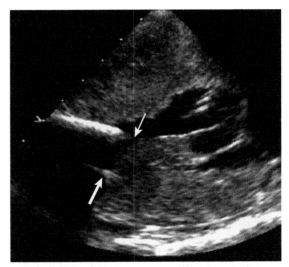

Figure 12-3. Inflow cannula orientation demonstrated by 2D and real-time 3D TEE. **A,** 2D TEE midesophageal long-axis view suggests that the inflow cannula (*thick arrow*) may abut the ventricular wall. **B,** 3D acquisition from the same position was performed. Looking from the perspective of the mitral valve annulus and into the LV apex, the LVAD inflow cannula (*thick arrow*) is shown to be oriented toward the anteroseptum, but the orifice (*thin arrow*) is not obstructed by trabeculation.

Diagnosis of the Cause of LVAD Dysfunction

Anatomic Imaging
Acquisition
- LV size (LVEDD) is measured in the parasternal long-axis view at the mitral valve leaflet tips.
- Degree and frequency of aortic valve opening is assessed by 2D and M-mode in the parasternal long-axis view.
- Cannulae are examined for vegetations, thrombi, and obstruction by papillary muscles or trabeculations in all views (parasternal long axis, parasternal short axis at the apex, and all apical views for the inflow cannula, and parasternal long axis and right upper parasternal for the outflow cannula).
- Chambers are examined for thrombi (including the aortic root).
- All valves are assessed for vegetations.
- TEE is usually necessary to investigate endocarditis on valves or cannulae, and for the detection of atrial thrombi (see Box 12-2).
- Real-time 3D TEE may better delineate the relationship of the cannula to adjacent structures (see Figure 12-3).
- In the presence of a pericardial effusion (including localized effusions), all chambers must be examined for collapse. TEE may be necessary to examine compression of the atria (especially in a total artificial heart), superior vena cava, and pulmonary veins (see Box 12-2).

Analysis
- In cannula obstruction, the LV becomes distended with the septum shifted into the RV.
- Spontaneous echocardiographic contrast may be seen.
- Alternatively, septal bowing into the RV may be caused by LVAD inflow or outflow cannula malposition or kinking.

Figure 12-4. "Suck-down" phenomenon. Transgastric TEE long-axis view of the LV demonstrates the anteromedial papillary muscle (*thin arrow*) being sucked into the opening of the LVAD inflow cannula (*thick arrow*).

- Aortic valve opening can be a marker of LV filling. By mechanically unloading the ventricle, LVADs prevent blood from being ejected through the aortic valve. Thus, the aortic valve may not open, or may open minimally and intermittently. Increased aortic valve opening may signal overfilling.
- Septal bowing into the LV may be caused by LV underfilling or elevated RV pressures.
- Chamber underfilling can lead to obstruction by walls, septae, papillary muscles, chordal apparati, ridges, or trabeculae ("suck-down" phenomenon) (Figure 12-4).
- Pericardial effusions can also reduce VAD preload through chamber collapse (Figure 12-5).
- Though the total artificial heart is opaque to ultrasound, the pericardium and portions of the

Figure 12-5. Pericardial hematomas. **A,** An apical 4-chamber view of large hematomas (*asterisk*) causing extrinsic compression of the LV and RA after LVAD and RVAD implantation. **B,** A short-axis view of the RV and LV. The *small arrows* demonstrate the invagination of the inferior and inferolateral walls of the LV by the hematoma.

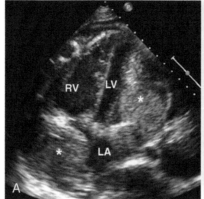 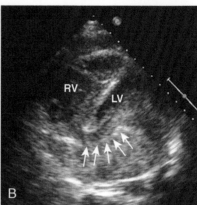

native atria, inferior and superior venae cavae, and pulmonary veins can sometimes be visualized and demonstrate collapse in tamponade.

- Endocarditis of internal VAD components or native or prosthetic valves can lead to VAD dysfunction and septic emboli, in addition to septic shock.

Pitfalls (see Box 12-1)

- Assessment of septal orientation and motion to assess LV filling can be complicated by acute pulmonary embolism, pulmonary arteriolar and venous hypertension, conduction delays/bundle branch blocks, pericardial tamponade and constriction, and post-sternotomy state.
- Although a marker for increased LV filling and cannula obstruction, increased aortic valve opening may, alternatively, be the result of ventricular recovery. Improved systolic function leads to increased ejection through the aortic valve. Aortic valve opening must therefore be interpreted in light of changes in ventricular function and size.

Physiologic Data
Acquisition

- Standard color and spectral Doppler assessment of all valves should be performed. (Even in the absence of aortic valve opening by 2D motion, continuous and pulsed wave [PW] Doppler interrogations through the ventricular outflow tract provide an assessment of residual cardiac function and/or quantify ventricular recovery).
- Standard echocardiographic assessment of right-sided pressures should be performed.
- Color and spectral Doppler (both PW and continuous wave) interrogation of the inflow cannula is performed. PW velocity profile should be recorded with the sample volume within the cannula and at the cannula orifice.

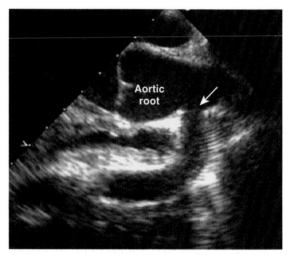

Figure 12-6. Midesophageal TEE demonstrating orientation of LVAD outflow cannula as it curves to its anastomosis with the proximal ascending aorta (*arrow*). This cannula orientation is difficult to image by TTE.

- The best angle of insonation is usually from an off-axis apical view, but the orientation of the cannulae is often variable, and the best Doppler alignment may be achieved from parasternal or even subcostal views.
- Color and spectral Doppler interrogation of the outflow cannula usually requires imaging from a right or left upper sternal window.
- Depending on the orientation of the cannulae, obtaining a parallel Doppler angle of insonation to measure velocities through cannulae may necessitate a TEE (Figure 12-6).

Analysis

- Thrombotic partial occlusion produces color Doppler aliasing at the cannula orifice and high Doppler velocities (>2.3 m/s inflow and >2.1 m/s outflow for pulsatile flow pumps, and >2 m/s for continuous flow pumps) (Figure 12-7).

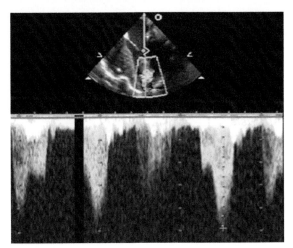

Figure 12-7. Continuous wave Doppler interrogation of the inflow cannula in this TEE midesophageal view demonstrates elevated velocities (4.3 m/s, well above the normal of 2.3 m/s for a pulsatile flow pump).

- High pulsatile velocities can also result from ventricular recovery.
- Kinking can be detected by a loss of Doppler flow signal within the LVAD cannulae.
- In continuous flow pumps, interruption of non-pulsatile (continuous diastolic) flow can also signal obstruction.
- Aortic regurgitation can be worsened by LVAD implantation (increased pressure and flow in the proximal aorta), creating a circuit—LV → VAD → aorta → LV—that excludes the systemic circulation.
- VAD regurgitation can be seen by color and spectral Doppler analysis of the cannulae. Inflow valve regurgitation manifests as decreased flows and velocities in the outflow cannula.
- In VAD regurgitation, there may be a high flow through the VAD compared with the unsupported ventricle.
- In pulsatile VADs, regurgitant volumes (RV_{VAD}) can be calculated by measuring the velocity-time integral (VTI) from PW Doppler examination within the inflow and outflow cannulae, and using the known cannula diameters (dia_{in}, dia_{out}), which are usually 12 to 25 mm:

$$RV_{VAD} = \pi(dia_{in}/2)^2\,VTI_{in} - \pi(dia_{out}/2)^2\,VTI_{out}$$

- For nonpulsatile VADs, PW VTI and diameters of the ascending aorta (dia_{asc}) and pulmonary artery (dia_{pa}) can be used to indirectly estimate VAD flows and regurgitant fractions (RF):

$$RF_{VAD} = \pi(dia_{asc}/2)^2\,VTI_{asc} - \pi(dia_{pa}/2)^2\,VTI_{pa}$$

- TR can increase post–LVAD placement due to tension on the tricuspid septal leaflet and annular distortion. Tricuspid repair may be considered if TR is moderate or greater.
- Doppler-based estimation of pulmonary pressures from the tricuspid and pulmonic regurgitant jets, as well as pulmonary vascular resistance estimates appear to be valid post–LVAD implantation in preliminary studies.

Pitfalls (see Box 12-1)

- Increases in the pulsatile velocities through the VAD cannulae suggest obstruction and overfilling but may also be seen in ventricular recovery. Velocities should therefore be interpreted in light of ventricular size and function.
- Though the aortic valve does not open or opens minimally with an LVAD, AS may or may not be present.
- Significant AI and AS have been reported months after LVAD implantation. The cause of AS is unclear (leaflets do not appear thickened or calcified but are nonetheless fused). AS may present a problem in the use of LVAD as a bridge to recovery.
- In continuous-flow LVADs, there is often some pulsatile flow through the aortic valve, but thrombus formation is a risk in pulsatile LVADs and on oversewn or stenotic aortic valves.
- After LVAD placement, color Doppler can still assess the degree of aortic and mitral valve regurgitation, but spectral Doppler gradients, other Doppler measures of valvular stenosis (such as mitral valve pressure half-time), and diastolic parameters (such as E and A velocities, tissue Doppler relaxation velocities at the mitral annulus) can be influenced by the LVAD. Normal values have not been established and likely depend on LVAD flow settings.
- Exaggerated flow paradox by spectral Doppler interrogation of valvular inflow or outflow is an unreliable marker of increased intra-pericardial pressure; therefore, chamber collapse becomes an important marker of tamponade.
- Some of the newer generation VADs create interference with Doppler signals (e.g., HeartWare, HeartWare, Inc).

Alternative Approaches

- Invasive measures of intracardiac hemodynamics may be necessary to establish accurate filling pressures, cardiac output, and pulmonary vascular resistance to guide therapy in the setting of LVAD dysfunction.

Echocardiography-Guided LVAD Optimization and Weaning

Anatomic Imaging
Acquisition
- At each different LVAD setting, echocardiographic measurements are performed.
- LV size (LVEDD) is measured as the largest cavity dimension in the parasternal long-axis view at the mitral valve leaflet tips by 2D or M-mode.
- The degree and frequency of aortic valve opening is assessed by 2D and M-mode (in the parasternal long-axis view) (Figure 12-8).

Analysis
- Neutral alignment of the interventricular septum indicates proper preload, whereas septal bowing into the RV suggests overfilling, and bowing into the LV suggests underfilling or high RV pressures (Figure 12-9).
- Quantitative and reproducible changes in LV filling in response to LVAD adjustments can be tracked by LVEDD.
- Increased aortic valve opening can signal ventricular recovery or overfilling.
- Rotor speed can be set to allow some valve opening in continuous-flow LVADs to prevent aortic root thrombosis.
- RV function and noninvasive pulmonary pressures can be assessed to examine the impact of LVAD settings on right-sided hemodynamics and function.
- Minimal change in LVEDD and increase in LVEF predicts ventricular recovery (LVEF > 45% and LVEDD < 5.5 cm in one study).
- Increase in LVEF in response to dobutamine stress testing suggests the presence of ventricular reserve.

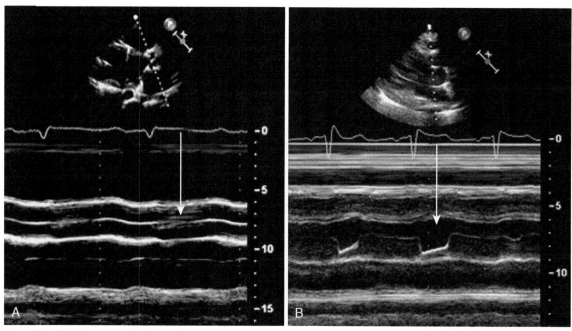

Figure 12-8. Aortic valve opening. **A,** A patient with a normally functioning pulsatile-flow LVAD with no aortic valve opening by M-mode in the parasternal long-axis view (*arrow*). **B,** A patient with a continuous flow LVAD and ventricular recovery. The aortic valve opens during systole with nearly every beat (*arrow*).

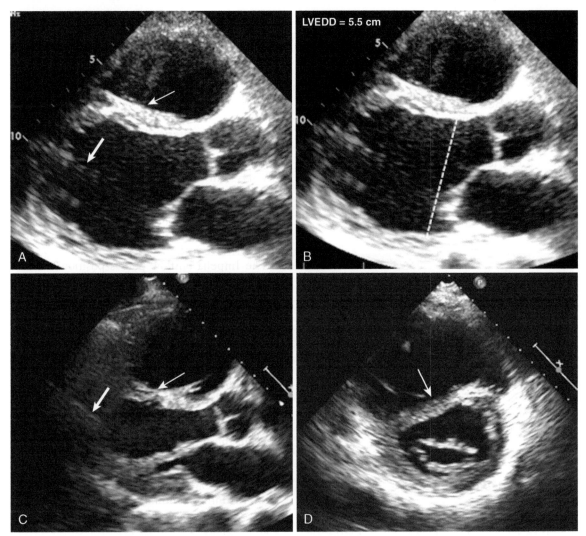

Figure 12-9. Septal change. **A** and **B,** Optimal VAD settings. **A,** A parasternal long-axis view of a patient with an LVAD (*thick arrow* delineates inflow cannula in LV) and a neutrally oriented septum (*thin arrow*). **B,** The LVEDD is normal at 5.5 cm. **C** and **D,** An underfilled LV in the same patient. The septum shifted toward the LV (**C** and **D**) and the LVEDD is reduced to 4.1 cm.

- Increased degree and/or frequency of aortic valve opening on full LVAD support suggests ventricular recovery.

Pitfalls (see Box 12-1)
- Care must be taken to measure chamber dimensions in precisely the same imaging plane each time, and to measure along an axis perpendicular to the septal and inferolateral walls.
- LVAD weaning/"turndowns" must be performed gradually and with careful monitoring to avoid acute decompensation. Invasive hemodynamic monitoring (arterial and venous) should be considered, in addition to echocardiography.

Physiologic Data
Acquisition
- Spectral Doppler measurements of the VTI in the left ventricular outflow tract from the apical 5-chamber view or apical long-axis view can be used to measure native cardiac output at different LVAD settings.
- Spectral and color Doppler can assess cannula regurgitation at different VAD settings, as described above.
- Color Doppler can be used to evaluate changes in aortic or mitral regurgitation at different LVAD settings.

Analysis

- In addition to optimizing ventricular size, shape, and aortic valve opening, adjustment of LVAD flow rates can reduce valvular regurgitation.

Pitfalls (see Box 12-1)

- Although increasing rotor speed may decompress the ventricle and lead to a reduction in mitral regurgitation, underfilling with "suck down" can lead to disruption of mitral valve chordal function and tethering of mitral valve leaflets, leading to an increase in mitral regurgitation.

KEY POINTS

- LVAD weaning and optimization can be directed by changes in LVEDD, septal orientation, aortic valve opening, and mitral regurgitation.
- Minimal change in LVEDD and increase in LVEF predicts ventricular recovery.
- Increase in LVEF in response to dobutamine stress testing suggests the presence of ventricular reserve.

Percutaneous Ventricular Assist Devices

Anatomic Imaging
Acquisition

- Standard echocardiographic imaging techniques are used preimplantation to perform a comprehensive 2D and Doppler examination.
- TEE is sometimes necessary to exclude LV thrombi prior to placement of the Impella Recover device, and left atrial and left atrial appendage thrombi prior to placement of a TandemHeart (see Box 12-2).
- Percutaneous VADs are usually placed under transthoracic echocardiographic (TTE), TEE, or intracardiac echocardiographic guidance, which can ensure proper placement of catheters, and can guide trans-septal puncture in TandemHeart placement.
- Real-time 3D imaging via TTE or TEE may be helpful in visualizing the orientation of the percutaneous VAD catheters in relation to other structures (e.g., tip of the Impella device in relation to the anterior mitral valve leaflet).
- TEE is often required to visualize the tip of the IABP, though it can sometimes be visualized in the suprasternal notch TTE view. The portions of the IABP in the descending and abdominal aorta are seen in the parasternal long-axis, modified apical 2-chamber, and subcostal views on TTE.

Analysis

- Aortic abnormalities, including extreme tortuosity, aneurysms, and protruding plaques, can complicate Impella Recover placement and function.
- A redundant anterior mitral valve leaflet can be drawn into and obstruct the Impella Recover inflow port.
- VSDs can cause systemic hypoxemia from right-to-left shunting.
- The inflow port of the Impella Recover device should be positioned 3 to 4 cm below the aortic valve, away from the septum and the anterior mitral valve leaflet.
- The Impella outflow port is positioned 1.5 to 2 cm above the sinuses of Valsalva.
- Echocardiographic guidance during transseptal puncture of the TandemHeart VAD can prevent inadvertent puncture of the aortic root, coronary sinus, right atrium, or left atrium.
- The TandemHeart inflow cannula should be positioned in the LA away from ridges, septae, atrial walls, and mitral valve leaflets.
- Echocardiography can confirm proper placement and diastolic inflation of the IABP, as well as diagnosing vegetations or thrombi on the IABP tip.
- Echocardiography can ensure proper placement of ECMO cannulae, particularly guiding the RA inflow cannula away from walls, ridges, valves, Chiari networks, and aneurysmal inter-atrial septae (Figure 12-10).

Pitfalls (see Box 12-1)

- The Impella Recover catheter can migrate forward, moving the outflow cannula below the aortic valve where it ejects blood into the LV, rather than the aorta (Figure 12-11).
- Alternatively, it may migrate backward, moving the inflow cannula above the aortic valve where it draws blood in from the aorta, rather than the LV.
- The TandemHeart inflow cannula can migrate into the left atrial appendage or pulmonary veins or across the mitral valve (potentially causing regurgitation).
- Catheters can become obstructed by thrombi or infected by vegetations.

Physiologic Data
Acquisition

- Standard echocardiographic imaging techniques are used, especially preimplantation, to

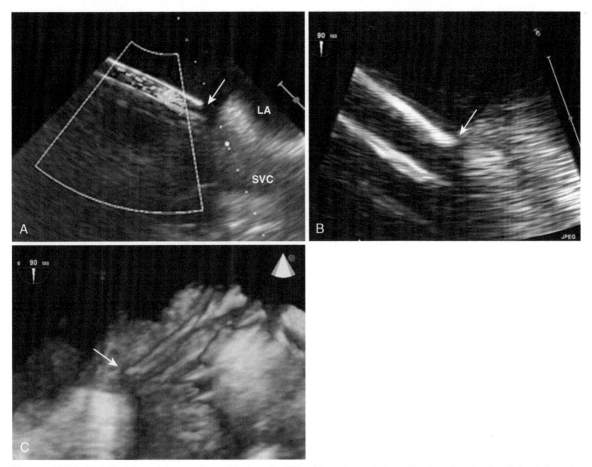

Figure 12-10. ECMO right atrial cannula positioning. **A,** TEE midesophageal view showing that the tip of the right atrial inflow ECMO cannula is positioned very near the superior aspect of the interatrial septum (*arrow*). Zoomed view confirms the location (**B**), as does real-time 3D TEE imaging (**C,** 3D dataset rotated 180 degrees from 2D orientation).

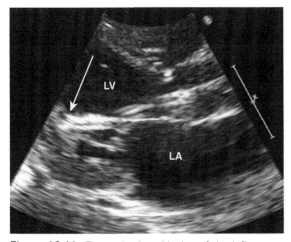

Figure 12-11. The optimal positioning of the inflow port of the Impella Recover is 3 to 4 cm below the aortic valve. In this parasternal long-axis view, the tip of the device abuts the anterolateral papillary muscle (*arrow*) and is located 6 cm below the aortic valve. In this patient, the outflow port was ejecting into the left ventricular outflow tract instead of the proximal ascending aorta.

perform a comprehensive spectral and color Doppler examination.

Analysis
- Aortic valve stenosis and regurgitation should be carefully assessed before placement of the Impella device.

Pitfalls (see Box 12-1)
- Moderate or great AS (valve area ≤ 1.5 cm^2) and more than moderate aortic regurgitation complicates placement and function of the Impella Recover device.
- Severe aortic regurgitation can cause diastolic LV pressure elevation and thereby augment the reduction in coronary perfusion pressure caused by the fact that the TandemHeart shunts blood from the left atrium to the outflow catheter in the distal aorta (bypassing the coronary ostia in the aortic root).

- Echocardiography can detect aortic stenosis or regurgitation, aortopathy, and VSD that complicate percutaneous VAD placement.
- Echocardiography directs positioning of the Impella Recover inflow port 3 to 4 cm below the aortic valve, away from the septum and the

anterior mitral valve leaflet, and also guides trans-septal puncture of the TandemHeart device.
- Echocardiography can assess for migration, infection, and obstruction of percutaneous VAD catheters.

Suggested Readings

1. Catena E, Milazzo F. Echocardiography and cardiac assist devices. *Minerva Cardiolangiol.* 2005;55:247-265.
   This paper provides a comprehensive overview of the use of echocardiography in mechanical cardiac support device imaging. The authors rely heavily on their experience.
2. Catena E, Milazzo F, Pittella G, et al. Echocardiographic approach in a new left ventricular assist device: Impella Recover 100. *J Am Soc Echocardiogr.* 2004;17: 470-473.
   This paper provides an overview of the early experience with the Impella device.
3. Catena E, Milazzo F, Montorsi E, et al. Left ventricular support by axial flow pump: The echocardiographic approach to device malfunction. *J Am Soc Echocardiogr.* 2005;18:1422e7-1422e13.
   This article was among the first to describe echocardiographic approaches to imaging patients suspected of LVAD malfunction, focusing on axial flow devices.
4. Chumnanvej S, Wood MJ, MacGillivray TE, Vidal Melo MF. Perioperative echocardiographic examination for ventricular assist device implantation. *Anesth Analg.* 2007;105: 583-601.
   This article reviews the use of TEE in the perioperative management of ventricular assist devices, including a discussion of the de-airing procedure.
5. Horton SC, Khodaverdian R, Chatelain P, et al. Left ventricular assist device malfunction: An approach to diagnosis by echocardiography. *J Am Coll Cardiol.* 2005;45:1435-1440.
   This article was among the first to describe echocardiographic approaches to imaging patients suspected of LVAD malfunction, focusing on axial flow devices.
6. John R, Mantz K, Eckman P, Rose A, May-Newman K. Aortic valve pathophysiology during left ventricular assist device support. *J Heart Lung Transplant.* 2010;29:1321-1329.
   This recent paper reflects the growing recognition of the important role that aortic pathology plays in patients with LVADs. It describes the impact of aortic disease preimplantation and the development of aortic disease after implantation.
7. Kirkpatrick JN, Wiegers SE, Lang RM. Left ventricular assist devices and other devices for end-stage heart failure: Utility of echocardiography. *Curr Cardiol Reports.* 2010;12: 257-264.
   This paper is a recent review of the literature describing the use of echocardiography in mechanical circulatory support.
8. Scalia GM, McCarthy PM, Savage RM, Smedira NG, Thomas JD. Clinical utility of echocardiography in the management of implantable ventricular assist device. *J Am Soc Echocardiogr.* 2000;13:754-763.
   This older paper was one of the first to highlight the important role that echocardiography can and should play in the management of LVAD patients.

Echocardiography in Cardiac Transplantation

Atif N. Qasim and Amresh Raina

13

Introduction

- Approximately 2200 heart transplantations are performed yearly in the United States, with a little over half of all transplantations performed for nonischemic causes of heart failure.
- In 2009, the 5-year survival rate post-transplantation was 73% for men and 67% for women.
- Echocardiography remains a principle diagnostic modality in the process of heart transplantation, and is particularly important in the stages shown below, which will form the focus of this chapter:
  - Assessing the appropriateness for transplantation in acute and chronic heart failure patients
  - Evaluating suitability of the donor heart
  - Assessing the transplanted heart postoperatively
  - Echocardiographic determinants of cardiac rejection
  - Long-term surveillance of heart transplantation survivors
  - Guidance of endomyocardial biopsy

Assessing the Appropriateness of Heart Transplantation in Acute and Chronic Heart Failure Patients

- Establishing the suitability of heart failure patients for heart transplantation is a multidisciplinary process incorporating a variety of medical and psychosocial factors.
- In general, patients eligible for heart transplantation are less than 65 years old and have systolic or diastolic heart failure with New York Heart Association (NYHA) functional class IIIb or IV symptoms despite optimal medical therapy.

- Exclusion criteria for cardiac transplantation include cancer within the past 5 years, significant obesity, irreversible pulmonary hypertension, and other organ dysfunction not attributable to cardiac dysfunction.
- Echocardiography is an essential test used to evaluate potential heart transplant recipients and may provide information with regard to the etiology of heart failure and severity of the cardiomyopathy (ejection fraction in systolic heart failure, diastolic parameters in restrictive cardiomyopathies).
- Transthoracic echocardiography can provide clues to other abnormalities that should be addressed prior to consideration for transplantation, such as severe valvular abnormalities or constriction.
- In rare instances, a screening echocardiogram can reveal conditions that might preclude transplantation without further investigation, such as severe pulmonary hypertension, endocarditis, or cardiac neoplasm.

Evaluating Suitability of the Donor Heart

- Initial extracardiac factors, beyond those which exclude organ donation in general, may exclude the cardiac donor.
- These include advanced age (typically >55 years), prolonged ischemic time, or inappropriate donor size.
- Male donors over 70 kg are usually suitable in most cases. Body mass index and height are more accurately used for matching heart size to body weight in small donors.
- Echocardiography is now the imaging modality of choice in the evaluation of a potential cardiac donor, and special attention should be given to the echocardiographic factors noted below.

Step-By-Step Approach
Step 1: Assessment of Left Ventricular Hypertrophy

KEY POINTS	
• Anything more than mild left ventricular hypertrophy (LVH) in the donor heart typically precludes transplantation. • It is important to obtain a true determination of LVH using both wall thickness criteria and, if possible, LV mass criteria. However, with poor acoustic windows, this may not always be feasible.	• Care should be taken to characterize the presence of LVH accurately because of pseudo-hypertrophy with an underfilled LV, or because of disproportionate upper septal thickening (which is a normal variant).

Step 2: Assessment of Valvular and Congenital Abnormalities

KEY POINTS	
• Complex congenital heart disease may occasionally exclude eligibility for transplant donation. • Simple repairs can be made to the donor heart during transplantation for some conditions, making the donor heart still useable; these include valvular repair for mild insufficiency in	select cases and repair of secundum atrial septal defects (ASDs). • Bicuspid aortic valves in the donor heart that function normally do not necessarily preclude transplantation.

Step 3: Careful Assessment of Ejection Fraction, and Dobutamine Challenge if Indicated

KEY POINTS	
• Many hearts in the United States are declined for transplantation because of abnormal LV function. • However, many young donor hearts that have depressed function resulting from secondary effects from brain death can recover normal function after transplantation.	• Those with mild LV dysfunction can be given a low-dose dobutamine infusion to see if LV function improves; appropriate augmentation of function suggests favorable transplantation outcome.

The Transplanted Heart in the Postoperative Period

Step-By-Step Approach
Step 1: Assessment of Atrial Structure and Function

KEY POINTS	
• Two major surgical approaches are used in heart transplantation that impact atrial structure and function: (1) the bi-atrial anastomosis (developed by Lower and Shumway), where recipient right and left atrial cuff tissue is left behind and sutured to the donor atria; and (2) the bicaval anastomosis, where a direct anastomosis is made to the venae cavae and a small portion of the recipient left atrium containing the pulmonary veins (Figure 13-1). • In both cases, the left atrium is a composite of donor and recipient tissue and may look enlarged, especially as seen in the apical 4-chamber view (Figure 13-2). • The right atrium, however, appears composite and enlarged only with the bi-atrial anastomosis.	• A dense ridge in the left atrium can be seen at the surgical anastomosis site and may be mistaken for a mass or thrombus, especially if a large cuff is present when there is donor and recipient size mismatch. This ridge otherwise allows discrimination between donor and recipient atrial tissue. • The bi-atrial technique is associated with an increased risk of atrial thrombus, abnormalities in atrial filling, and poor LV hemodynamics. Hence the bicaval approach is now the technique of choice. • Studies have shown that the bicaval anastomosis is associated with improved atrial geometry, decreased valvular insufficiency, decreased risk of arrhythmias, and decreased hospital stay.

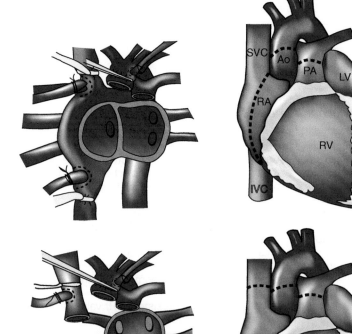

Figure 13-1. Bi-atrial anastomosis (*top panels*) and bicaval anastomosis (*bottom panels*). The left atrial suture line is not readily visible on this anterior view of the heart.

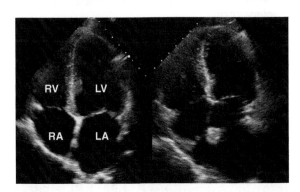

Figure 13-2. Left atrial surgical cuff variants in two examples of bicaval anastomosis. *Left panel:* There is a barely recognizable suture line along the left atrium. *Right panel:* The left atrial cuff is quite marked. This should not be confused with a cardiac mass or thrombus.

Step 2: Assessment of Right Ventricular Dysfunction

KEY POINTS

- Right ventricular dilatation and dysfunction are common immediately post-transplantation. The cause is multifactorial.
- In part this is related to chronic pulmonary venous hypertension and mild pulmonary vascular disease that may occur pre-transplantation in patients with chronic heart failure. There may also be associated ischemia and reperfusion injury during the process of transplantation.

- RV dysfunction is estimated to account for up to 50% of all cardiac transplantation complications and 20% of causes of early death after transplantation, as the donor ventricle cannot accommodate the acute increase in workload.
- The majority of cases of RV dilatation and dysfunction are treated medically and begin to improve over the course of 1 week post-transplantation.

Continued

- In the case shown in Figure 13-3, the marked RV dysfunction seen immediately postoperatively, with associated tricuspid regurgitation (TR), resolved with recovery to completely normal RV function and minimal TR within 1 month.

- Cases in which there is persistent RV dysfunction post-transplantation are associated with increased mortality.

Step 3: Assessment for Presence and Mechanism of TR

- Significant TR is the most common valvular abnormality after orthotopic heart transplantation (OHT). Significant regurgitation of the mitral and aortic valves, in contrast, is rare in the donor heart post-transplantation, unless there is acute rejection or prolonged ischemic time.
- Causes of TR early after transplantation include pulmonary hypertension, elevated pulmonary vascular resistance, and atrial dysfunction (more commonly seen with bi-atrial anastomosis). Typically TR improves with time as the pulmonary artery pressures normalize, usually over the first month after transplantation.

- Causes of TR that occur later include injury to the tricuspid valve and chordal apparatus by repeated endomyocardial biopsies, as well as allograft rejection. The TR from biopsy-related injury is usually more eccentric, and flail tricuspid valve leaflets may be seen (Figure 13-4).
- Bicaval anastomoses result in less TR, suggesting preservation of atrial structure and function and of tricuspid valve geometry are important in preventing TR.
- In cases of severe persistent TR, valve repair or replacement need to be considered.

Step 4: Assessment for Presence and Etiology of Pericardial Effusions

- Pericardial effusions are common immediately post-transplantation, especially in patients with significant mismatch in size between donor and recipient.
- The differential diagnosis for an effusion postoperatively, however, includes acute allograft

rejection and even purulent pericarditis, as these patients are immuno-compromised.
- Most postoperative effusions resolve within 1 month after transplantation without specific intervention.

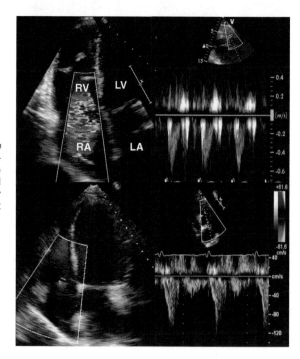

Figure 13-3. RV dysfunction post-transplantation. *Top panel:* There is significant RV dilatation with TR at 1 day post-transplantation. *Bottom panel:* After 1 week, note that the size of the RV has decreased to normal and there is only mild TR. Note also the RV velocity-time integral (VTI) has markedly improved (see also Videos 13-8 and 13-9 on the Expert Consult website).

KEY POINTS—cont'd

- An enlarging pericardial effusion more than 1 month post-transplantation should raise concern for rejection or other causes, such as infection. Constriction is a rare complication post-transplantation, but has been reported.

- In cases in which the pericardial effusion is large and impairs RV or LV filling, percutaneous or surgical drainage may be necessary.

Step 5: Assessment of Left Ventricular Function and Mass

KEY POINTS

- LV systolic function should be preserved immediately postoperatively unless there is prolonged ischemic time for the donor heart or there is acute allograft rejection.
- Frequently, transplant recipients are placed on a combination of inotropic drugs such that hyperdynamic function may occur.
- Over time (months to years), it is common to have an increase in LV mass and wall thickness.

- The cause of LVH post-transplant is multifactorial, involving: post-transplantation hypertension, repeat episodes of rejection, effect of the immunosuppression regimen (especially calcineurin inhibitors), effects of chronic tachycardia, or injury and remodeling of the donor heart at the time of transplantation.

Step 6: Assessment for Possible Technical Complications of Surgery

KEY POINTS

- Echocardiography in the transplant recipient is very useful to examine the sites of anastomosis, using color and spectral Doppler interrogation, in areas that may otherwise be overlooked in a routine echocardiogram of the native heart.
- In bicaval anastomosis, increased gradients across the inferior vena cava (IVC) and superior vena cava (SVC) should be assessed as these have adverse long-term hemodynamic consequences, including hepatic dysfunction.
- It is less common to encounter problems with the anastomosis of the great arteries, however, pulsed wave (PW) and continuous wave (CW) Doppler should be used to interrogate the pulmonary artery and aorta, especially in cases of donor-recipient size mismatch.
- Additional attention should be paid to detect ASDs at the site of atrial anastomosis.

Echocardiographic Determinants of Cardiac Rejection

- Acute allograft rejection is common in the first year after OHT.
- At present, endomyocardial biopsy remains the gold standard in the diagnosis of acute rejection.
- However, profiling of inflammatory gene expression in combination with echocardiography may prove to be equivalent to routine scheduled biopsies in the diagnosis of rejection.
- Multiple echocardiographic techniques, including M-mode, two-dimensional (2D) echocardiography, conventional Doppler, and other indices of systolic and diastolic function, have correlated with episodes of biopsy-proven rejection.
- Unfortunately, no single echocardiographic technique to date has proved to have sufficient sensitivity and negative predictive value to be used as a sole predictor of acute rejection.

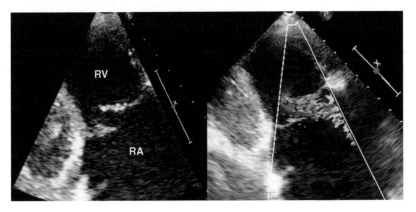

Figure 13-4. TR caused by injury from endomyocardial biopsy. *Left panel:* A parasternal RV inflow view showing significant prolapse of the septal leaflet caused by trauma from repeated biopsy. Note the eccentric TR jet (*right panel*) (see also Videos 13-3 and 13-4 on the Expert Consult website).

Step-By-Step Approach
Step 1: M-mode and 2D
Echocardiography of the Left Ventricle

KEY POINTS

- Acute allograft rejection is characterized by a cellular infiltrate in the myocardium, resulting in myocyte inflammation, edema, and ultimately contractile dysfunction.
- M-mode of the left ventricle can detect the resulting increase in LV wall thickness, rise in LV mass, and decrease in LV fractional shortening and ejection fraction (Figure 13-5).
- 2D echocardiography complements M-mode findings but can also reveal an increase in myocardial echogenicity and the presence of an associated pericardial effusion (Figure 13-6).
- Unfortunately, neither M-mode nor 2D echo findings are specific for acute rejection; increases in wall thickness and LV mass can also occur as sequelae of hypertension, immuno-suppression, and chronic tachycardia post-transplantation.
- In the current era of potent immuno-suppression, acute rejection may present in a subtle fashion without frank symptoms or as a decline in LV systolic function until late in the course.
- Because decreases in M-mode and 2D measures of systolic function, such as fractional shortening and ejection fraction, may not occur until later in the presentation of acute rejection, these techniques are not sufficiently sensitive alone to exclude an episode of rejection.

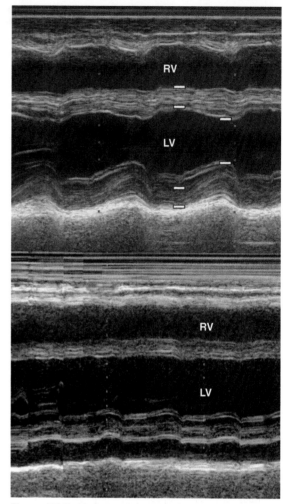

Figure 13-5. M-mode of the left ventricle at baseline (*top panel*) and during an episode of acute rejection (*bottom panel*). Note the marked decrease in systolic thickening of the septum and posterior wall, with a decrease in fractional shortening during the episode of rejection. Also note the presence of a posterior pericardial effusion.

Step 2: Evaluation of Diastolic Function Using Standard Doppler Echocardiography

KEY POINTS

- Diastolic function is typically impaired at an earlier stage than systolic function during episodes of acute rejection.
- Measurement of standard Doppler indices of diastolic function and correlation of changes in diastolic function with episodes of rejection is therefore an appealing strategy for the detection of acute rejection.
- From the apical views, PW Doppler of the LV inflow allows measurement of E- and A-wave velocities, isovolumic relaxation time (IVRT), and E-wave deceleration times.
- Of these measures, rise in E-wave velocity, shortened IVRT and E-wave deceleration time have correlated best with episodes of rejection (Figure 13-7).

- However, these parameters have proved to have relatively low specificity for rejection episodes due to their dependence on loading conditions and heart rate.
- The myocardial performance index is theoretically a load- and heart rate–independent composite measure of systolic and diastolic function derived from standard Doppler of LV inflow and outflow: (IVCT + IVRT)/ET, where IVCT is the isovolumic contraction time and ET is the ejection time.
- Unfortunately, small echocardiographic studies evaluating episodes of acute rejection have yielded conflicting results with regard to the effect of rejection on the myocardial performance index.

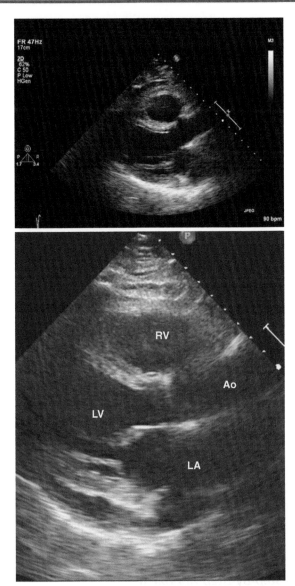

Figure 13-6. 2D echocardiogram of the left ventricle from the parasternal long-axis view of the same patient at baseline (*top panel*) and during an episode of acute rejection (*bottom panel*). Notice the increased thickness and echogenicity of the myocardium in rejection and the presence of a significant pericardial effusion. (See also Videos on the Expert Consult website.)

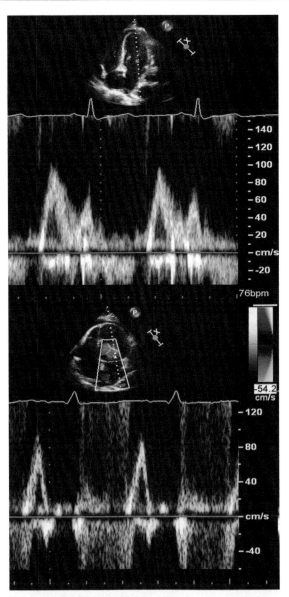

Figure 13-7. PW Doppler of mitral inflow at baseline (*top panel*) and during an episode of acute rejection (*bottom panel*). Note the increase in the E/A ratio and decrease in the E-wave deceleration time during the rejection episode.

Step 3: Use of Tissue Doppler, Strain Imaging, and Advanced Techniques as Needed

KEY POINTS

- Tissue Doppler imaging (TDI) conveys a major advantage over conventional Doppler of being much less dependent on heart rate and LV loading conditions.
- Studies of TDI of the mitral annulus have shown that a reduction in early diastolic velocities (E′) and lower systolic velocities (S) correlate well with acute episodes of rejection seen on endomyocardial biopsy (Figure 13-8).
- Myocardial strain and strain-rate imaging measure the actual deformation of the myocardium and have the promise of being significantly more sensitive than other indices for detecting early or subclinical rejection.

Continued

- Small, single-center studies have shown that reduced longitudinal peak systolic strain and reduced strain rate are predictive of episodes of acute rejection confirmed on endomyocardial biopsy.
- Contrast echocardiography of the left ventricle using leukocyte-targeted microbubbles is another promising technique in which a rise in myocardial signal intensity has correlated with episodes of acute rejection in animal studies, reflecting myocardial infiltration with leukocytes.
- Both myocardial strain/strain-rate imaging and contrast echocardiography need further validation in large, human studies.

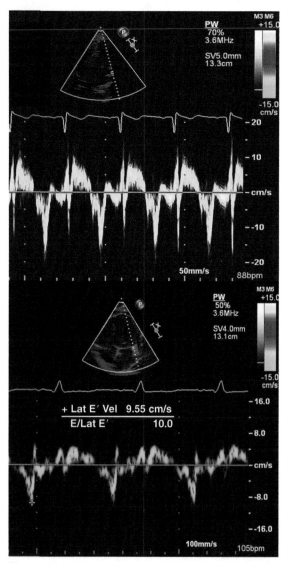

Figure 13-8. TDI of the lateral mitral annulus at baseline (*top panel*) and during an episode of acute rejection (*bottom panel*). During rejection, there is a marked decrease in early diastolic velocities (E′) and systolic velocities.

Long-Term Surveillance of Heart Transplantation Survivors

- Patients post-transplantation are at risk for a wide spectrum of complications, including systemic hypertension, diabetes, side effects of repeated biopsies, episodes of acute rejection, and chronic allograft vasculopathy (CAV).
- Invasive angiography is the current gold standard for the detection of CAV.
- The sensitivity of conventional angiography is improved with the addition of intravascular ultrasound due to the diffuse nature of graft vasculopathy.
- Routine resting echocardiography and dobutamine stress echocardiography (DSE) both play an important role in monitoring for complications related to therapy for OHT and for the detection of CAV.

Step-By-Step Approach
Step 1: Use of Serial Resting 2D and Doppler Echocardiography

KEY POINTS

- A new resting wall motion abnormality (WMA) on 2D echocardiography has a poor sensitivity but a relatively high specificity for detecting the presence of CAV.
- Although resting echocardiography cannot replace an invasive angiographic evaluation for the presence of CAV, a new WMA seen on resting 2D echocardiography should prompt further assessment with coronary angiography.
- Serial 2D transthoracic echocardiography is nevertheless useful in the post-transplantation patient for detecting the sequelae of episodes of asymptomatic rejection, potential side effects of procedures such as biopsy, and development of LVH and diastolic dysfunction.

Step 2: Use of DSE for Evaluation of CAV

Guidance of Endomyocardial Biopsy

- Routine endomyocardial biopsies are common in the first several years post-transplantation, even in asymptomatic patients, due to the inability of a noninvasive means to reliably diagnose rejection.
- The most common complications of endomyocardial biopsy include cardiac tamponade and damage to the tricuspid valve or chordal apparatus/papillary muscles, resulting in significant TR. Echocardiography can be used to quickly diagnose both of these conditions.
- Several centers use transthoracic echocardiography to help guide the bioptome, in addition to fluoroscopy, to lower the risk of these complications as well as radiation dose. Standard 2D transthoracic echocardiography from the apical 4-chamber view can ensure appropriate position of the bioptome toward the ventricular septum, and across the tricuspid valve.
- Emerging real-time three-dimensional (3D) techniques allow better visualization (see example shown in Figure 13-9) of the bioptome, and in some series have demonstrated that the bioptome was not in an ideal septal position for biopsy when guided conventionally by fluoroscopy alone.
- Larger prospective studies are needed to determine whether echocardiographic guidance of endomyocardial biopsy reduces long-term procedural complications.

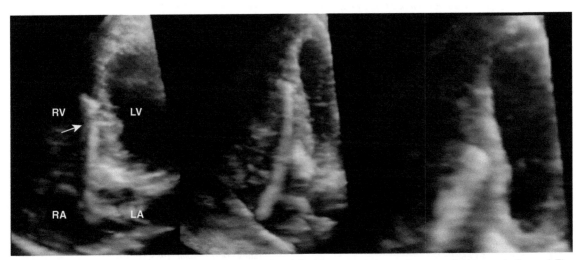

Figure 13-9. Real-time 3D transthoracic echocardiography of the bioptome during endomyocardial biopsy. *Left panel:* The 3D echocardiogram is used to assist in proper placement of the bioptome. *Middle panel:* The bioptome is shown in the correct position along the septum. *Right panel:* The view used while the biopsy is taken. In this case the biopsy was done on a native heart (see also Videos 13-5 to 13-7 on the Expert Consult website). *(Courtesy of Frank Silvestry and Daniel Kolansky, the Hospital of the University of Pennsylvania.)*

Suggested Readings

1. Aggarwal M, Drachenberg C, Douglass L, deFilippi C. The efficacy of real-time 3-dimensional echocardiography for right ventricular biopsy. *J Am Soc Echocardiogr.* 2005; 18:1208-1212.
   Fifteen patients underwent 32 right ventricular biopsies, half with real-time 3D echocardiography alone and half with biplane fluoroscopy. All 3D echocardiography–guided biopsy specimens were comparable to fluoroscopic samples with respect to interpretability for rejection.

2. Akosah KO, McDaniel S, Hanrahan JS, Mohanty PK. Dobutamine stress echocardiography early after heart transplantation predicts development of allograft coronary artery disease and outcome. *J Am Coll Cardiol.* 1998;31: 1607-1614.
   In this small study of 22 new heart transplant subjects, dobutamine stress echocardiography testing was predictive of worse outcome only for those who developed persistent wall motion abnormalities during testing.

3. Akosah KO, Mohanty PK, Funai JT, et al. Noninvasive detection of transplant coronary artery disease by dobutamine stress echocardiography. *J Heart Lung Transplant.* 1994;13:1024-1038.
   Dobutamine stress echocardiography in this study of heart transplant recipients (on average 5 years out from transplant) had the following characteristics for detection of transplant coronary artery disease: sensitivity, 95%, specificity, 55%, positive predictive value, 69% and negative predictive value, 92%.

4. Aranda JM Jr, Weston MW, Puleo JA, Fontanet HL. Effect of loading conditions on myocardial relaxation velocities determined by Doppler tissue imaging in heart transplant recipients. *J Heart Lung Transplant.* 1998;17:693-697.
   Twenty transplant subjects were given nitroglycerin for preload and afterload reduction with tissue Doppler imaging performed pre and post. There was no significant change in myocardial relaxation velocities despite significant reductions in PCWP and mean arterial blood pressure suggesting loading conditions on the heart have little influence on relaxation velocities in transplant recipient, perhaps making it useful for the diagnosis of rejection.

5. Aziz TM, Burgess MI, Rahman AN, Campbell CS, Deiraniya AK, Yonan NA. Risk factors for tricuspid valve regurgitation after orthotopic heart transplantation. *Ann Thorac Surg.* 1999;68:1247-1251.
   Tricuspid regurgitation was assessed in 249 heart transplant subjects with color Doppler. Those with greater early TR tended to be those who did not have a bicaval technique, episodes of ≥ grade 2 rejection, an increased transpulmonary gradient preoperatively and elevated PVR. The number of biopsies was also correlated with increased TR farther out from transplant.

6. Bacal F, Moreira L, Souza G, et al. Dobutamine stress echocardiography predicts cardiac events or death in asymptomatic patients long-term after heart transplantation: 4-year prospective evaluation. *J Heart Lung Transplant.* 2004;23:1238-1244.
   Thirty-nine subjects an average of 86 months after transplant underwent thallium scintigraphy, treadmill stress testing, dobutamine stress echocardiography (DSE), and coronary angiography to detect allograft vasculopathy. Both positive DSE results and positive angiography were associated with cardiac events across 4 years of follow-up and in the absence of coronary angiography. DSE was a unique independent predictor of cardiac events.

7. Bedanova H, Necas J, Petrikovits E, et al. Echo-guided endomyocardial biopsy in heart transplant recipients. *Transpl Int.* 2004;17:622-625.
   In a single series of 1262 endomyocardial biopsies in transplant subjects obtained using echocardiography guidance, the success rate of obtaining 4-5 specimens was 96% with few complications overall and the need for conversion to X-ray guidance occurred in only 11 subjects.

8. Bhatia SJ, Kirshenbaum JM, Shemin RJ, et al. Time course of resolution of pulmonary hypertension and right ventricular remodeling after orthotopic cardiac transplantation. *Circulation.* 1987;76:819-826.
   In 24 transplant recipients studied with serial echocardiography and right heart catheterizations, the right and left heart filling pressures declined together and reached a range near the upper limit of normal by 2 weeks. An increase in right ventricle size was seen on day 1 after surgery, and this size increase was maintained at 1 year follow-up although the incidence of tricuspid regurgitation decreased.

9. Bolad IA, Robinson DR, Webb C, Hamour I, Burke MM, Banner NR. Impaired left ventricular systolic function early after heart transplantation is associated with cardiac allograft vasculopathy. *Am J Transplant.* 2006;6:161-168.
   Quantitative coronary angiography (QCA) was performed on 121 heart transplant subjects at baseline and at 1 year and found that echocardiographic fractional shortening was inversely related to mean coronary artery lumen diameter loss, suggesting ventricular systolic dysfunction early after heart transplantation may be associated with subsequent development of allograft vasculopathy.

10. Ciliberto GR, Mascarello M, Gronda E, et al. Acute rejection after heart transplantation: Noninvasive echocardiographic evaluation. *J Am Coll Cardiol.* 1994;23: 1156-1161.
    Various echocardiographic measurements were taken over 1400 serial echocardiograms among 130 transplant recipients within 24 hours of endomyocardial biopsy. Overall echocardiography had a poor sensitivity for mild rejection but was better (80%) for signs of moderate rejection.

11. Dandel M, Hummel M, Muller J, et al. Reliability of tissue Doppler wall motion monitoring after heart transplantation for replacement of invasive routine screenings by optimally timed cardiac biopsies and catheterizations. *Circulation.* 2001;104(suppl I):I184-I191.
    Echocardiography with tissue Doppler imaging was performed just prior to 408 endomyocardial biopsies in heart transplant recipients to assess diagnostic value for rejection. In those without any significant diastolic parameter changes, acute rejection was unlikely with negative and positive predictive values of 96% and 92%.

12. Desruennes M, Corcos T, Cabrol A, et al. Doppler echocardiography for the diagnosis of acute cardiac allograft rejection. *J Am Coll Cardiol.* 1988;12:63-70.
    Same day Doppler echocardiography was performed on 55 heart transplant subjects undergoing endomyocardial biopsy. Those with mild or moderate rejection had decreased isovolumic relaxation time and pressure half-time without change in heart rate or peak early mitral flow velocity. These changes recovered after immunosuppressive therapy. Those without rejection had Doppler indexes that remained unchanged.

13. El Gamel A, Yonan NA, Grant S, et al. Orthotopic cardiac transplantation: A comparison of standard and bicaval Wythenshawe techniques. *J Thorac Cardiovasc Surg.* 1995;109:721-729; discussion 729-730.
    Seventy-five patients were randomized to either the bicaval or conventional bi-atrial technique during orthotopic heart transplantation. Overall the bicaval technique implantation was associated with lower right atrial pressures, a lower incidence of atrial tachyarrhythmias, less need for pacing, less mitral regurgitation, lower doses of diuretics and a shorter length of hospital stay.

14. French JW, Popp RL, Pitlick PT. Cardiac localization of transvascular bioptome using 2-dimensional echocardiography. *Am J Cardiol.* 1983;51:219-223.
    This article contains one of the initial case series in which 2D echocardiography was added to fluoroscopy for guidance of bioptome. Eight children underwent 12 biopsies, all without complications, with the advantage of reducing radiation exposure.

15. Fyfe DA, Ketchum D, Lewis R, et al. Tissue Doppler imaging detects severely abnormal myocardial velocities that identify children with pre-terminal cardiac graft failure after heart transplantation. *J Heart Lung Transplant.* 2006;25:510-517.
Among 53 heart transplantation recipients in children, tricuspid, but not mitral, S and E tissue Doppler imaging velocities deteriorated to low levels 3 to 6 months before the terminal graft failure. Right ventricular deterioration occurred during the final 3 months before death and severely reduced left ventricular velocities.

16. Grande AM, Minzioni G, Martinelli L, et al. Echo-controlled endomyocardial biopsy in orthotopic heart transplantation with bicaval anastomosis. *G Ital Cardiol.* 1997;27:877-880.
Among 38 transplant recipients with bicaval anastomosis, 339 endomyocardial biopsies were performed, 309 under echocardiographic guidance and 30 under fluoroscopy. Echocardiographic guidance allowed for better choice of biopsy site, reduced the risk of damaging cardiac structures, and allowed immediate monitoring of heart performance. Complications overall were rare.

17. Kato TS, Oda N, Hashimura K, et al. Strain rate imaging would predict sub-clinical acute rejection in heart transplant recipients. *Eur J Cardiothorac Surg.* 2010;37: 1104-1110.
Statistically significant differences in systolic and diastolic strain rate were found among a group of 35 transplant recipients across 396 endomyocardial biopsies for those with (45) and without (351) acute rejection (considered to be grade 1b or higher in this study).

18. Kociolek LK, Bierig SM, Herrmann SC, Labovitz AJ. Efficacy of atropine as a chronotropic agent in heart transplant patients undergoing dobutamine stress echocardiography. *Echocardiography.* 2006;23:383-387.
In this retrospective review of 68 OHT subjects, 21 required atropine in an attempt to reach target heart rate during a standard DSE protocol. Only half of those receiving atropine actually reached target HR. No clear risk factors predicted responsiveness to atropine. Those however with a high resting heart rate appeared to have a better response to dobutamine.

19. Kono T, Nishina T, Morita H, Hirota Y, Kawamura K, Fujiwara A. Usefulness of low-dose dobutamine stress echocardiography for evaluating reversibility of brain death-induced myocardial dysfunction. *Am J Cardiol.* 1999;84:578-582.
Serial changes in LV fractional shortening (FS) was measured in 30 brain-dead patients. Twenty-three patients had ≥ 30% fractional shortening and seven had < 30% fractional shortening. Dobutamine stress echocardiography was performed in this latter group. Of the seven, four showed no response to dobutamine as FS remained decreased whereas in the three dobutamine-responsive wall motion FS became normal at 7 days after brain death. This suggests that some brain death-induced myocardial dysfunction is reversible and can be detected by low dose dobutamine infusion.

20. Leonard GT Jr, Fricker FJ, Pruett D, Harker K, Williams B, Schowengerdt KO Jr. Increased myocardial performance index correlates with biopsy-proven rejection in pediatric heart transplant recipients. *J Heart Lung Transplant.* 2006;25:61-66.
Left ventricular myocardial performance index (LVMPI), the sum of the isovolumic contraction time and isovolumic relaxation time divided by aortic ejection time, was measured in 21 heart transplant subjects across 36 echocardiography studies at the time of endomyocardial biopsy. Significant differences were noted between those without rejection (n = 23), those with moderate to severe rejection (n = 5) and those with focal moderate rejection (n = 8). The LVMPI was 0.42 ± 0.03 (mean ± SEM) for the group without rejection, 0.57 ± 0.06
for those with Grade 2 rejection and 0.73 ± 0.05 for those with Grade 3 rejection.

21. Lewis JF, Selman SB, Murphy JD, Mills RM Jr, Geiser EA, Conti CR. Dobutamine echocardiography for prediction of ischemic events in heart transplant recipients. *J Heart Lung Transplant.* 1997;16:390-393.
Dobutamine stress echocardiography (DSE) was performed in 63 consecutive heart transplant recipients as part of routine yearly evaluation. Twenty-one patients had abnormal wall motion at baseline or during dobutamine infusion. Over a mean follow-up of 8 months five major adverse cardiac events occurred in those with abnormal results; whereas one event occurred in those with a normal DSE, suggesting that normal wall motion during DSE are at lower risk for development of cardiac events.

22. Mahle WT, Cardis BM, Ketchum D, Vincent RN, Kanter KR, Fyfe DA. Reduction in initial ventricular systolic and diastolic velocities after heart transplantation in children: Improvement over time identified by tissue Doppler imaging. *J Heart Lung Transplant.* 2006;25:1290-1296.
Tissue Doppler imaging studies were serially performed during 6 months post-heart transplantation in 13 children and demonstrated a steady increase in both systolic tissue velocities at the tricuspid annulus, systolic tissue velocities at the mitral annulus as well as early diastolic (E) velocities at the tricuspid annulus and mitral annulus. The systolic and diastolic velocities were reduced in children after heart transplantation when compared with controls.

23. Mankad S, Murali S, Kormos RL, Mandarino WA, Gorcsan J 3rd. Evaluation of the potential role of color-coded tissue Doppler echocardiography in the detection of allograft rejection in heart transplant recipients. *Am Heart J.* 1999; 138:721-730.
Seventy-eight consecutive transplant recipients underwent 89 echocardiography exams with tissue Doppler imaging within 1 hour of endomyocardial biopsy. Significant rejection was seen in 14 by biopsy. A tissue Doppler peak-to-peak mitral annular velocity >135 mm/s had 93% sensitivity, 71% specificity, and 98% negative predictive value for detecting rejection.

24. Mannaerts HF, Balk AH, Simoons ML, et al. Changes in left ventricular function and wall thickness in heart transplant recipients and their relation to acute rejection: An assessment by digitised M mode echocardiography. *Br Heart J.* 1992;68:356-364.
M-mode echocardiography was used for measuring left ventricular wall thickness, internal dimension, and fractional shortening across 4-6 consecutive expiratory beats in 32 transplant recipients and 10 healthy volunteers. Two hundred and sixty-three consecutive M-mode studies were examined in relation to concurrent biopsy results. While M-mode echocardiography did not predict acute rejection, most patients with rejection had a slow left ventricular relaxation pattern.

25. Mannaerts HF, Simoons ML, Balk AH, et al. Pulsed-wave transmitral Doppler does not diagnose moderate acute rejection after heart transplantation. *J Heart Lung Transplant.* 1993;12:411-421.
The value of pulsed-wave transmitral Doppler for the diagnosis of moderate acute rejection was examined across 347 recordings in 32 transplant recipients. There was significant overlap of common pulsed-wave Doppler measurements among those with or without rejection.

26. Marciniak A, Eroglu E, Marciniak M, et al. The potential clinical role of ultrasonic strain and strain rate imaging in diagnosing acute rejection after heart transplantation. *Eur J Echocardiogr.* 2007;8:213-221.
Among 31 consecutive heart transplant recipients who underwent 106 routine follow-up endomyocardial biopsies, strain and strain rate imaging appeared to be a good technique for detecting > or =IB grade of acute rejection.

27. McCreery CJ, McCulloch M, Ahmad M, deFilippi CR. Real-time 3-dimensional echocardiography imaging for right ventricular endomyocardial biopsy: A comparison with fluoroscopy. *J Am Soc Echocardiogr.* 2001;14: 927-933.
    Among 63 routine right ventricular biopsy procedures (total of 315 biopsy attempts) in 33 cardiac allograft recipients, the use of real-time 3-dimensional (RT3D) echocardiography helped guide the bioptome against the intraventricular septum along with biplane fluoroscopy. Bioptome visualization in multiple planes helped with localization of the biopsy site.

28. Mena C, Wencker D, Krumholz HM, McNamara RL. Detection of heart transplant rejection in adults by echocardiographic diastolic indices: A systematic review of the literature. *J Am Soc Echocardiogr.* 2006;19: 1295-1300.
    This systematic review looked at the quality of published data that included diastolic indices to predict heart transplant rejection. Nineteen studies fit the inclusion criteria, although they had widely varying quality. Diastolic indices included E-wave pressure half-time, IVRT, and E′ and A′ velocities. Sensitivity of these parameters was inconsistent, as was the quality of studies, making it difficult to recommend these parameters as a routine screening test for allograft rejection without additional, more rigorous study.

29. Mondillo S, Maccherini M, Galderisi M. Usefulness and limitations of transthoracic echocardiography in heart transplantation recipients. *Cardiovasc Ultrasound.* 2008; 6:2.
    This general review discusses the major uses of Doppler echocardiography in heart transplant recipients and discusses the normal findings in the transplant recipient as well as the limitations in diagnosing acute allograft rejection. It also nicely reviews the use of stress echocardiography for the detection of cardiac graft vasculopathy.

30. Morgan JA, Edwards NM. Orthotopic cardiac transplantation: Comparison of outcome using biatrial, bicaval, and total techniques. *J Card Surg.* 2005;20:102-106.
    This review provides a discussion of three different surgical techniques for heart transplantation described in 39 comparative studies published since 1994. The authors conclude that the bicaval technique has several anatomic and functional advantages in addition to decreasing valvular regurgitation, arrhythmias, and length of hospital stay. However, the studies included were quite heterogeneous and this paper was not a formal meta-analysis.

31. Palka P, Lange A, Galbraith A, et al. The role of left and right ventricular early diastolic Doppler tissue echocardiographic indices in the evaluation of acute rejection in orthotopic heart transplant. *J Am Soc Echocardiogr.* 2005; 18:107-115.
    This study of 44 consecutive transplant patients with and without rejection suggests that for those with acute rejection, abnormal tissue Doppler indices suggests that late isovolumic relaxation myocardial velocity gradient and early diastolic timing intervals are markers that may be useful for surveillance of acute rejection.

32. Peteiro J, Redondo F, Calvino R, Cuenca J, Pradas G, Castro Beiras A. Differences in heart transplant physiology according to surgical technique. *J Thorac Cardiovasc Surg.* 1996;112:584-589.
    Twenty subjects with biatrial anastomosis were compared to 11 with bicaval anastomosis and with the use of quantitative echocardiography, those with bicaval anastomosis had lower right sided filling pressures, improved right atrial contraction and lower left atrial dimension in the bicaval approach. There were no differences in left ventricular end-diastolic pressure or cardiac index.

33. Pham MX, Teuteberg JJ, Kfoury AG, et al. Gene-expression profiling for rejection surveillance after cardiac transplantation. *N Engl J Med.* 2010;362:1890-1900.
    Six hundred and two transplant patients were randomly assigned to either gene-expression profiling (which looks at expression levels of 11 informative genes and generates a score) or the use of routine endomyocardial biopsy for the monitoring of rejection in addition to usual care. The composite primary outcome of first occurrence of rejection with hemodynamic compromise, graft dysfunction from other causes, death, or re-transplantation was similar between groups, as was the 2-year death rate. Those in the gene-expression profiling arm had fewer biopsies per patient-year.

34. Prakash A, Printz BF, Lamour JM, Addonizio LJ, Glickstein JS. Myocardial performance index in pediatric patients after cardiac transplantation. *J Am Soc Echocardiogr.* 2004;17:439-442.
    Myocardial performance index (MPI) was found to be higher in 41 children post cardiac transplantation who had no evidence of microscopic rejection compared to 31 pediatric control subjects. Isovolumic relaxation time was higher in the transplant group but isovolumic contraction time was similar between groups, suggesting the difference may be due to abnormal diastolic function.

35. Rodney RA, Johnson LL. Myocardial perfusion scintigraphy to assess heart transplant vasculopathy. *J Heart Lung Transplant.* 1992;11:S74-S78.

36. Roshanali F, Mandegar MH, Bagheri J, et al. Echo rejection score: New echocardiographic approach to diagnosis of heart transplant rejection. *Eur J Cardiothorac Surg.* 2010;38:176-180.
    This paper derives an echo rejection score from 50 endomyocardial biopsy specimens in transplant recipients who also had preprocedure transthoracic echocardiography. Important predictors of rejection appear to be peak systolic strain at the lateral left ventricular base and interventricular septal base as well as posterior wall thickness, and left ventricular mass index. However the score needs validation in other cohorts.

37. Santos-Ocampo SD, Sekarski TJ, Saffitz JE, et al. Echocardiographic characteristics of biopsy-proven cellular rejection in infant heart transplant recipients. *J Heart Lung Transplant.* 1996;15:25-34.
    In a pediatric population of 32 consecutive heart transplantations performed in infants <20 months old and followed over 2.5 years with concurrent endomyocardial biopsy and M-mode echocardiography, left ventricular mass index appeared to increase in cellular rejection but were only significant when more than 1 month from transplantation. Measurements were compounded by significant inter-observer and intra-observer variability.

38. Scheurer M, Bandisode V, Ruff P, Atz A, Shirali G. Early experience with real-time three-dimensional echocardiographic guidance of right ventricular biopsy in children. *Echocardiography.* 2006;23:45-49.
    Real-time transthoracic 3D echocardiography was used in endomyocardial right ventricular biopsies in 28 consecutive biopsy procedures in a pediatric population and was found to be safe without any complication, with decreased need for fluoroscopic guidance of the bioptome into the right ventricle.

39. Spes CH, Mudra H, Schnaack SD, et al. Dobutamine stress echocardiography for noninvasive diagnosis of cardiac allograft vasculopathy: A comparison with angiography and intravascular ultrasound. *Am J Cardiol.* 1996; 78:168-174.
    Fifty-six transplant recipients with normal coronary angiograms an average of 41 months out from transplantation underwent both DSE and intravascular ultrasound. Seventy percent of patients had abnormal findings by either one or both tests (six were abnormal by DSE alone), suggesting only a minority of patients several years out are free of pathologic coronary artery changes when assessed by these techniques.

40. Stork S, Behr TM, Birk M, et al. Assessment of cardiac allograft vasculopathy late after heart transplantation: When is coronary angiography necessary? *J Heart Lung Transplant.* 2006;25:1103-1108.
Fifty-four consecutive transplant recipients were studied with 1) intravascular ultrasound (IVUS), 2) angiography, 3) dobutamine stress echocardiography and 4) immunofluorescence staining against anti-thrombin III (AT-III) in endomyocardial biopsies. The authors found that when compared with IVUS, cardiac transplant vasculopathy was reliably identified using a combination of information on donor age, wall motion score at rest and AT-III staining late after transplant.

41. Sun JP, Abdalla IA, Asher CR, et al. Non-invasive evaluation of orthotopic heart transplant rejection by echocardiography. *J Heart Lung Transplant.* 2005;24: 160-165.
This study of 406 transplant patients undergoing biopsy and echocardiography on the same day attempted to generate a predication model for rejection. Although Doppler E/A ratio, IVRT, recipient age, and the presence of a pericardial effusion were predictors of acute allograft rejection, no single predictor was strong enough to be able to eliminate the need for surveillance biopsies.

42. Sundereswaran L, Nagueh SF, Vardan S, et al. Estimation of left and right ventricular filling pressures after heart transplantation by tissue Doppler imaging. *Am J Cardiol.* 1998;82:352-357.
Fifty transplant patients had right-sided cardiac catheterization and Doppler echocardiography simultaneously and found that mean wedge pressure and mean right atrial pressure can be estimated in heart transplants with reasonable accuracy using the ratio of E/Ea.

43. Thorn EM, de Filippi CR. Echocardiography in the cardiac transplant recipient. *Heart Fail Clin.* 2007;3: 51-67.
This article reviews the spectrum of echocardiographic findings in the adult heart transplant patient. Appreciation of typical alterations from "normal" allows the transplant physician to identify clinically significant changes and to avoid unnecessary invasive procedures based on misinterpretation of these differences. Though abnormalities of systolic and diastolic function correlate with episodes of acute rejection, the primary diagnostic usefulness of echocardiography in acute rejection is guiding the endomyocardial biopsy. Additionally, echocardiography has found a role as a supplement to invasive angiography in the diagnosis of cardiac allograft vasculopathy.

44. Tona F, Caforio AL, Montisci R, et al. Coronary flow reserve by contrast-enhanced echocardiography: A new noninvasive diagnostic tool for cardiac allograft vasculopa-thy. *Am J Transplant.* 2006;6:998-1003.
The authors assessed coronary flow reserve (CFR) by contrast-enhanced transthoracic echocardiography in the left anterior descending coronary artery of 73 transplants who were 8±4.5 years post transplant. CFR was found to be lower in patients with graft vasculopathy but the sensitivity varied widely based on where the CFR cutpoint was taken.

45. Tona F, Caforio AL, Montisci R, et al. Coronary flow velocity pattern and coronary flow reserve by contrast-enhanced transthoracic echocardiography predict long-term outcome in heart transplantation. *Circulation.* 2006;114(suppl I):I49-I55.
This study of 66 consecutive transplant patients primarily compared coronary flow reserve measured by contrast-enhanced echocardiography against a qualitative angiographic grading system found CFR to be an independent predictor of major adverse cardiac events.

46. Valantine HA, Fowler MB, Hunt SA, et al. Changes in Doppler echocardiographic indexes of left ventricular function as potential markers of acute cardiac rejection. *Circulation.* 1987;76(suppl V):V86-V92.
Serial Doppler echocardiography measurements were made in 23 normal volunteers and in 22 transplant subjects within 24 hours of endomyocardial biopsy. Heart rate and mean arterial pressure were significantly higher in transplant recipients than in normal subjects. Left ventricular filling dynamics were markedly different: IVRT and PHT were significantly longer and mitral flow velocity was similar.

47. Valantine HA, Yeoh TK, Gibbons R, et al. Sensitivity and specificity of diastolic indexes for rejection surveillance: Temporal correlation with endomyocardial biopsy. *J Heart Lung Transplant.* 1991;10:757-765.
This study looked at Doppler echocardiographic indexes of diastolic function among sequential endomyocardial biopsies (114 Doppler echocardiographic studies and biopsies done in 39 transplant recipients) to assess for possible factors accounting for false-positive and false-negative results seen in prior studies.

48. Vandenberg BF, Mohanty PK, Craddock KJ, et al. Clinical significance of pericardial effusion after heart transplanta-tion. *J Heart Transplant.* 1988;7:128-134.
Fifty-two consecutive patients undergoing heart transplantation were evaluated with echocardiography at frequent intervals for 12 weeks after transplantation and at three monthly intervals for one year. In a selective group of 38 of 52 patients with adequate 2D echocardiograms performed serially post transplant over the first year, a common finding was pericardial effusion (40%) which was moderate in two (5%) and small in seven patients (18%). A large pericardial effusion was seen in six of 38 patients (16%) and three (8%) developed cardiac tamponade physiology leading to prompt pericardiocentesis. The presence of pericardial effusion was not independently correlated with cyclosporine therapy, acute rejection, level of blood urea nitrogen (BUN), infection or preoperative diagnosis of idiopathic dilated cardiomyopathy.

49. Venkateswaran RV, Townend JN, Wilson IC, Mascaro JG, Bonser RS, Steeds RP. Echocardiography in the potential heart donor. *Transplantation.* 2010;89:894-901.
This study looked at echocardiographic parameters in 66 donor hearts in which both echocardiography and right heart catheterization were performed. Fifty-eight percent had abnormal LV systolic function on initial evaluation, but in over half of the cases, LV function and invasive hemodynamics improved upon repeat assessment after careful management. Therefore, low or borderline ejection fraction on initial evaluation does not always preclude suitability as a donor.

50. Weller GE, Lu E, Csikari MM, et al. Ultrasound imaging of acute cardiac transplant rejection with microbubbles targeted to intercellular adhesion molecule-1. *Circulation.* 2003;108:218-224.
This animal study took contrast microbubbles targeted to the endothelial cell (EC) inflammatory marker intercellular adhesion molecule-1 (ICAM-1) and found preferential adherence to rejecting versus nonrejecting rat cardiac transplant myocardium as seen by ultrasound.

51. Wong RC, Abrahams Z, Hanna M, et al. Tricuspid regurgitation after cardiac transplantation: An old problem revisited. *J Heart Lung Transplant.* 2008;27: 247-252.
This article provides a useful review of TR in the transplanted heart and discusses functional and anatomic causes of this condition post-transplantation. Management strategies, including the possibility of valve repair or replacement, are discussed, as well as the concept of prophylactic donor heart tricuspid valve annuloplasty.

52. Yankah AC, Musci M, Weng Y, et al. Tricuspid valve dys-function and surgery after orthotopic cardiac transplanta-tion. *Eur J Cardiothorac Surg.* 2000;17:343-348.

In a study of 647 of 889 patients who survived heart transplantation for more than 30 days, mild, moderate and severe tricuspid regurgitation was seen in 14.5%, 3.1% and 2.5%, respectively. Severe tricuspid regurgitation in transplanted hearts was associated mainly with biopsy-induced injury or endocarditis. Valvular surgery in these cases had acceptable mortality, low morbidity and excellent intermediate-term clinical results without significant detrimental effect on the right ventricular performance.

53. Zaroff JG, Rosengard BR, Armstrong WF, et al. Consensus conference report. Maximizing use of organs recovered from the cadaver donor: Cardiac recommendations. *Circulation.* 2002;106:836-841.
This statement provides recommendations for improving evaluation and utilization cardiac donors and describes the utility of echocardiography in the assessment of donor heart function before recovery.

Index

Printed and bound by CPI Group (UK) Ltd, Croydon, CR0 4YY

03/10/2024

01040303-0002